W0255485

Durchführung des Seminars und Drucklegung der Referat
erfolgte mit Unterstützung der Beiersdorf AG Hamburg.

Überreicht
mit freundlicher Empfehlung

BDF ●●●●
Beiersdorf AG Hamburg

N. Rietbrock, B. G. Woodcock, G. Neuhaus

Methods in Clinical Pharmacology

Methods in Clinical Pharmacology

The Proceedings of an International Symposium held in Frankfurt/M. 6-8 May 79

General Editors:

Norbert Rietbrock (Frankfurt)

Barry G. Woodcock (Frankfurt)

Günter Neuhaus (Berlin)

Springer Fachmedien Wiesbaden GmbH

1980

Ursprünglich erschienen bei Friedr. Vieweg & Sohn Verlagsgesellschaft mbH, Braunschweig 1980

Produced by Mohndruck Graphische Betriebe GmbH, Gütersloh

ISBN 978-3-528-07902-4 ISBN 978-3-663-14027-6 (eBook)
DOI 10.1007/978-3-663-14027-6

Contents

Foreword

"We pharmacologists must acquire a knowledge of the tools we use... Fortunately a surgeon who uses the wrong side of a scalpel cuts his own fingers and not the patient; if the same applied to drugs they would have been investigated very carefully a long time ago... More *ceterum censeo* is perhaps necessary in order to rouse pharmacology from its sleep. The sleep is not a natural one since pharmacology, as judged by its past accomplishments, has no reason for being tired."

From R. Buchheim

Beiträge zur Arzneimittellehre, Voss, Leipzig, 1849.

Chapter 1

Preface and introduction

Methods, clinical pharmacology and the clinical pharmacologist

In this book are brought together the proceedings from lecures and poster-demonstrations at the International Symposium on Methods in Clinical Pharmacology held in Frankfurt, May 6th—8th 1979.
The symposium provided a forum for a group of invited clinical pharmacologist to speak on a topic of their own selection. They were asked to place special emphasis on the methodological aspects of their work they considered to be important. Seventeen of the speakers came from overseas. The symposium was thus an attempt to establish a methodological basis for further advancements in clinical pharmacology. This book, we hope, will be recognised as documentary evidence that this has been done.
Owing to the considerable advancements that have been achieved, it may be forgotten or not realised that clinical pharmacology is a relatively young discipline (7 to 10 years at the most). In this respect a striking parallelism can be drawn between the clinician's point of view and the position in our society today of children.
Although no-one can dispute the significance of children for the continuation of our world, in the 'International Year of the Child,' throughout the world, attention is being drawn at great expense to their importance. Many state and private organisations are devoting great material and personnel resources to projects which should produce an improvement in the children's situation. No-one making a claim to moral quality and progressiveness will stand aloof from such claims.
The position here is quite similar with regard to clinical pharmacology: state authorities and the responsible scientific societies emphasise its necessity and support the advancement of young scientists, for example through the Paul Martini Foundation and the German Research Association. These efforts and encouragement will, however, always be in vain unless it is possible to provide definite and independent possibilities of employment in the clinics for the trained clinical pharmacologists. In the past this has been realised in too few places. The State—as supporter of the universities—at all events has not fulfilled this requirement, and has not adequateley continued the preliminary work done as a result of private initiative.
Instead, a great deal of time and effort has been devoted to the usual business for institutionalising clinical pharmacology between clinic and pharmacology—including the efforts to develop the curriculum for training clinical pharmacologists.
But with regard to their children, fathers and mothers are prisoners of their dimensions, in which not only their dreams and expectations, but also their status anxieties, develop. As the 'mothers' and 'fathers' of clinical pharmacology, the same applies to the established subjects of pharmacology and clinical medicine. Both are trying to give the child which is slowly approaching adulthood what are—in their view—favourable conditions for development without, however, loosening their parental tie too much.

This symposium of Methods in Clinical Pharmacology signifies, to quote Professor E. HABERMANN who spoke at the opening ceremony of the symposium and who is President of the German Pharmacological Society, that "clinical pharmacology comes of age and is no longer driven by the urgency of problems to be solved. Instead it catches for a solid background reaching beyond the actual needs . . .". Professor HABERMANN thought it significant that the title of the symposium was Methods *in* (not *of*) Clinical Pharmacology and pointed out that clinical pharmacology, like pharmacology and toxicology is a discipline without methods of its "own." It is united by a goal: to study the interactions between drugs and man and has to assimilate techniques currently offered by the basic sciencies, mainly physics, chemistry, mathematics and certain biosciences. Selection takes place according to usefulness in problem solving.

The use and development of the scientific method is one of clinical pharmacology's most important functions since it provides information about drugs based on sound factual evidence rather than on clinical impressions. It is important however that new techniques are properly used, not only to ensure that the investigator gets the best return for the time and effort he has devoted to his observations but also that high standards of investigation are maintained.

In daily work with sick people, it is not only the specialist in internal medicine who makes use of the special skills, experience and knowledge on the effects of drugs, which are the clinical pharmacologist's speciality as a result of his training. He can be of service to clinical colleagues in giving expert advice on all problems connected with drug therapy. Professor MICHAEL RAWLINS described this advisory relationship briefly and aptly as follows: "Just as there are patients with cardiac, endocrine or neurological problems, there are also patients in whom clinico-pharmacological problems occur—problems which can often be solved by reasonable application of the knowledge of modern pharmacology, pharmacokinetics or metabolic behaviour of the drug" (J. Royal Soc. Med. *71* [1978] 556). It is precisely these clinico-pharmacological problems occurring at the sick-bed in the day-to-day work, that result in scientific projects, in the solution of which the clinical pharmacologist as a *researcher* makes his contribution to a more rational and safer drug therapy. Clinical pharmacology has thus developed because of the increasing realisation that the optimum use of drugs requires a level of expertise which has in the past only been demanded in the diagnosis of disease. Without this expertise, both the efficacy and safety of drug therapy is jeopardized.

The clinical pharmacologist advises the clinician on the basis of his special knowledge and skills; usually he will not himself be the physician in charge of treatment. There is the opinion that he can only satisfy these tasks as an equal partner to the clinician if he has previously done clinical work for a sufficient period on his own responsibility. The knowledge gained through his own experience at the sick bed about the diseases, the value and the risks of diagnostic procedures, about the organisation of everyday life in the clinic, and not least the depressing experiences at the limits of our therapeutic possibilities, give the prospective clinical pharmacologist the medical reference without which he remains a theoretician when he concerns himself scientifically with clinical problems.

On the other hand, the clinician who, without comprehensive theoretical and practical training as a pharmacologist, describes himself as a clinical pharmacologist is in an even worse position. He lacks the strong foundation which provides the solid basis for him being able to advise the clinician about all aspects and problems of drug therapy as a result of his specialist knowledge and experience.

Unlike KALCHAS between the Greeks and the Trojans, the clinical pharmacologist cannot enjoy independence—he is involved and affected as a *doctor*. However, he considers the clinical problems in his own way, from his special point of view, that of *pharmacology*.

In this position, between the clinical treatment on one side and pharmacology on the other, clinical pharmacology, as an own discipline, takes its place. In order to maintain its power to support patient therapy in the future, it must continue to obtain its energy from pharmacology. Without keeping together with pharmacology, the energy supply would swiftly become exhausted. Without modulation through contact with other clinical disciplines, clinical pharmacology would be dispossessed of that body of information which is obtained from therapeutics involving the patient, and which it extends by being involved in it. It is thus indispensible that both disciplines work together on therapeutic problems and progress.

One of the tasks of clinical pharmacology is the development of new methods, which are then offered to the clinic and then jointly with the clinician, examined for their application and usefulness. Concomitant with this task is the necessity that the number of redundant diagnostic procedures ap-

plied in therapy does not grow larger. An essential task for the clinical pharmacologist and the attending doctor is drug analysis during treatment of the illness and an analysis of the data in order to demonstrate and critically assess novel avenues and approaches in therapy. The clinician can then select therapeutically sensible measures at any point in time during the course of treatment of a defined illness. In this way only will clinical pharmacology remain as a real consultant partner and in this way only will clinicians and pharmacologists be able to fulfil their mission for the patient.
Few would deny the comment that clinical pharmacology is no easy discipline—it has perhaps its greatest role to play in those who are most sick—it has to unify intangible events (the therapeutic response) with invisible existance (the drug and its receptor). It must strive to bring mathematical clarity to a mess of facts. The product of these efforts must be immediately dispensible, metaphorically speaking, as quanta, for the healing of the sick and the elimination of suffering. In this task clinical pharmacology has a noble partner in the pharmaceutical industry who have been responsible for the discovery and development of most of our current drugs. You will not be surprised to learn that without their financial support this symposium could never have taken place. An acknowledgement to those companies who have given support is given below. The editors are particularly grateful to Beiersdorf AG, Hamburg, who supported the symposium and the proceedings publication far beyond their call.
Thanks is given to Vieweg Verlag/Wiesbaden, the publishers and to Mrs. S. Seltmann, Dr. N. Heinz, Dr. B. Hemmer, Dr. H. Schmitz (Beiersdorf), Dr. G. Leopold (Merck), Dr. A. S. E. Fowle (Wellcome), and Dr. H. Staib (Frankfurt/Main) for the personal effort they gave so generously.

N. Rietbrock
B. G. Woodcock
G. Neuhaus

The symposium has received financial support from:

Bundesministerium für Forschung und Technologie, Bonn
Asta-Werke, Bielefeld
Beiersdorf AG, Hamburg
Biotest-Serum-Institut GmbH, Frankfurt
Biotronik GmbH, Frankfurt
Boehringer Mannheim, Mannheim
Byk Gulden, Konstanz
Cassella, Frankfurt
Chemische Werke Minden GmbH, Minden
Colora Messtechnik GmbH, Lorch/Württ.
Deutsche Abbott GmbH, Ingelheim am Rhein
Deutsche Wellcome GmbH, Burgwedel
Giulini-Pharma GmbH, Hannover
Gödecke AG, Berlin
LKB Instrument GmbH, Gräfelfing b. München
Dr. Madaus & Co, Köln
Medice GmbH, Iserlohn
Merck, Darmstadt
Dr. Willmar Schwabe, Karlsruhe
Winthrop GmbH, Neu-Isenburg
Verla-Pharm, Tutzing
Paul-Martini-Stiftung der Medizinisch-Pharmazeutischen Studiengesellschaft e.V., Mainz

Chapter 2

Advances in pharmacodynamic assessment of drugs

Techniques for studying the pharmacodynamic effects of cardiac glycosides on patients' own tissues during glycoside therapy

J. K. Aronson
MRC Unit and University Department of Clinical Pharmacology, Radcliffe Infirmary, Oxford, U. K.

Introduction

Since the advent of fast immunoassay techniques for measuring the concentrations of cardiac glycosides in body tissues a vast literature has accumulated concerning numerous different aspects of the relationships between plasma and tissue glycoside concentrations on the one hand and the therapeutic or toxic effects of cardiac glycosides on the other. Concentration measurements, however, relate only to the *distribution* of the drug in body tissues and give no direct information about the *effects* of drug in those tissues.
The pharmacological events following the administration of a cardiac glycoside may be considered schematically as follows:

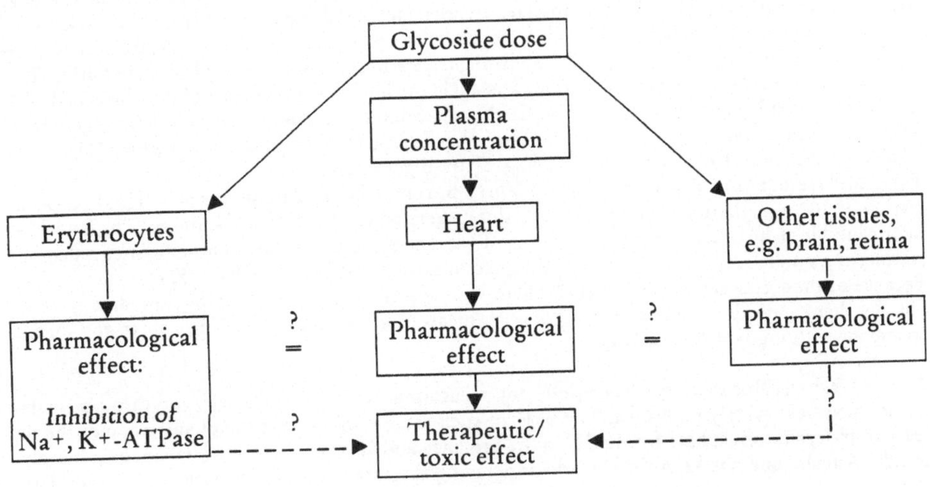

Following administration, cardiac glycosides are distributed first throughout the plasma and then to almost all body tissues. In erythrocytes cardiac glycosides are known to inhibit the cation transport enzyme, Na^+,K^+-ATPase and the effects of that inhibition are measurable in several ways as will be discussed below. In the heart pharmacological effects occur, resulting in therapeutic or toxic effects and, although it is by no means proven, there is a great deal of circumstantial evidence linking those pharmacological effects either directly or indirectly to inhibition of Na^+,K^+-ATPase [1]. Pharmacological effects in other (*e.g.* central or peripheral nervous) tissues may also be related to the therapeutic or toxic effects in the heart but the pharmacological mechanisms of those effects are not well characterized. Pharmacological effects in the tissues of the eye may result in impairment of colour visual discrimination and the relevance of that effect will be discussed below.
I shall first describe the techniques available for measuring the pharmacological effects of cardiac glycosides on human tissues, restricting myself to a discussion of digoxin with which the majority of studies have been concerned. I shall then show that such measurements may be related to therapeutic or toxic events in the heart.

Techniques

A. Erythrocyte measurements

The course of events following the exposure of digoxin to erythrocytes is presumed to be as follows:
1. Digoxin binds to the erythrocyte membrane.
2. Na^+,K^+-ATPase activity is inhibited.
3. Transmembrane sodium and potassium fluxes are inhibited.
4. Intracellular sodium and potassium concentrations alter accordingly.

The following measurements may be carried out related to each part of this sequence:
1. The ability of the erythrocyte membrane to bind digoxin (as 12-α-^{3}H-digoxin) specifically (^{3}H-digoxin binding).
2. Erythrocyte membrane Na^+,K^+-ATPase activity.
3. The ability of the erythrocyte to transport potassium from outside to inside the cell. In practice it is much simpler to use radioactive rubidium (^{86}Rb uptake) which is handled in the same way as potassium by the erythrocyte membrane and which has a longer half-life than ^{42}K.
4. Intraerythrocytic sodium and potassium concentrations.

1. *^{3}H-digoxin binding* Erythrocytes are prepared from whole venous blood by centrifugation, separation of plasma and buffy coat and washing three times by alternate suspension in 112 mM $MgCl_2$ and recentrifugation. The erythrocytes are then incubated at a haematocrit of 10% in a potassium-free Ringer solution at 37° for 2h in the presence or absence of 12-α-^{3}H-digoxin in varying concentrations. After further washes the erythrocytes are haemolysed with a phosphate buffer. The membranes are prepared by centrifugation, washed in the buffer, solubilized and then bleached with hydrogen peroxide. The amount of 12-α-^{3}H-digoxin bound to the membranes is determined by liquid scintillation counting. The exact technique has been described in detail elsewhere [2].
The characteristics of the membrane binding of ^{3}H-digoxin are:
Time- and temperature-dependency; saturability (maximum binding occurring at a digoxin concentration of 100 ng/ml after a 2h incubation); slow reversibility ($T_{\frac{1}{2}}$ of dissociation = 17h); stoichiometric inhibition by other cardiac glycosides and potassium; only one class of binding sites is demonstrable; the number of receptors per erythrocyte in normal subjects is 339 (± 52).
Because of these characteristics it is possible to measure the number of receptor sites already occupied by therapeutically administered digoxin by measuring ^{3}H-digoxin binding before and during treatment with digoxin (see below).

2. *Na^+,K^+-ATPase activity* Technique for measuring Na^+,K^+-ATPase in erythrocyte membranes have been widely published. The basis of such assay techniques is the quantitation of the release of inorganic phosphate from ATP in the presence and absence of excess ouabain or other glycoside. A technique has been developed for assaying the extent of inhibiton of Na^+,K^+-ATPase

activity in the erythrocyte membranes of patients receiving digoxin by rapidly reversing the inhibition and comparing inhibited and non-inhibited activities [3]. The technique involves the pre-incubation of the membranes with Na+ and ATP in the absence of Mg++ for 15 min followed by conventional assay of enzyme activity. This 'regenerated' activity may then be compared with the activity in membranes assayed conventionally and percentage inhibition of activity calculated.

3. ^{86}Rb *uptake* Erythrocytes are prepared as described under '^{3}H-digoxin binding' above, incubated with ^{86}Rb for 1h at 37°, washed three times and the accumulated radioactivity in the erythrocytes detected by a γ-counter. ^{86}Rb uptake is then expressed as the amount accumulated within the cells as a percent of total ^{86}Rb in the original incubation. Full details of the method have been published elsewhere [4].

4. *Intraerythrocytic sodium and potassium concentrations* Erythrocytes, prepared as described above, are haemolysed in distilled water and cation concentrations measured by flame photometry or atomic absorption spectrophotometry.

Effects of digoxin in vitro

If one incubates intact erythrocytes for 2h with unlabelled digoxin in varying concentrations and then carries out any of the four measurements described above, dose-related changes are observable. Such changes are illustrated for ^{86}Rb uptake in Figure 1 and similar changes occur in respect of ^{3}H-digoxin binding ATPase activity and intraerythrocytic Na+ concentrations.

B. Colour vision measurement

It is not possible to measure directly the pharmacodynamic effects of digitalis on the eye. Retinal tissue is rich in Na+,K+-ATPase and it has been suggested that inhibition of retinal ATPase activity may be linked to digitalis-induced colour visual abnormalities [5]. Thus, an indirect assessment of the effects of digitalis on the eye may be obtained by measuring colour vision and I shall show below that changes in colour vision relate both to clinical digoxin toxicity and to the pharmacological effects on patients' erythrocytes described above.

Colour vision is quantitated using the Farnsworth-Munsell 100-Hue test. Subjects are presented with a series of 85 coloured buttons which form a one-dimensional, roughly circular section of the entire colour spectrum. The differences in wavelength between adjacent buttons are just detectable by the perfect eye and subjects are required to arrange the buttons in order of wavelength. A score in obtained by adding up the differences between each button's correct position (from 1 to 85) and the position assigned to it by the subject. Scores are corrected for the subject's age on the basis of published data [6]. The 85 buttons are exhibited to the subject in four sections with a reference button at either end of each section to indicate starting colours. Each test is performed in duplicate and the whole procedure takes about 20 minutes at the bedside.

Clinical applications

A. Erythrocyte measurements

When digoxin is administered therapeutically to patients in either atrial fibrillation or cardiac failure in sinus rhythm there are falls in ^{3}H-digoxin binding and ^{86}Rb uptake and rises in intraerythrocytic Na+ concentration. Such changes are illustrated in the case of a patient in sinus rhythm in Figure 2. In the first few days of treatment ^{3}H-digoxin binding and ^{86}Rb uptake fell while intraerythrocytic Na+ concentrations rose. Other workers have shown that during the early stages of digitalization there is also a fall in intraerythrocytic K+ concentrations [7, 8]. At the same time there was a fall in the systolic time intervals, the QS_2I (total electromechanical systole corrected for heart rate) and also (not shown) the LVETI (left ventricular ejection time corrected for heart rate). After a few days,

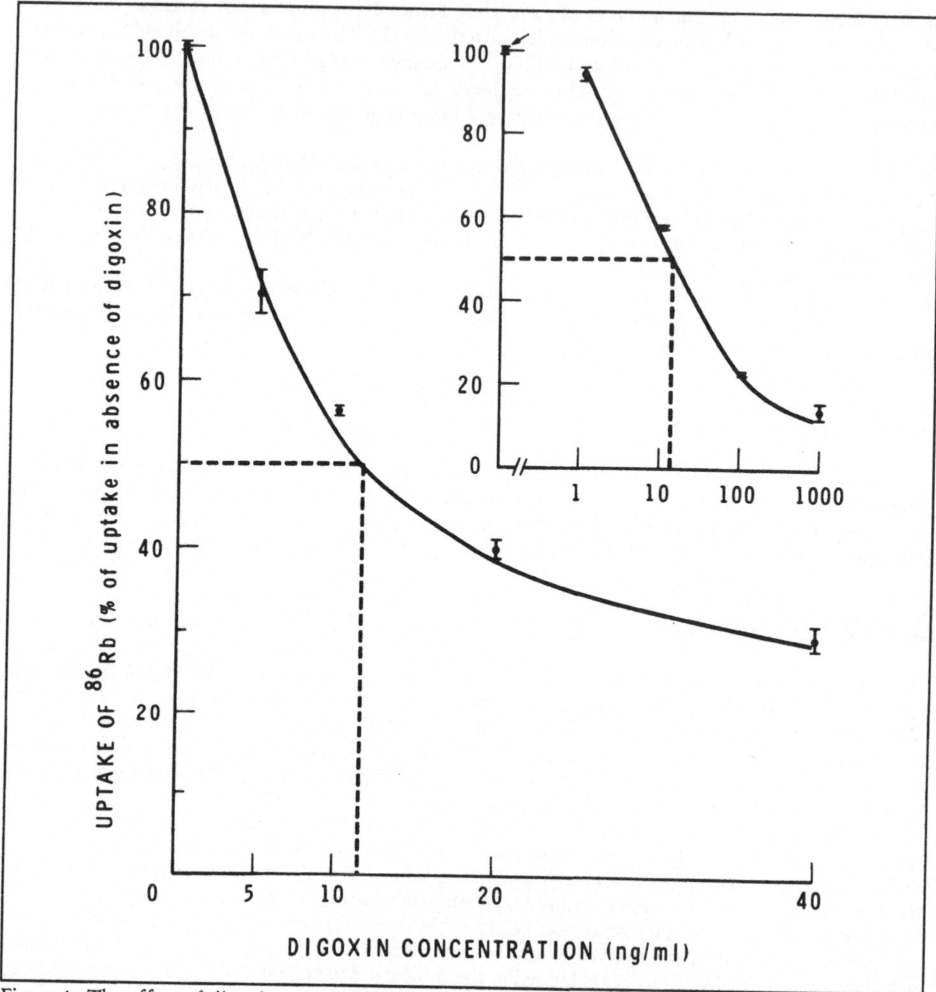

Figure 1: The effect of digoxin on *in vitro* ^{86}Rb uptake by normal human erythrocytes.

however, fluctuations started to occur in ^{3}H-digoxin binding and ^{86}Rb uptake (concomitant with each other) but not in intraerythrocytic Na^{+} concentration or QS_2I. The possible relevance of these fluctuations has been discussed elsewhere [9]. Similar changes have been seen in patients in atrial fibrillation [4].

In Figure 3 are illustrated the relationships between, on the one hand, the QS_2I and, on the other, each of the three red cell measurements.

In each case there is a significant correlation in the expected direction of change. Similar, although weaker, correlations were found with the LVETI (not illustrated). In contrast there was no correlation between QS_2I and plasma digoxin concentrations (not illustrated, see [9]). In patients in AF there were correlations between the slowing of ventricular rate and both ^{86}Rb uptake and plasma digoxin concentrations (not illustrated, see [4]).

After several months of continuous treatment, however, (Figure 2) all three red cell measurements returned to pre-treatment values as did a single measurement of QS_2I. Although the plasma digoxin concentration had fallen a little by that time it was no lower than it had been during the first two or so days when maximum changes in the red cell measurements had occurred.

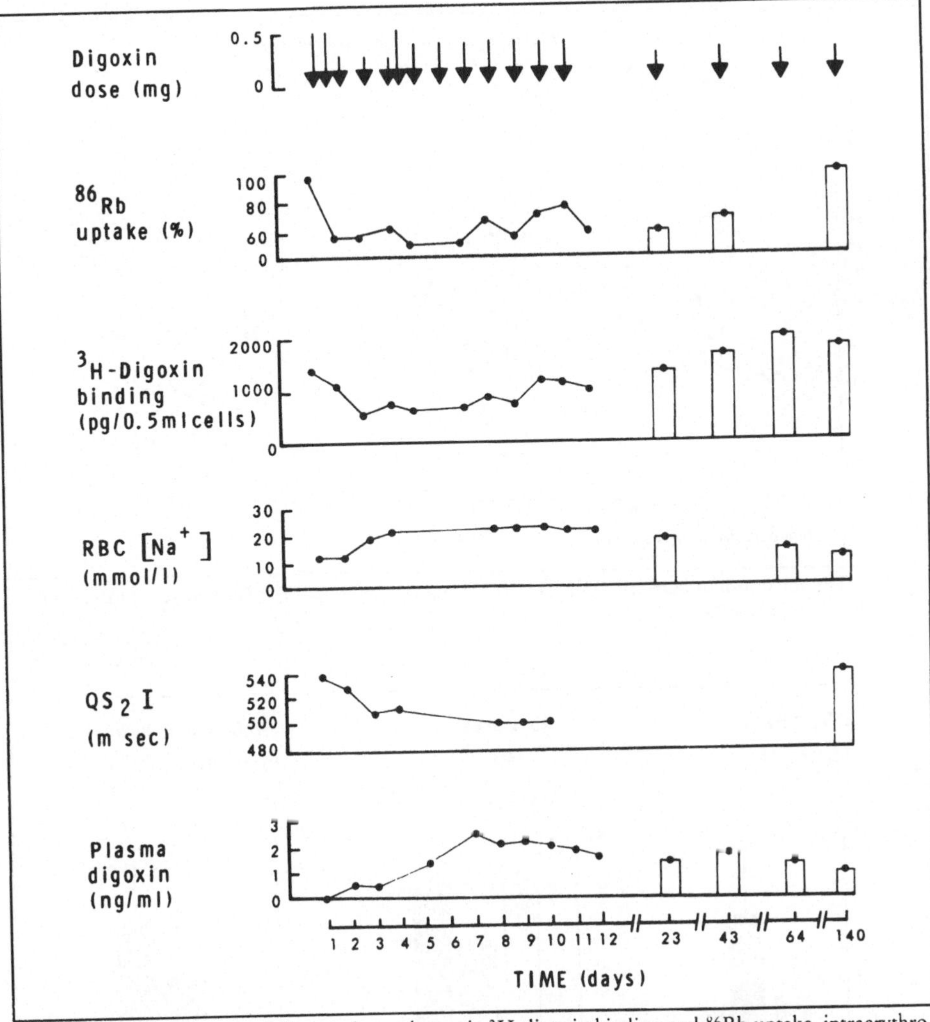

Figure 2: The time-course of changes in erythrocytic ^{3}H-digoxin binding and ^{86}Rb uptake, intraerythrocytic sodium and plasma digoxin concentrations, and QS_2I during treatment with digoxin in a patient with cardiac failure in sinus rhythm.

In Figure 4 are illustrated the grouped data (mean + lsd) for all patients studied. There was overall a significant fall in ^{3}H-digoxin binding and in ^{86}Rb uptake and a rise in intraerythrocytic Na^+ concentrations during short-term tratment (< 10 days). Others have shown that inhibition of Na^+,K^+-ATPase activity occurs in erythrocyte membranes in treated patients as compared with untreated [10]. However there was no difference between the values of these measurements in untreated patients and in patients treated in the long-term (> 2 months). This lack of difference between untreated and treated (long-term) subjects was not attributable to differences in plasma digoxin concentrations. This apparent pharmacological tolerance to effects of digoxin, at least in the erythrocyte, has been discussed in detail elsewhere and has been suggested to be due to the development of an increased number of glycoside receptors in erythrocyte membranes during long-term treatment [11]. There is other experimental evidence that the number of receptor sites in tissues may be

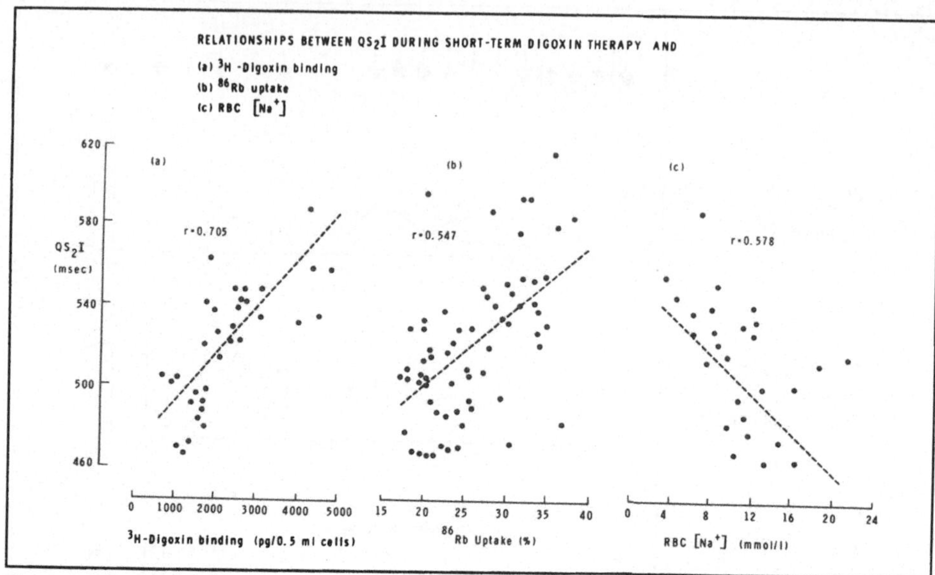

Figure 3: The relationships between QS2I and (a) ^{3}H-digoxin binding, (b) ^{86}Rb uptake (c) intraerythrocytic sodium concentrations.

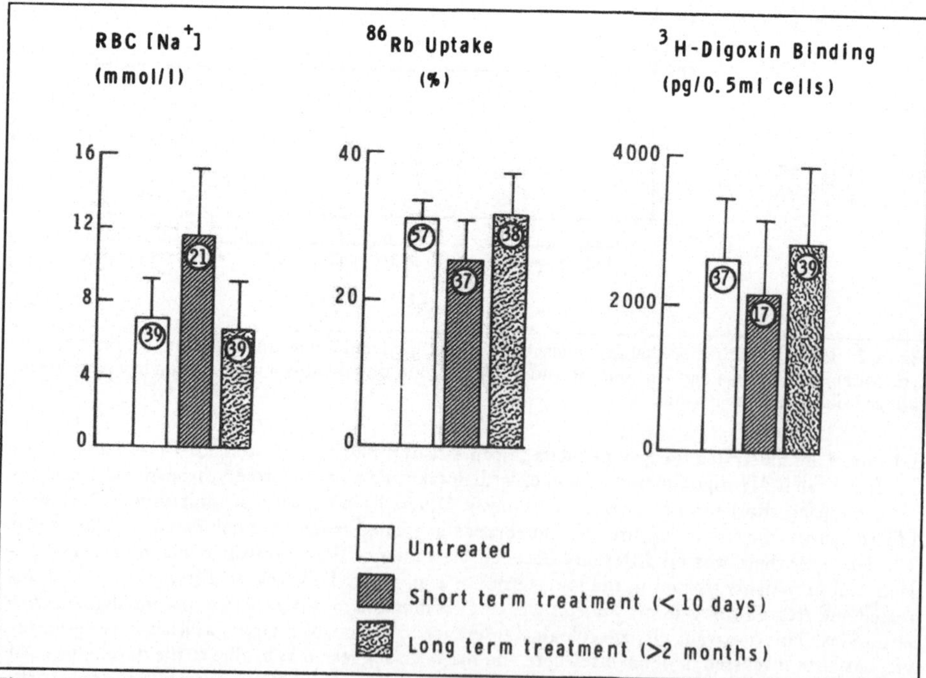

Figure 4: Values of ^{3}H-digoxin binding, ^{86}Rb uptake and intraerythrocytic sodium concentrations in untreated patients, patients during short-term treatment and patients during longterm treatment.

increased following exposure to cardiac glycosides and in particular it has been shown that guinea-pig heart muscle ATPase activity increases during long-term digitalis administration [12]. Assuming that the changes which occur in erythrocytes in man also occur in the heart then a question arises concerning the long-term clinical efficacy of cardiac glycosides. There is a growing body of data showing firstly that the clinical effects of cardiac glycosides, measurable during the early stages of therapy may not be present during more long-term administration and, secondly, that in some patients on established long-term treatment withdrawal of digitalis results in no apparent deterioration of clinical condition over a period of weeks or months (for references and discussion see [13]). The data presented here lend support to those clinical observations and clearly the problem requires further investigation.

B. Colour vision measurements

Patients with digitalis toxicity occasionally experience colour visual disturbances (notably xanthopsia) as well as other visual disturbances. However in patients without visual symptoms colour visual discrimination may be impaired and such impairment may be detected with the 100-Hue test [14]. In Figure 5 are shown the colour vision scores (as median values) and plasma digoxin and intraerythro-

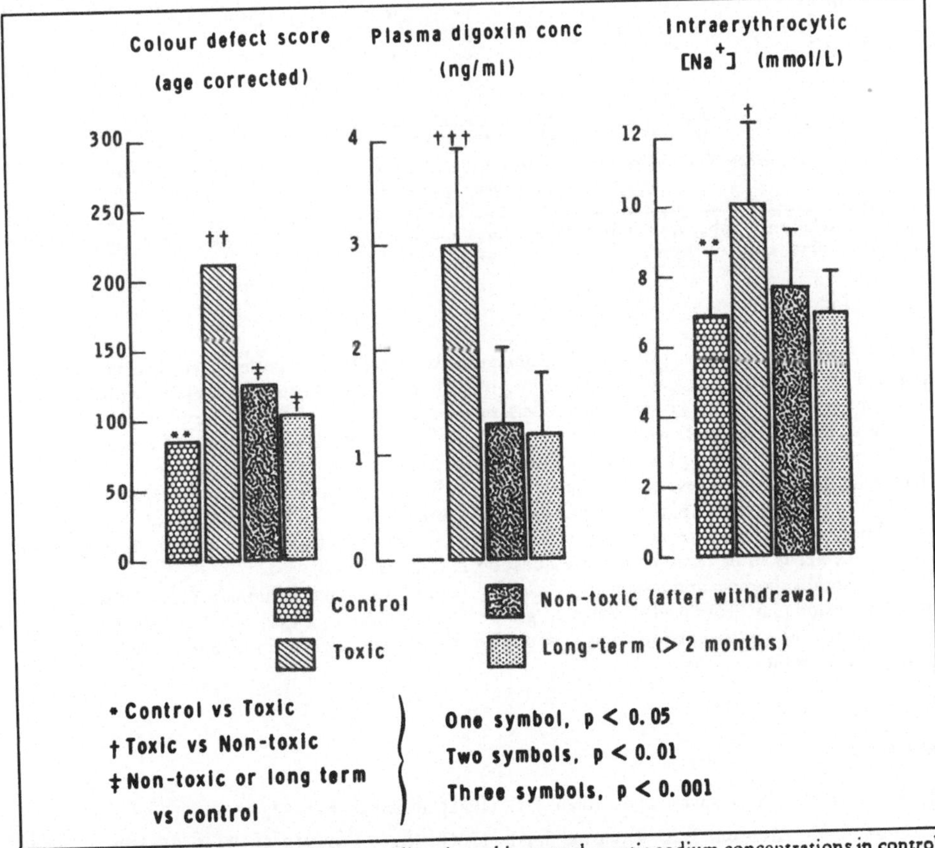

Figure 5: Colour vision scores, and plasma digoxin and intraerythrocytic sodium concentrations in control subjects, patients with digoxin toxicity, the same patients when no longer toxic after withdrawal of digoxin and patients on long-term therapy.

cytic Na+ concentrations (as mean + sd) in four groups of subjects—untreated, toxic, non-toxic (after withdrawal of digoxin) and non-toxic (long-term treatment).
In toxic subjects colour vision is impaired (high scores) and improves following withdrawal but some impairment remains compared with untreated subjects. In patients on long-term treatment there is similar mild impairment. The changes in plasma digoxin and intraerythrocytic Na+ concentrations need no further discussion here.
In Figure 6 are shown the relationships between, on the one hand, colour vision scores and, on the other, the three red cell measurements. There are significant rank correlations in the expected directions of change. There is a similar correlation between colour vision score and log plasma digoxin concentration (not illustrated).

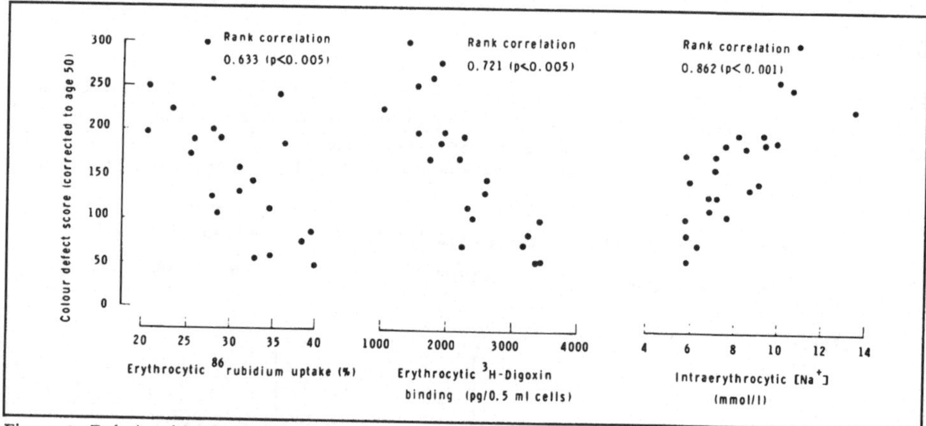

Figure 6: Relationships between colour vision scores and ^{3}H-digoxin binding, ^{86}Rb uptake and intraerythrocytic sodium concentrations.

Conclusions

I have demonstrated that the pharmacodynamic effects of digitalis on patients' erythrocytes may be detected *in vitro* using several simple techniques; that during short-term therapy with digoxin, changes occur in patients' erythrocytes consistent with inhibition of membrane Na+,K+-ATPase; that those changes correlate well with some clinical effects on the heart (slowing of ventricular rate in AF, shortening of systolic time intervals in sinus rhythm); and that during long-term therapy those changes do not persist. These data suggest that while digitalis may be of value in short-term tratment its value in the long term (particularly in cardiac failure in sinus rhythm) must be called into question. There is some evidence to suggest that not all patients benefit from long-term treatment but more work needs to be done before the question is fully resolved.
During digitalis therapy, and especially in toxicity, colour vision may be impaired and measurement of colour vision may prove useful in studying the effects of digitalis on yet another tissue besides the heart during both routine therapy and in patients with digitalis toxicity, in whom it may prove to be of diagnostic value.

References

[1] Schwartz, A., Lindenmayer, G. E., Allen, J. C. (1975). Pharmac. Rev. 27, 3-134.

[2] Ford, A. R., Aronson, J. K., Grahame-Smith, D. G., Rose, J. A. (1979). Br. J. Clin. Pharmac. 8, 115—124.

[3] Huang, W.-H., Askari, A. (1975). Life Sci. 16, 1253—1263.

[4] Aronson, J. K., Grahame-Smith, D. G., Hallis, K. F., Hibble, A., Wigley, F. (1977). Br. J. Clin. Pharmac. 4, 213—221.

[5] Robertson, D. M., Nollenhorst, R. W., Callahan, J. A. (1966). Arch. Ophthal. 76, 852—857.

[6] Verriest, G. (1963). J. Opt. Soc. Amer. 53, 185—195.

[7] Astrup, J. (1974). Scand. J. Lab. Clin. Invest. 33, 231—237.

[8] Kettlewell, M., Nowers, A., White, R. (1972). Br. J. Pharmac. 44, 165—167.

[9] Ford, A. R., Aronson, J. K., Grahame-Smith, D. G., Carver, J. G. (1979). Br. J. Clin. Pharmac. 8, 125—134.

[10] Huang, W., Forney, R. B., Patrick, J. R., Askari, A. (1977). Life Sci. 20, 2037—2040.

[11] Ford, A. R., Aronson, J. K., Grahame-Smith, D. G., Carver, J. G. (1979). Br. J. Clin. Pharmac. 8, 135—142.

[12] Greef, K. (1976). Eur. J. Pharmac. 37, 189—191.

[13] Aronson, J. K. (1980). In Meyler's Side Effects of Drugs Annual IV. Chapter 18.

[14] Aronson, J. K., Ford, A. R. (1978). 7th International Pharmacology Congress, Paris. Abstract No. 2894 and (1980) Quart. J. Med. In press.

Methods for measuring changes in alertness induced by drugs and associated effects on human performance

A. W. Peck and A. S. E. Fowle

Over the past ten years we have been interested in measuring changes in alertness and drowsiness and associated changes in performance tests induced by drugs. The subjects have been healthy volunteers, recruited from the Wellcome Research Laboratories at Beckenham. The most useful measure of subjective effects proved to be the series of visual analogue scales described by LADER and NORRIS (1969), and the most useful objective test that of auditory vigilance, described by WILKINSON (1968). Aspects of the use of these two measures will be considered in detail later, but before doing that it is necessary to describe briefly the experimental design and conditions in which the measures have been used.

The investigations to be described have usually used a crossover type design involving 12 subjects receiving 6 treatments at weekly intervals. Treatments were administered according to a balanced Latin square design in order to minimize the effects of learning or boredom during the course of the study. Treatments have always included lactose dummies and double blind conditions used, with testing conducted in a sound-proof air-conditioned room at 20° C. Four subjects were tested on each day, and the groups kept the same throughout the course of the study. The subjects spent the whole day in the laboratory, and for most of this were engaged in test procedures. They were not given knowledge of their results during the course of the study, and were paid a small gratuity on completion of the study. The results were analysed by analysis of variance, and values of $p < 0.05$ regarded as significant.

Subjective measurements of alertness

The series of 16 visual analogue scales described by LADER and NORRIS (1969) was used plus two more subsequently added by LADER. The 18 scales used were lines connecting adjectives indicating the extremes of one particular dimension of feeling. They were: alert-drowsy; calm-excited; strong-feeble; muzzy-clearheaded; well co-ordinated-clumsy; lethargic-energetic; contented-discontented; troubled-tranquil; mentally slow-quick witted; tense-relaxed; attentive-dreamy; incompetent-proficient; happy-sad; antagonistic-amicable; interested-bored; withdrawn-sociable; depressed-elated; selfcentred-outgoing.

Subjects were instructed to make a vertical mark along the 100 mm line to indicate how they felt at that particular moment, bearing in mind that the ends of the lines represented the absolute extremes of their experience of these feelings. This obviously deterred them from using the extreme ends of the scale, but they were also asked to avoid using only the central portion of the line. Obviously while subjects have to make an absolute rating of their feelings at the particular moment of the test session, the position they mark will be influenced by previous ratings during the course of the study, both at different times of day, and following different treatments. Mean ratings by 12 subjects after various doses of tricyclic antidepressants (BYE, CLUBLEY, and PECK, 1978) are shown in Figure 1A. It can be seen that the drowsiness produced by amitriptyline was rapid in onset and considerably greater than that produced by nortriptyline in approximately equal dosage. The effects of the secondary amine appeared later and were only significant at the highest dose. Protriptyline by contrast failed to produce any change.

AITKEN (1969) drew attention to the fact that at times subjects tended to mark the extreme ends of particular lines and thus produce skew distributions. He advocated the use of arc-sine transformation to produce a more normal distribution and we began to use this routinely. This procedure of taking the arc-sine of the square root (SNEDECOR and COCHRAN, 1976) effectively increases differences in high and low ratings, and decreases differences in the middle ratings. The wisdom of arc-sine transformation however, has recently been questioned by MAXWELL (1978) on the grounds that it might produce erroneous results. In view of this we analysed the results of several studies both as raw scores and after arc-sine transformation. The three studies each involved 12 subjects receiving 6 treatments, and visual analogue scales were completed before treatment, and twice after it. Drugs administered were the three tricyclic anti-depressants mentioned previously, and cyclizine and caffeine in various dosages and combinations in two other studies involving the same number of subjects and design (CLUBLEY, BYE, HENSON, PECK, and RIDDINGTON, 1979). A total of 162 scales (18 lines, 3 for each occasion, and 3 investigations) were examined for drug effects by analysis of variance. Of these 49 showed F values indicating significant drug effects ($p < 0.05$) on both untransformed data and arc-sine transformed data. On 112 analses F values did not indicate a significant drug effect, in either method of data handling. On only 1 analysis was there a discrepancy between the two methods, untransformed data giving a p value of < 0.05 while after arc-sine transform p was > 0.05. DUNCAN's test was then used to evaluate the significance of drug effects in the fifty analyses where F values suggested effects existed. Six different treatments produced fifteen treatment pairs for examination, making a total of 750 comparisons. Of these 237 showed significant drug effects, and 497 failed to show drug effects on both untransformed and arc-sine transformed data. Three pairs were significant after transformation, but not on the raw data, and 13 pairs were significant on the raw data, but failed to reach significance after arc-sine transformation. It would seem from this, that in our hands transformation of the data makes very little difference to the final result, but may give a slightly more conservative analysis.

In their earlier papers LADER and NORRIS empirically grouped lines which they felt might indicate similar feelings, and analysed them together to give ratings of mental sedation, physical sedation, tranquillisation, and various attitudes. In a more recent paper, BOND and LADER (1974) submitted the data on 500 subjects to a factor analysis which indicated that three factors could represent all the scales. Alertness was measured by nine of the scales, and possible differences between mental and physical sedation were not seen. Another five of the scales indicated contentment, and two calmness. The authors explain that theoretically it would be possible to devise an abbreviated scale involving only three lines. They do not recommend this, however, because the present scale is easy and quick to administer and score, and they feel that changing the instrument might reduce its reliability.

We have long suspected that the ability of the visual analogue scales to detect drug effects in our hands when it appeared less sensitive in work published by other investigators, might be due in part to the type of volunteer participating in our investigation. Subjects are almost entirely drawn from technical, scientific and secretarial personnel, and as a result are both literate and capable of understanding the attempt to measure aspects of a mental state. It was, therefore, with some pleasure that we saw the investigation by SCHROGIE, HENSLEY, DIGIORE, and HARRIS (1977) in which they compared the value of prison immates and students as subjects in drug assessment. Part of the paper describes a study in which the effects of a new benzodiazepine, Halazepam, were assessed using the NORRIS (1971) visual analogue scales. The ratings of prison inmates shown in Figure 2 were very similar on all measures both before and at 2 and 4 hours after administration of drug. By contrast, both mental and physical sedation increased in the students after administration of the drug. This could be explained as a failure of the drug to change the state of alertness of prisoners, but a failure of this group to record any change using visual analogue scales is a more plausible explanation. Tranquilli-

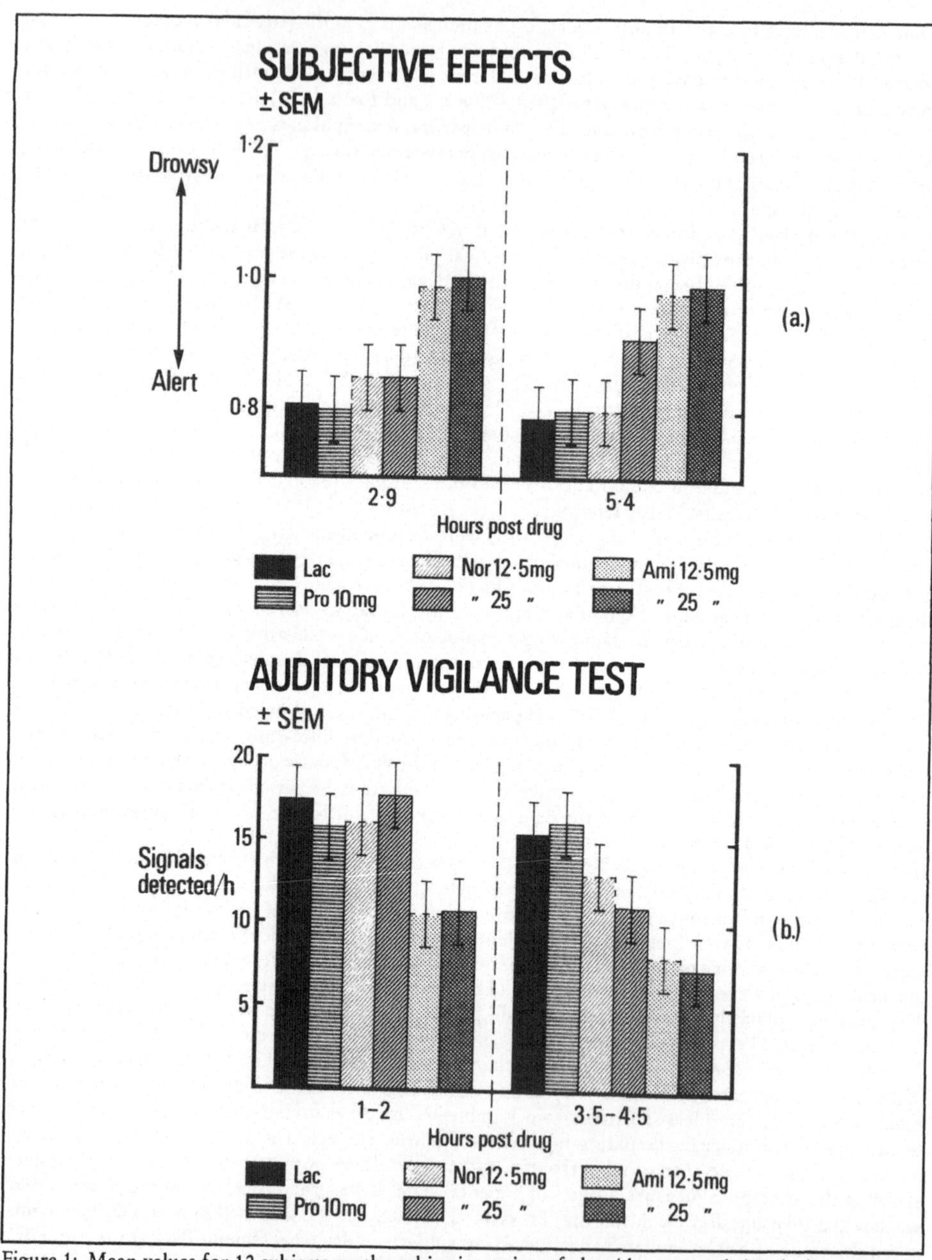

Figure 1: Mean values for 12 subjects on the subjective rating of alert/drowsy, and signals detected in an auditory vigilance test after treatment with tricyclic antidepressants are shown. Abbreviations for treatments: lactose dummy, LAC; amitriptyline hydrochloride 12.5 and 25 mg (base), AMI12.5 and AMI25 respectively; nortriptyline 12.5 and 25 mg (base), NOR12.5 and NOR25 respectively; protriptyline hydrochloride 10 mg (base), PRO10. The visual analogue scale ratings shown on the ordinate of A have been transformed by arc-sine transformation. The standard errors shown are derived from the analysis of variance.

sation scores remained very similar in the student population, presumably indicating that they were fully relaxed at all times. While the authors do not comment on this, it is likely that the students were more familiar both with the words on the scales and with the experimental aims, and probably more co-operative.

The Wilkinson auditory vigilance test

Vigilance tests were selected as the most likely objective tests to be affected by drugs varying the subjects' alertness or drowsiness. These tests are prolonged and monotonous and a degree of performance possible over 5 or 10 minutes often falls off with time. One of the earliest vigilance tests was that described by MACKWORTH (1950) and required subjects to watch a clock face of 100 divisions with the hand progressing discontinously by one division per second. Signals to be detected consisted of the hand jumping two divisions at a time. The test lasted 2 hours, and performance was evaluated every half hour. In all vigilance tests, a decrement in signals detected occurs with time as seen in Fig. 3. Administration of amphetamine (benzedrine) 10 mg, however, largely abolished this

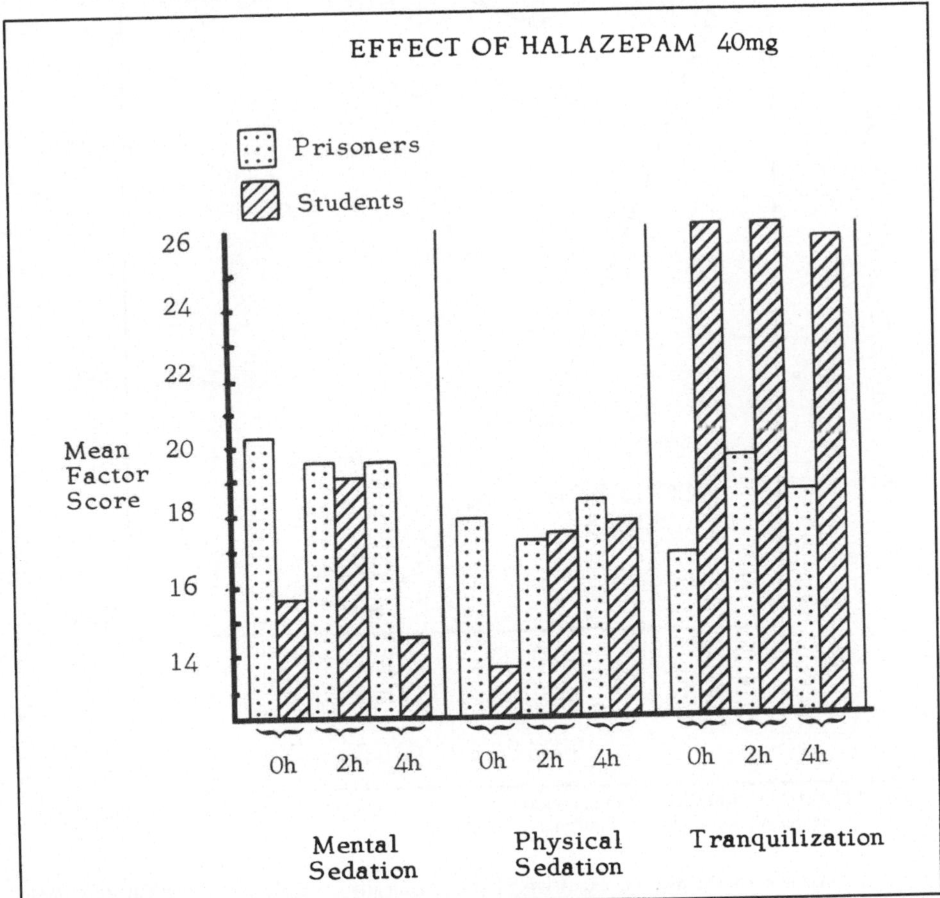

Figure 2: Subjective effects before and after Halazepam 40 mg as recorded by groups of students and prisoners using groups of visual analogue scales are shown. (Redrawn from Schrogie et al, 1977, with the permission of the Journal of Clinical Pharmacology and Therapeutics.)

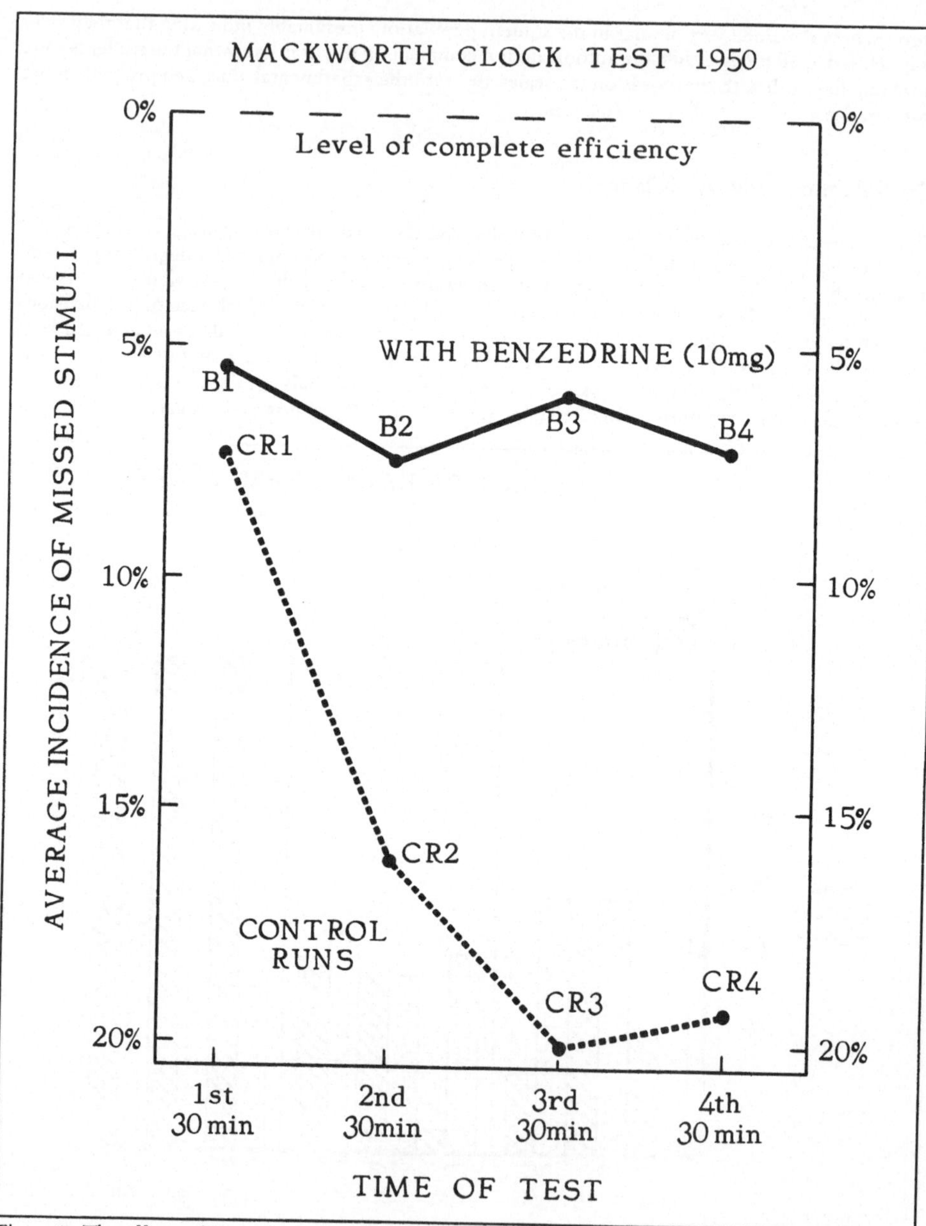

Figure 3: The effects of benzedrine in preventing performance decrement (Mackworth, N. 1950. Reproduced with the permission of H. M. Stationery Office).

decrement. For our use the test was excessively long, technically difficult to set up when studying a group of subjects, and by using a visual stimulus suffered from the fact that signals could be missed, by the subject's gaze straying from the clock face.

Wilkinson (1968) devised a test sensitive to relatively small amounts of sleep deprivation on the previous night. The test lasts 1 hour and consists of short tones 1 kHz frequency and mostly 0.5 s in duration, presented every 2 seconds against a background of white noise. Signals to be detected consist of slightly shorter tones, 0.4 seconds in duration. These occur randomly with the constraint that 10 occur in each consecutive 15 minutes of test i. e. 40 in 1 hour. On hearing a signal the subject records his detection by pressing a button. The test is administered by head phones, and this avoids inattention due to movements of the head. The test proved useful in detecting amphetamine-like activity in a study in which benzylpiperazine, a potential anti-depressant, was compared with dexamphetamine (Bye, Munro-Faure, Peck, and Young, 1973) illustrated in Figure 4. After dexamphetamine the number of signals detected during the test was significantly increased by doses as low as 2.5 mg at the end of the first test and beginning of the second. Subjects received a meal between the two tests. Similarly benzylpiperazine increased detections and its further clinical evaluation was abandoned. By contrast the number of signals detected fell significantly after amitriptyline (Figure 1B), and also, though at a later time, after the higher doses of nortriptyline (Bye, Clubley, and Peck, 1978). No changes followed protriptyline. These objective findings closely mirrored the subjective effects measured using the visual analogue scales. Similar changes have been found in various studies involving effects of sedatives and tranquillisers (Hart, Hill, Bye, Wilkinson, and Peck, 1976), and the hangover effects of hypnotics (Peck, Bye, and Claridge, 1977; Oswald, Adam, Borrow, and Idzikowski, 1979). Assessment of impairment following antihistamine drugs was particularly easy by this test, and enabled different doses of established drug (triprolidine) and a newly introduced drug (clemastine) to be compared, and their respective time course also to be examined (Peck, Fowle, and Bye, 1975). The degree of drowsiness and impairment was related to the antihistamine effect measured as flares and weals in response to minute intradermal histamine injections.

Those psychopharmacologists who subscribe to modern signal detection theory, can investigate further the mechanism by which drugs impair or improve vigilance performance (Swets, Tanner, and Birdsall, 1961; Broadbent and Gregory, 1963). Consider the situation illustrated in Figure 5A in which a subject listens to a series of short tones interspersed among longer tones. Obviously, on hearing each tone an event occurs within the nervous system, and the subject decides on the magnitude of this event, whether they are long or short. Signal detection theory postulates that the size of these events even in response to fixed constant stimuli, will vary from time to time within a subject, and will follow a Gaussian distribution. The theory also postulates that the two distributions will have the same variance. In a situation illustrated in Figure 5A when there is a large difference in the size of the two tones, 0.5 seconds, and 0.1 seconds, the subject will have no difficulty in distinguishing them, and will be able completely to separate the signal tones from the unwanted or "noise" tones. Consider now the situation illustrated in Figure 5B when the duration of the two tones is much closer, as in the Wilkinson test. Most of the tones are 0.5 seconds in duration, and constitute the noise to be rejected. The signal tones are 0.4 seconds in duration and must be reported. In this situation subjects cannot always distinguish the shorter signal from the longer noise and the two distributions now overlap. The subject, however, has to make a decision after every tone, and the decision point it usually designated as beta. All events to the right of beta are reported as signals, while all events to the left are rejected as noise. It can be seen that the signals reported are in fact composed in part of correct detections, but are also in part false reports. Similarly the rejected noise is mainly unwanted 0.5 second tones, but also includes some missed signals.

How then might drugs affect performance in signal detection tests of this type? Fig. 5C and 5D illustrate two possible ways. Firstly, the subject may change his willingness to report, effectively moving beta along the abscissa. Moving from beta 1 to beta 2 the number of correct detections will fall, but the number of false reports will also fall. In effect, the subject becomes more cautious. Conversely a move in the opposite direction increases correct detections at the expense of more false reports. The second way in which performance could change arises from changes in the ability of the subject to discriminate between the two tones. This is illustrated in the lower diagram, where the decision point remains the same, but the Gaussian distributions are closer together. In this situation correct detections will fall, while false reports remain the same or could increase if the left distribution moved to the right. In signal detection theory, the distance between the two means, d′ has fallen, and "detectability" is reduced. Conversely, drugs could produce increased separation of the distributions with an increased d′ resulting in an increase in correct detections, and a fall in false reports. Obviously there is a third possibility in that changes in both d′ and beta may occur in varying degress.

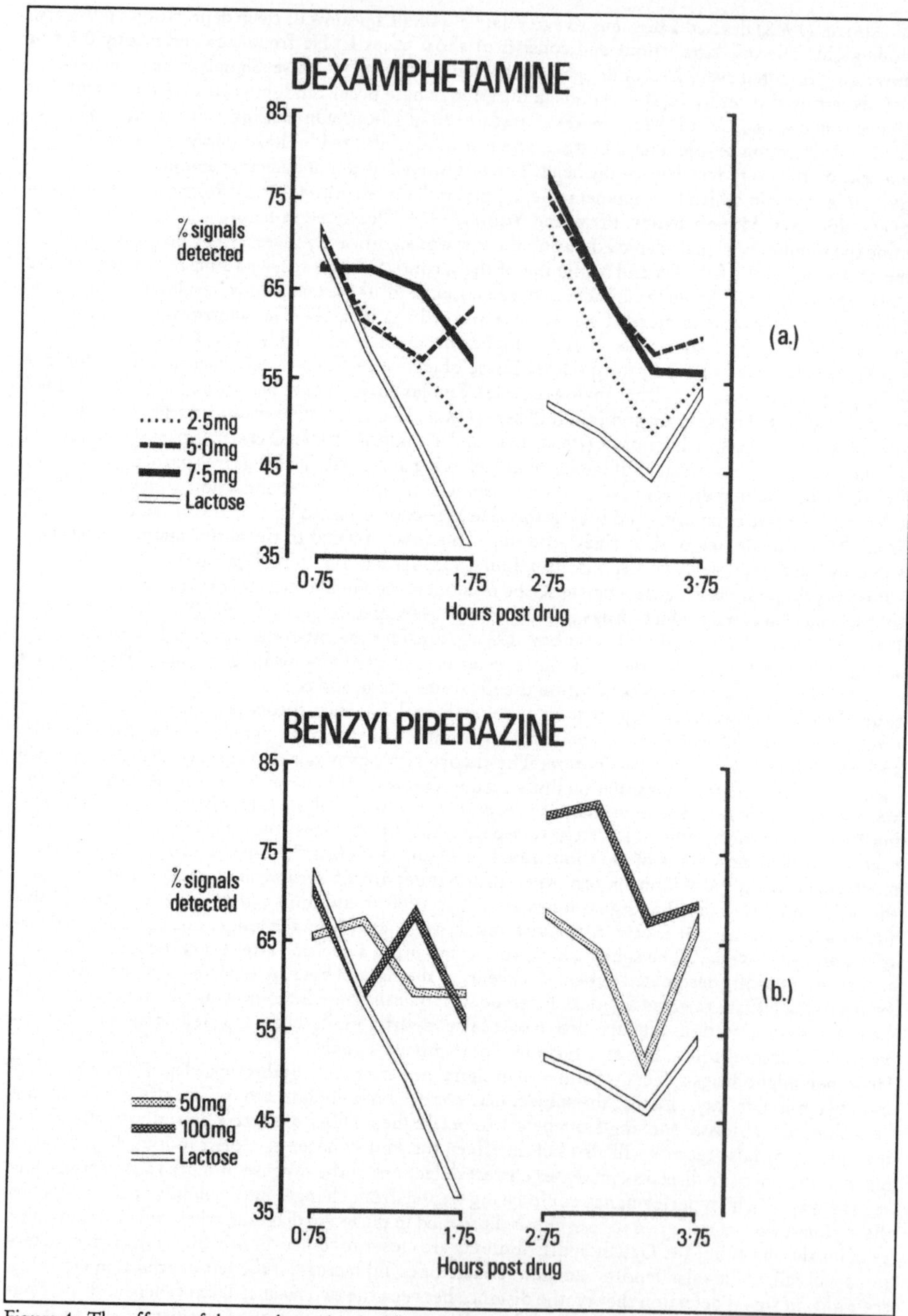

Figure 4: The effects of dexamphetamine and benzylpiperazine on the auditory vigilance performance of 12 subjects.

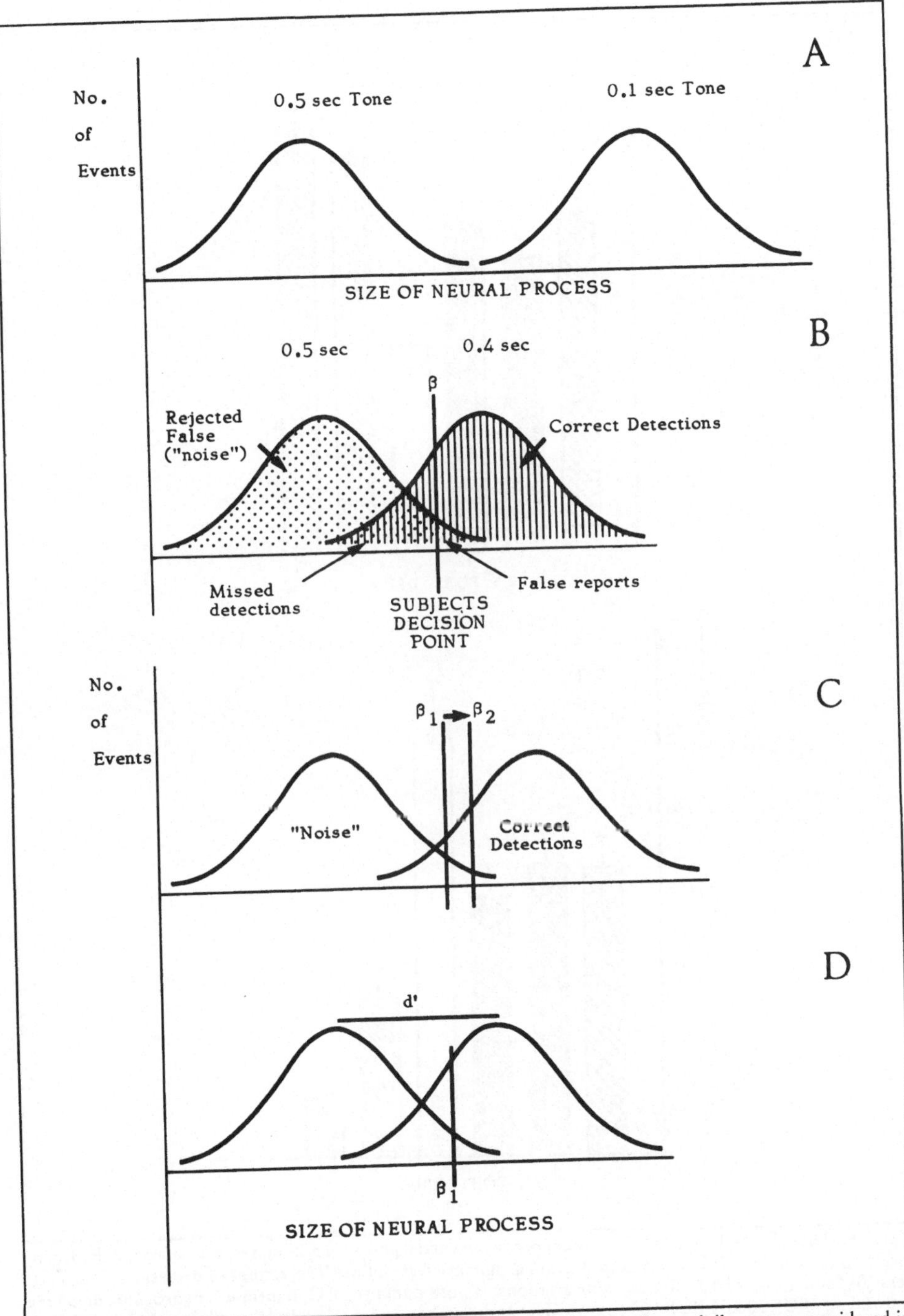

Figure 5: Possible ways in which drugs may affect performance in an auditory vigilance test considered in relation to signal detection theory. For discussion see text.

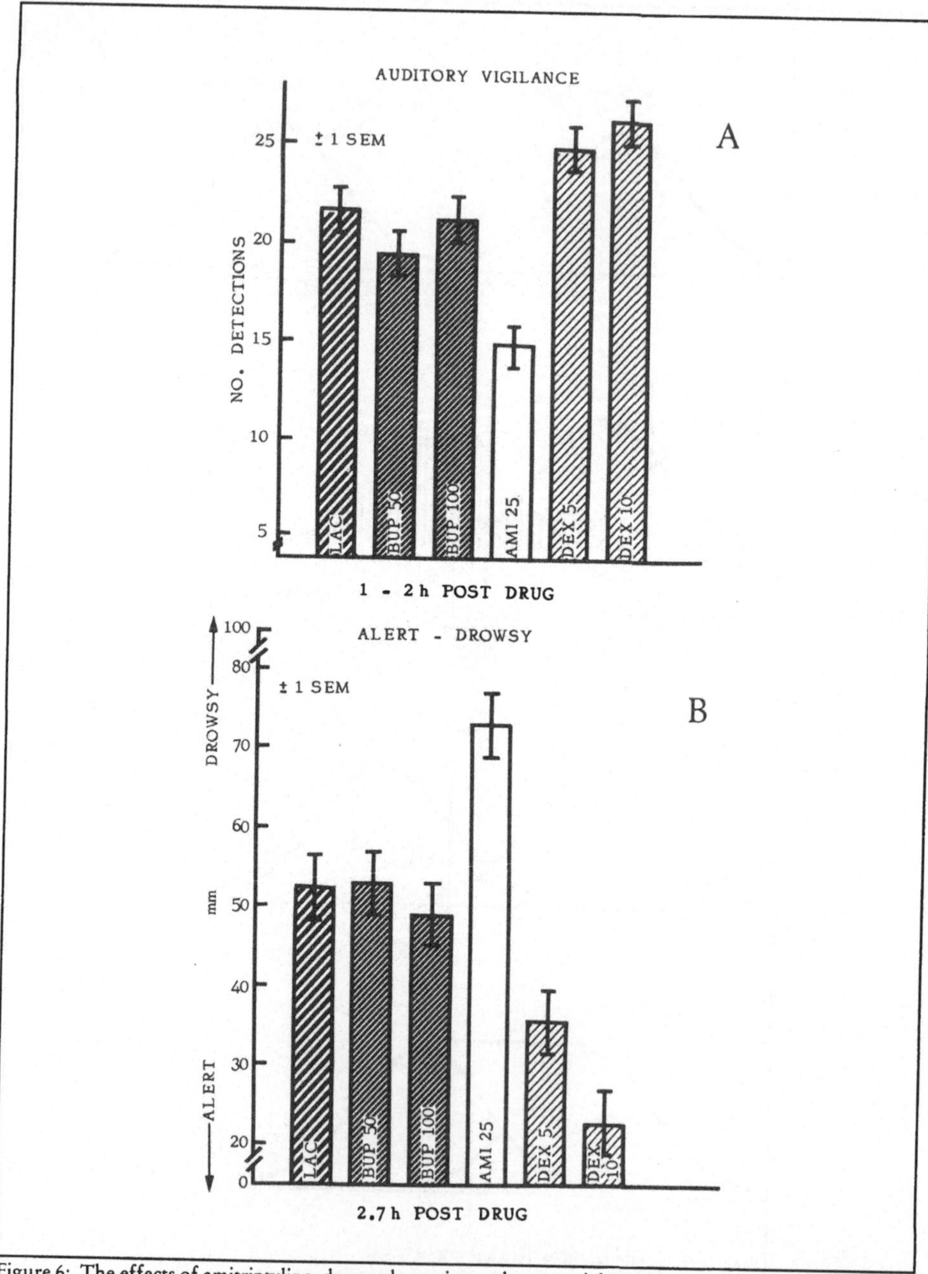

Figure 6: The effects of amitriptyline, dexamphetamine and a potential antidepressant bupropion hydrochloride on the number of signals detected (A) in a vigilance test and the VAS ratings of drowsiness and alertness (B) for a group of 12 subjects. Abbreviations: lactose dummy, LAC; bupropion hydrochloride 50 mg and 100 mg, BUP 50 and BUP 100 respectively; amitriptyline hydrochloride 25 mg (base), AMI25; dexamphetamine sulphate 5 and 10 mg, DEX5 and DEX10 respectively. The visual analogue ratings have been plotted as raw scores. The standard errors shown are derived from the analysis of variance.

It is possible to calculate changes in d′ and beta from the four measures obtained in the test: signals detected (total 40); missed signals; false reports; and rejected noise (total 1760). The main problem in analysing our data, is that our subjects make very few false reports. This may result from their scientific background; an unwillingness to report except when certain. The pattern contrasts vividly with the performance of the young sailors who participated in Wilkinson's original sleep deprivation studies, who made many false reports, and whose philosophy towards signal detection could be quite different by virtue of their training. When a subject has failed to make a single false report, it is of course impossible to calculate d′ and beta, and we have used two procedures to achieve an approximation. Firstly, it is possible to take the lowest level of false reporting in the tables of d′ and beta, compiled by FREEMAN (1973), this is a rate of 1 false report in 10,000. An alternative approach that we have used is to add one false report to the score of each subject. Both methods give very similar results. While this may not be strictly valid it seems to give results which at least appear sensible.
A final example describes an investigation comparing the effects of a new anti-depressant with dexamphetamine, and amitriptyline on subjective effects and vigilance performance. Bupropion has a chemical resemblance to amphetamine, and while the animal studies of SOROKO, MEHTA, MAXWELL, FERRIS, and SCHROEDER (1977) suggest that the compound is not amphetamine-like, it is important to examine and compare the effects in man. Dexamphetamine 10 mg produced a significant increase in correct detections compared with lactose, during the test period one to two hours after treatment, and the 5 mg dose produced a similar trend (Figure 6A). Amitriptyline 25 mg, as expected, significantly reduced the number of correct detections during the test period, but bupropion at either the 50 or 100 mg dose produced no significant difference. A similar pattern occurred four hours after administration of the treatments. Signal detection analysis shown in Table 1, revealed no significant difference in beta, but there were significant differences in the values of d′. Amitriptyline significantly reduced d′, whereas dexamphetamine 10 mg increased it. No significant difference from lactose occured after either dose of bupropion or dexamphetamine 5 mg. Analysis of the visual analogue scales (Figure 6B) largely mirrored that of vigilance correct detections; amitriptyline made the subjects more drowsy, while dexamphetamine made them more alert. No changes followed bupropion. A similar pattern was seen on the visual analogue scales reflecting happiness and sociability. Subjects rated themselves as more withdrawn after amitriptyline, and more sociable after amphetamine. Fortunately no changes occurred after bupropion.
In conclusion we propose that used in conjunction with a suitable experimental design, and standardization of conditions, the Lader and Norris visual analogue scales provide simple and useful means for assessing feelings of subjects involved in drug experiments, while the Wilkinson vigilance test provides an objective measure of their performance, and may give some indication of how the drug affects the central processing of information.

d′

AMI25	LAC	B100	B50	DEX5	DEX10
2.02	2.70	2.77	2.89	2.90	3.07

β

AMI25	DEX5	B100	LAC	DEX10	B50
61.2	73.6	76.0	78.4	80.8	83.6

Values shown are means for 12 subjects who each received six treatments. The abbreviations are: lactose dummy—LAC; dexamphetamine sulphate 5 and 10 mg respectively—DEX5 and DEX10; bupropion hydrochloride 50 and 100 mg respectively—B50 and B100; amitriptyline hydrochloride 25 mg—AMI 25. Values have been ranked in ascending order and means not differing significantly ($P > 0.05$) have been underlined. Means not underlined by a common bar differ significantly ($P < 0.05$). Values shown occurred 3h 50 min to 4h 50 min post-treatment. Values are approximate and were calculated by the addition of one false report to all scores. This was necessitated because occasional subjects made no false reports.

References

Aitken, R. C. B. (1969). A growing edge of measurement of feelings. Proc. Roy. Soc. Med., *62*, 989—993.

Bond, A., and Lader, M. (1974). The use of analogue scales in rating subjective feelings. Br. J. Med. Psychol., *47*, 211—218.

Broadbent, D. E., and Gregory, M. (1963). Vigilance considered as a statistical decision. Br. J. Psychol., *54*, 309—323.

Bye, C. E., Clubley, M., and Peck, A. W. (1978). Drowsiness impaired performance and tricyclic antidepressant drugs. Br. J. clin. Pharmac., *6*, 155—169.

Bye, C. E., Munro-Faure, A. D., Peck, A. W., and Young, P. A. (1973). A comparison of the effects of 1-benzylpiperazine and dexamphetamine on human performance tests. Eur. J. clin. Pharmac., *6*, 163—169.

Clubley, M., Bye, C. E., Henson, T. E., Peck, A. W., and Riddington, C. J. (1979). Effects of caffeine and cyclizine alone and in combination on human performance, subjective effects and EEG activity. Br. J. clin. Pharmac., *7*, 157—163.

Freeman, P. R. (1973). Table of d′ and β (Tracts for computers XXX). Cambridge University Press.

Hart, J., Hill, H. M., Bye, C. E., Wilkinson, R. T., and Peck, A. W. (1976). The effects of low doses of amylobarbitone sodium and diazepam on human performance. Br. J. clin. Pharmac., *3*, 289—298.

Lader, M. H., and Norris, H. (1969). The effects of nitrous oxide on the human auditory evoked response. Psychopharmacologia (Berl), *16*, 115—127.

Mackworth, N. (1950). Researches on the measurement of human performance. Med. Res. Council Special Report Series, No. 268, H. M. Stationery Office, London.

Maxwell, C. (1978). Sensitivity and accuracy of the visual analogue scale: a psycho-physical classroom experiment. Br. J. clin. Pharmac., *6*, 15—24.

Norris, H. (1971). The actions of sedatives on brain stem oculomotor systems in man. Neuropharmacology, *10*, 181—189.

Oswald, I., Adam, K., Borrow, S., and Idzikowski, C. (1979). Effects of two hypnotics on sleep, subjective feelings and skilled performance. In: Pharmacology of the States of Alertness. Ed. P. Passquant and I. Oswald. Oxford, Permagon.

Peck, A. W., Bye, C. E., and Claridge, R. (1977). Differences between light and sound sleepers in the residual effects of nitrazepam. Br. J. clin. Pharmac., *4*, 101—108.

Peck, A. W., Fowle, A. S. E., and Bye, C. (1975). A comparison of triprolidine and clemastine on histamine antagonists and performance tests in man: implications for the mechanism of drug induced drowsiness. Eur. J. clin. Pharmac., *8*, 455—463.

Schrogie, J. J., Hensley, M. J., Digiore, C., and Harris, S. (1977). Evaluations of prison inmate as a subject in drug assessment. Clin. Pharm. and Therap., *21*, 1—8.

Snedecor, G. W., and Cochran, W. G. (1967). Stastical Methods. 6th ed., p. 327. Iowa: Ames.

Soroko, F. E., Mehta, N. B., Maxwell, R. A., Ferris, R. M., and Schroeder, D. H. (1977). Bupropion hydrochloride (dlα-t-butylamino-3-chloropropiophenone HCl), a novel antidepressant agent. J. Pharm. Pharmac., *29*, 767—770.

Swets, J. A., Tanner, W. P., and Birdsall, T. G. (1961). Decision processes in perception. Psychol. Rev., *68*, 301—340.

Wilkinson, R. T. (1968). Sleep deprivation: performance tests for partial and selective sleep deprivation. Prog. Clin. Psychol., *8*, 28—43.

Colour vision deficiencies in patients under long term-treatment with digitalis as detected by an Automated Farnsworth's Munsell 100 Hue-Test

R. G. Alken, N. Rietbrock
Klinikum der Johann Wolfgang Goethe-Universität, Frankfurt,
Abteilung für Klinische Pharmakologie

Summary: Evaluating anamnestic data of digitalis-intoxicated patients, rates of general disorders of vision between 6 and 20% have been reported. As a psychophysical method, an automatically evaluated Farnsworth's Munsell 100 Hue-Test was performed to detect colour vision deficiencies in patients who received β-methyldigoxin or β-acetyldigoxin for at least four weeks under maintenance therapy. Patients were subgrouped according to serum digoxin concentrations measured by radioimmunoassay. There was a significant correlation between extent and rate of colour vision dificiencies and serum digoxin concentrations. About 80% of the intoxicated patients showed generalized colour vision deficiencies.

Introduction

Digitalis is widely used in the treatment of congestive heart failure and certain cardiac arrhythmias despite a rather high incidence of digitalis toxicity. Intoxication rates of about twenty per cent have been reported by several groups in prospective studies on hospitalized patients [20].
Many toxic events from digitalis treatment are attributable to a direct effect on the myocardium. Others such as nausea and vomiting, some arrhythmogenic and even some antiarrhythmogenic effects of digitalis glycosides are attributable to actions in the CNS. Three neural effects of digitalis have been well documented in animal studies and have their counterpart in man: 1) vagomimetic actions, 2) sensitization of baroreceptors, 3) sympathetic stimulation at higher doses [8]. Furthermore the reported sensitization of the chemoreceptor trigger zone as well as the interaction with the retina-cortex system ("retinex") from LAND [12] should be considered as manifestations of neurotoxic activity of digitalis.
In severe intoxication by chronic ingestion of digitoxin, "a remarkable finding was the high rate (95%) of visual complaints." Various types of reading difficulties and complaints of colour vision deficiencies have been reported [13]. In suicidal intoxication by Digitaline Nativelle (digitoxin) solution in France (reported in two large series) complaints of visual disturbances were present in 6% of intoxicated patients [7,15]. In reports on acute intoxications, complaints of visual disturbances were present in 11 to 20% of intoxicated patients [13].

Information on visual disturbances associated with digoxin are less well documented. DUBNOW and BURCHELL [5] found more complaints of visual disturbances after digitoxin than after digoxin overdosage. But there have been no reports showing qualitatively different patterns of visual complaints between digoxin and digitoxin. A report on one severe case of digoxin intoxication describes the presence of central scotomas apparently due to retrobulbar neuritis—like manifestations of digitoxin poisoning [14].
Farnworth's Munsell 100 Hue-Test [6] has proved to be outstanding as a means of detecting acquired defects of colour vision of different types. Automatic processing and polar plotting [4] has made it suitable for wider application. In this study the possible value of this test in detection of digitalis-induced colour vision deficiencies has been examined. The incidence of colour vision deficiencies detected by the test was compared to serum digoxin concentrations under steady state conditions. The possibility of differences in side effects between β-methyldigoxin and β-acetyldigoxin was investigated.

Methods

A total of 47 hospitalized patients were studied. Of these, 35 were diagnosed as having congestive heart failure, 12 carcinomas, 18 gastrointestinal, and 11 respiratory disease. Patients on cardiac glycoside therapy, were under maintenance therapy with β-methyldigoxin or β-acetyldigoxin for treatment of congestive heart failure. Control patients were not suffering from cardiac failure, and had not received cardiac glycosides for at least four weeks. Patients with ocular diseases, or receiving drugs with known interference with digoxin pharmacokinetics and pharmacodynamics, or receiving drugs with known cross reactivity in the radioimmunoassay were excluded. Patients suffering from diabetes mellitus or hypertension were also excluded.
Patients were subgrouped according to serum digoxin concentrations estimated by radioimmunoassay (Digoxin RIA NEN). Average age of patients was 60 ± 11 years, average serum potassium concentration was 4.25 ± 0.47 mM, average creatinine clearance was 59.7 ± 19.3 ml/min with no significant difference between the subgroups when categorised according to serum digoxin concentration.
Blood samples were taken in the morning prior to the daily dose of cardiac glycoside. On the same day, in the afternoon, the Farnsworth's test was performed twice as a bedside test under daylight conditions, checked by Macbeth Daylighting Metamerism Test Kit 2. Results of first and second turn did not differ significantly (Wilcoxon test for paired groups).
In the Farnsworth's Munsell 100 Hue-Test patients had to assort 84 coloured buttons partitioned into four boxes. Each button was numbered on its back, corresponding to continously changing hue in a Munsell design. The total error score was equal to the sum for all buttons of the sums of the differences between the number on the back of the button and those of its two neighbours. These calculations and the polar plotting were carried out by computer. The degree of deficiency is determined by the total error score. The polar plotting allows evaluation for type of colour vision deficiency by inspection of the *shape* of the plot and by calculating the angle produced by the diameter drawn through the regions of maximal errors. This will correspond in general to wavelengths where maximal colour vision deficiency occurs.

Results

Three typical data plots are presented in Figure 1. The minimal sum of the difference is $1 + 1 = 2$ for each button, if they all lie between their regular neighbours. This result would be plotted as a circle (radius = 2 units) in a polar plot. Higher sums of differences give greater than 2 units and would result in extensions of radii corresponding to the particular wavelength. The first example (0 ng/ml) showed some errors, but the total error score is within normal biological variation. The patient (No. 39) with a digoxin serum level (0.74 ng/ml) in the therapeutic range shows evidently more errors than the control group with no preponderance for a particular wavelength except for some higher errors in the bluish-green wavelength range. The third plot for a patient (No. 45) in the toxic range

(3.97 ng/ml) shows generalized colour vision deficiencies (total error score: 364), which resemble scotoma—like colour vision deficiencies. At digoxin levels (1.5—2.5 ng/ml) we observed specific types of colour vision deficiencies in some patients although the wavelength ranges involved tended to vary from patient to patient.

The mean plots for each serum digoxin concentration group were derived by calculating the mean error for each button. In Figure 2 the mean plots of β-acetyldigoxin according to serum concentration ranges are presented in comparison to the mean plot of the control group. No significant difference could be obtained between β-methyl- and β-acetyldigoxin. They show an increase of single errors over the whole spectrum corresponding to serum digoxin concentration ranges, with slightly more errors in the bluish range of the spectrum at toxic levels.

As can be seen in Figure 3 total error scores were dependent on steady state digoxin serum concentration. A linear regression of $r = 0.6887, p < 0.01$ and loglinear regression of $r = 0.7016$ was found. Comparison of linear as well as log-linear regression analysis gave no significant difference between β-methyl- and β-acetyldigoxin, although this requires confirmation with larger numbers of patients.

In Figure 4 total error scores corresponding to serum concentrations for the combined data of both digoxin derivatives are presented. The control group showed total error score (71.6 ± 35.0 [S.D.]) which was consistant with results expected in a elderly group of patients [9]. The mean total error scores show increases corresponding to digoxin concentration ranges from subtherapeutic to toxic ranges.

The percentage of patients, grouped according to serum levels, with total error scores above the confidence interval (two standard deviations) of the control group, is presented in Figure 5. The incidence of colour vision deficiencies rises from about 20% in the therapeutic range (0.5–1.5 ng/ml) to 50% in the range (1.5–2.5 ng/ml), and to 80% in the toxic range (2.5 ng/ml). Only two of all the patients tested had complained of disturbed colour vision.

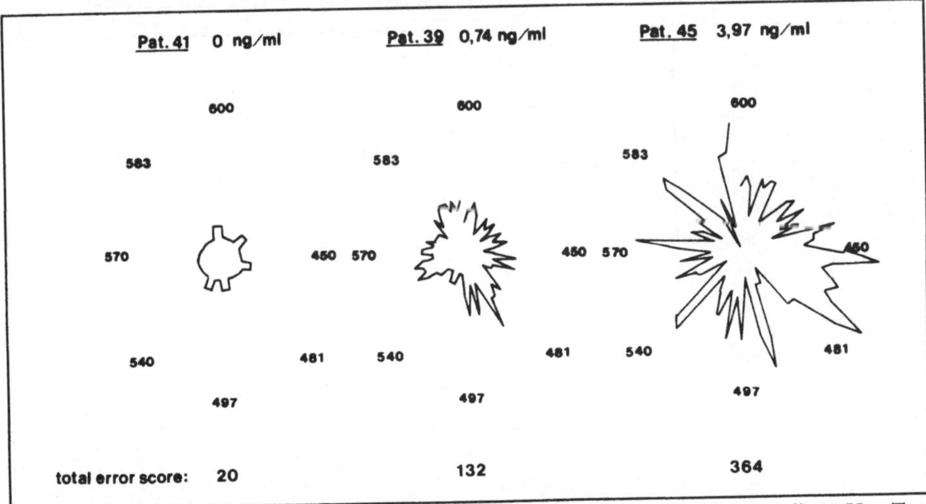

Figure 1: Original data plots obtained from automatically evaluated Farnsworth's Munsell 100 Hue-Test of three different patients (No. 41, 39, 45) at different digoxin serum levels (0.0, 0.74, 3.97 ng/ml); total error scores (20, 132, 364) show corresponding increase; circular arranged numbers (italics) give the wavelength (nm) corresponding to direction of radii in each polar plot.

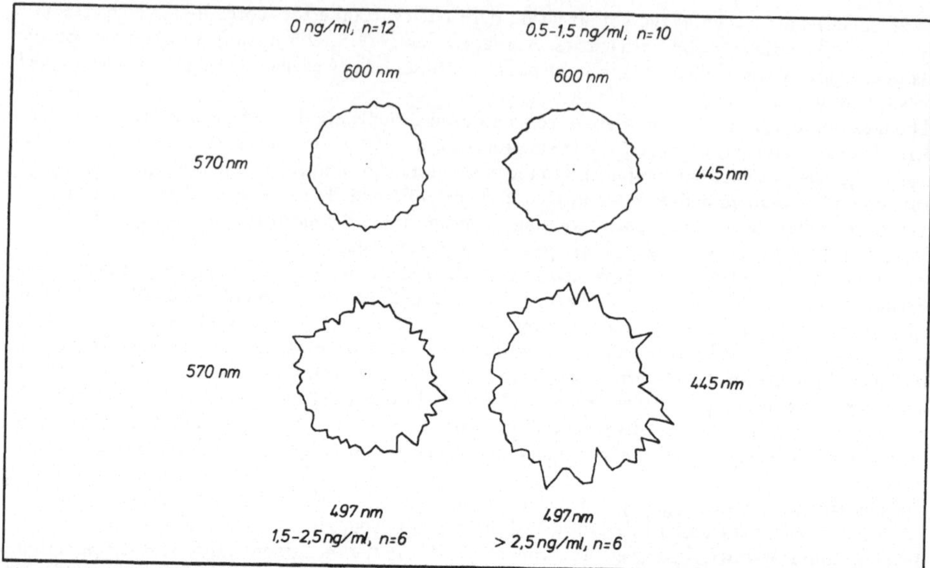

Figure 2: Mean polar plots according to digoxin serum concentration ranges obtained from Farnsworth's Munsell 100 Hue-Test by calculating the average error for each button. Numbers (nm) give the wavelength corresponding to direction of radii in each polar plot. All patients were treated with β-acetyldigoxin.

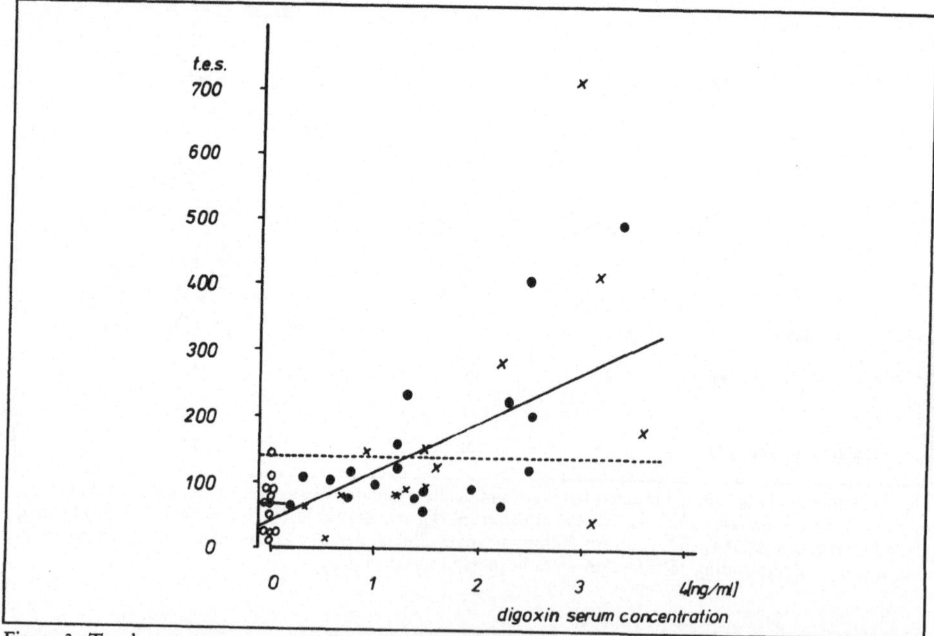

Figure 3: Total error scores (t.e.s., ordinate) vs. steady state digoxin serum concentration (abscissa). Single values of t.e.s. given as open circles (control group), crosses (β-methyldigoxin-treated group), dots (β-acetyldigoxin-treated group); straight line gives the linear regression over all points ($r = 0.6887$), dotted line gives the confidence interval (two standard deviations) above the average total error score of the control group (short straight line).

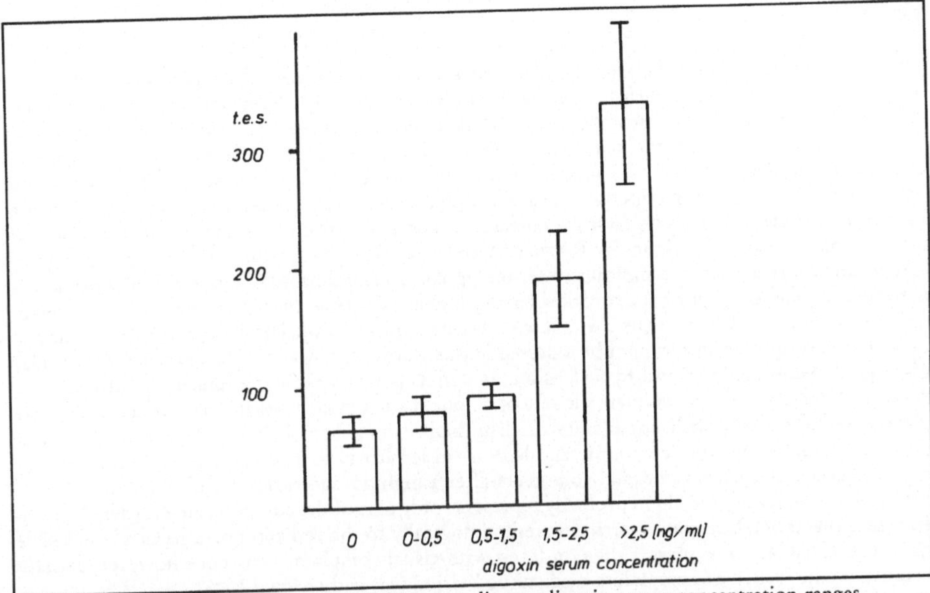

t.e.s.
300
200
100
0
0-0,5
0,5-1,5
1,5-2,5
>2,5 [ng/ml]
digoxin serum concentration
Figure 4: Mean total error scores (±S.D.M.) according to digoxin serum concentration ranges.

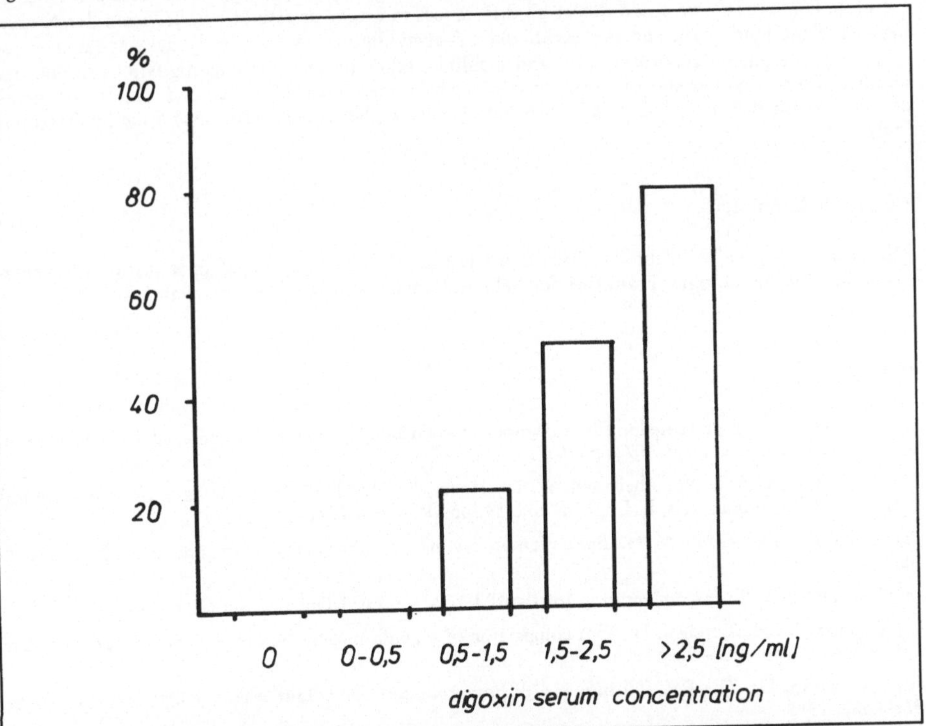

%
100
80
60
40
20
0
0-0,5
0,5-1,5
1,5-2,5
>2,5 [ng/ml]
digoxin serum concentration
Figure 5: Incidence of colour vision deficiencies (percentage of patients with total error score above mean total error score of the control group plus two standard deviations) according to digoxin serum concentration.

Discussion

The Farnsworth's Munsell 100 Hue-Test has proved to be a good method for detection of digoxin-induced colour vision deficiencies. The observations confirm earlier reports that these deficiencies resemble those produced by retrobulbar neuritis. In agreement with previous studies on digitoxin by LELY and VAN ENTER [13] a high incidence of colour vision deficiencies in chronically digoxin-intoxicated patients has been observed. In the present study however, it has been shown that colour vision deficiencies occur even at therapeutic levels of the glycosides. Such a relationship is reminiscent of a figure by AUGSBERGER [1], who found a correlation between expected compensation and expected intoxication and also of a figure by RIETBROCK and coworkers [17], who correlated percentage of cardiac and central toxicity symptoms to serum digoxin concentrations. Colour vision deficiency is therefore a common sign of intoxication having higher incidence than any single symptom diagnosed from ECG, and is as frequent as *overall* cardiac symptoms [20]. The predictive value of the test in diagnosis of intoxication cannot be assessed in this study, since we excluded patients with ocular diseases, diabetes mellitus, and hypertension, as well as patients receiving interfering drugs.
A few authors have tried to estimate the rate of colour vision deficiencies and have tried to correlate plasma digitalis levels with complaints of disturbed vision. Towbin and coworkers [21] using NAGEL's anomaloscope found a significant decrease in sensitivity to green light in nine patients after digitalization, and in twelve normal volunteers after a high dosage regimen with digoxin. This decrease in sensitivity to green light probably represents only part of the colour vision deficiencies present, since the anomaloscope is restricted methodologically to the red and green parts of the visible spectrum. Correlation of plasma digoxin levels with visual complaints was poor however, perhaps because the incidence of complaints of disturbed vision was rather low [2, 18].
Although β-methyldigoxin shows a 5-fold higher concentration than digoxin in various regions of the brain [10, 11, 16], we could detect no differences in extent or rate of colour vision deficiencies between β-methyldigoxin and β-acetyldigoxin. β-acetyldigoxin is completely desacetylated in the mucosa of the gut on absorption [19] and would be taken up into brain as digoxin. Although the number of β-methyldigoxin-intoxicated patients was limited, it can be concluded, that the incidence of colour vision deficiencies does not correspond to the higher concentrations of β-methyldigoxin in brain.

Acknowledgements

The authors are greatly indebted to Miss BAIER and Dr. KLINGAMAN, Max-Planck-Institut für Experimentelle Ophthalmologie, Frankfurt for help and advice on the automatic evaluation of data.

References

[1] Augsberger, 1951, presented in Pharmakologie und Grundlagen der Toxikologie, ed. by F. Hauschild, Leipzig, VEB Georg Thieme, 1973, p. 1057.

[2] Beller, G., Smith, T. W., Abelmann, W. H., Haber, E., Hood, W. B.: Digitalis intoxication: clinical correlation with serum levels, N Engl J Med, 284, pp 989—997, 1971.

[3] Cockroft, D. W., Gault, M. H.: Prediction of creatinine clearance from serum creatinine, Nephron 16, pp. 31—41, 1976.

[4] Donaldson, G. B.: Instrumentation for the FM 100 hue test, J Opt Soc Am 67, p. 248—254, 1977

[5] Dubnow, M. H., Burchell, H. B.: A comparison of digitalis intoxication in two separate periods, Ann Intern Med 62, pp. 956—965, 1965.

[6] Farnsworth, D.: The FM-100 hue and dichomotous test for colour vision, J Opt Soc Am 33, pp. 568—582, 1943.

[7] Gaultier, M., Fournier, E., Efthymiou, M. L., Frejaville, J. P., Jouanot, P., Deutan, M.: Intoxication digitalique aigue (70 observations), Soc Med Hop de Paris 119, pp. 247—274, 1968.

[8] Gillis, R. A., Pearle, D. L., Levitt, B.: Digitalis: a neuroexcitatory drug, Circulation 52, pp. 739—742, 1975.

[9] Klingaman, D.: personal communication, 1979.

[10] Kuhlmann, J., Erdmann, E., Rietbrock, N.: Tissue distribution of various glycosides in steady state and their affinity to the Na-K-ATPase, Naunyn-Schmiedebergs Arch Pharmacol in press.

[11] Kuhlmann, J., Rietbrock, N., Schnieders, B.: Tissue distribution and elimination of digoxin and methyldigoxin after single and multiple doses in dogs, J Cardiovasc Pharmacol 1, pp. 219—234, 1979.

[12] Land, E. H.: The retinex theory of colour vision, Scient Am 237, pp. 108—129, Dec 1977.

[13] Lely, A. H., Enter, C. H. J. van: Non-cardiac symptoms of digitalis intoxication, Am Heart J 83, pp. 149—152, 1972.

[14] Moore, C. E., Gilliland, J. M.: Central scotomas due to digoxin toxicity, Austral J Ophth 1, pp. 76—79, 1973.

[15] Potter, B. J., Perrot, L., Vechinne, J., Restoy, R.: L'intoxication digitalique massive, Masson et Cie, Paries, 1964.

[16] Rietbrock, N., Kuhlmann, J., Voehringer, H. F.: Pharmacokinetik von Herzglykosiden und klinische Konsequenzen, Forschr Med 95, pp. 909—915, pp. 951—954, 1977.

[17] Rietbrock, N., Kuhlmann, J., Voehringer, H. F.: Klinisch-pharmakologische Therapie mit Herzglykosiden, Therapiewoche, 27, 2325—2538, 1977.

[18] Rietbrock, N., Oeff, F., Maertin, K., Kuhlmann, G.: Glykosidkonzentration im Plasma und Intoxikationshäufigkeit nach β-Methyldigoxin und β-Acetyldigoxin unter standardisierten Bedingungen, Herz/Kreislauf 10, pp. 267—273, 1978.

[19] Ruiz-Torres, A., Burmeister, H.: Stoffwechsel und Kinetik von β-Acetyldigoxin, Klin Wschr 50, pp. 191—195, 1972.

[20] Schueren, K. P., Rietbrock, N.: Klinische Aspekte der Digitalisintoxikation, anaesth. praxis 15, pp. 99—115, 1978.

[21] Towbin, E. J., Pickens, W. S., Doherty, J. E.: The effects of digoxin upon colour vision and the electroretinogram, Clin Res 15, p. 60, 1967.

Pharmacodynamics and pharmacokinetics of a new aryl-alkylamine with negative chronotropic effects in man

Lothar Benedikter, Hermann Trouvain, Arno Zimmer,
Dr. Karl Thomae GmbH, Birkendorfer Straße 65, D-7950 Biberach an der Riß 1

Introduction

AQ-A 39 CL decreases heart rate in anaesthetized and conscious laboratory animals. Doses showing negative chronotropic action show no effect on cardiac contractility or peripheral resistance. The drug does not stimulate muscarinic receptors nor does it block beta adrenergic receptors.
Since the compound does not dilate coronary or peripheral vessels and has no intrinsic negative inotropic activity its hemodynamic profile is markedly different from that of Verapamil or Nifedipine. In this study the drug was shown to be also active in man.

Method

Four cross-over double blind studies were performed. In each study 12 healthy male volunteers took part. With 2 exceptions always the same persons were employed. Each subject had an individually allocated work load programme which guaranteed a heart rate of 150. This heart rate was attained after 5 increases of 25 watt in the load at intervals of 2 minutes. The starting work load ranged between 50 and 200 watt. Before starting peddling subjects sat on the bicycle for 15 minutes. The drug was then injected intravenously within 1 minute. The heart rate was recorded every 30 seconds by means of ECG tracing. The effect was measured by calculating the linear regression coefficient of the increase of heart rate between the second and fifth load level. In every subject there was a significant linear increase of heart rate ($p < 0.001$).
The statistical calculation was done by analysis of variance for latin squares.

Result

Treatment		Study 1	Study 2	Study 3	Study 4
Placebo		12.0	—	—	12.4
AQ-A 39 CL	25 mg	—	11.7	—	—
	50 mg	—	11.2	—	—
	75 mg	—	10.7	10.9	—
	100 mg	9.9	—	—	—
	150 mg	—	—	10.4	10.1
Pindolol	0.4 mg	—	—	—	9.3
	p	<.01	<.05	N.S.	<.001

Table 1: Increase of heart rate per 25 watt increase of work load.

Study 1 shows a significant reduction in heart rate after 100 mg *i. v.*
Study 2 shows a significant dose response relation of 25, 50, and 75 mg. *i. v.*
Study 3 shows that 150 mg is not significantly different from 75 mg.
In Study 4 the high significance is due to the difference between placebo and the two substances. There is no significant difference between AQ-A 39 and pindolol ($0.05 < p < 0.10$).

Treatment		Trial 1	Trial 2	Trial 3	Trial 4
Placebo		155	—	—	156
AQ-A 39 CL	25 mg	—	156	—	—
	50 mg	—	150	—	—
	75 mg	—	144	143	—
	100 mg	136	—	—	—
	150 mg	—	—	138	137
Pindolol	0.4 mg	—	—	—	137

Table 2: Heart rate at the end of exercise

The table shows that there is no effect below 50 mg (AQ-A 39 given *i. v.*) and that there is no further reduction in heart rate above 100 mg. It also can be concluded from this study that there is no difference between AQ-A 39 150 mg *i. v.* and pindolol 0.4 mg *i. v.*

The parotid gland as an "isolated organ" *in vivo*—Organ-specific determination of β-adrenergic stimulation in man

G. Schultze-Werninghaus, R. Merget, G. Fachinger, G. Kaiser, D. Palm
Zentrum der Inneren Medizin, Abt. für Pneumologie und Zentrum der Pharmakologie
Klinikum der Johann Wolfgang Goethe-Universität, Frankfurt am Main

This work was supported by a grant from the Deutsche Forschungsgemeinschaft

Introduction

Effects of β-sympathomimetic drugs in man can be measured indirectly, *e. g.* by determination of changes of cardiovascular parameters, or by measuring changes of biochemical parameters, *i. e.* increases of the concentrations of lactate or free fatty acids in blood. A more direct indicator for β-adrenergic stimulation would be the measurement of increased concentrations of cAMP in plasma. However, such changes would reflect only an overall stimulation of β-adrenoceptors in the organism.

It would be desirable, however, to have methods available for determination of organ-specific reactions in response to a β-adrenergic stimulator as is possible *in vitro* in isolated organs. It has been suggested by Schmid *et al.* (1975) that an increase of cAMP concentrations in the saliva of the parotid gland should provide a direct measure for β-adrenergic stimulation in man. If salivary cAMP originated from the parotid gland itself by a secretion process, and not from the intravasal compartment via a filtration process, it should be possible to measure directly an organ-specific stimulation of β-adrenoceptors in man. Furthermore, such an *in vivo* model of an "isolated organ" would offer the possibility to detect changes in sensitivity of organ-specific β-adrenoceptors in man. It has been suggested by Szentivanyi (1968) that in atopic patients there might be a functional imbalance between the parasympathetic and sympathetic system due to a defect on the level of the β-adrenoceptors, at least in the bronchial tract.

Recently, several authors have observed a desensitiziation of β-adrenoceptor-effector systems in man after chronic treatment with β-adrenoceptor agonists (for references, see Conolly and Greenacre, 1976; Galant *et al.*, 1978).

It was the aim of our study 1st to give experimental proof for the organspecific origin of salivary cAMP from the parotid gland (after stimulation by a β-adrenoceptor agonist) and 2nd to find out whether differences exist between asthmatic patients and healthy volunteers with respect to the response to a β-adrenergic stimulus.

Methods

The investigations were performed in 6 healthy volunteers (27.0 ± 2.7 years) and patients (31.2 ± 3.74 years) with extrinsic allergic bronchial asthma. The patients had been without any therapy for at least four weeks. Parotid saliva was collected through a polyethylene catheter in the parotid duct during stimulation of secretion by 5% citric acid solution dropping onto the tongue. cAMP-concentrations in the saliva and in the plasma were determined as described by STEINER *et al.* (1972). Salivary protein concentration was measured according to LOWRY *et al.* (1951). All experiments were performed at 9 *a. m.*; after a resting period of 30 min in supine position, saliva and blood samples were obtained simultaneously 15 and 5 min before and immediately and 3 to 60 min after slow *i. v.* injection of 0.01 mg/m² fenoterol and 0.04 mg/kg cAMP respectively.

Results

After *i. v.* injection of the β_2-sympathomimetic compound fenoterol, cAMP concentrations in parotid saliva were increased about 5 fold. Peak values were reached within 3 min after slow *i. v.* injection (Table 1). Normal values were reached again 10 to 20 min after injection. Similar changes were observed with respect to protein concentrations in the same salivary samples.
When the changes in cAMP concentrations in plasma were compared to those occurring in the saliva, plasma peaks appeared after a lag phase of 6 to 10 min after the *i. v.* injection of fenoterol. This might indicate that salivary cAMP originates from the parotid gland itself and not from the blood.
Direct evidence for this assumption came from experiments in which 0.04 mg/kg cAMP were injected slowly *i. v.* Immediately after injection, a 35 fold increase of cAMP concentrations in plasma could be measured; enhanced concentrations could be detected up to 6 min after injection (Table 2). Despite these pronounced increases of plasma cAMP there occured no significant alterations of salivary cAMP concentrations. From these results it can be concluded that salivary cAMP originates from the parotid gland and not from the blood. Thus it can be assumed that enhancement of cAMP concentrations in saliva after *i. v.* injection of fenoterol is the consequence of the stimulation of β-adrenoceptors in the parotid gland itself.
When the effects of fenoterol on cAMP and protein concentration in saliva from healthy volunteers were compared to those occurring in untreated asthmatic patients, no significant differences could be shown. Similar results were obtained with respect to the changes of cAMP concentrations in plasma. This holds true also for the small changes in heart rate after *i. v.* injection of fenoterol (Table 1).

Time (min)	−15	−3	0	+3	+6	+10	+20	+30	+60
Plasma cAMP (pmoles/ml)	14.7 ± 0.3	13.7 ± 0.8	493.3 ± 31	293.3 ± 75.1	221.3 ± 25	152 ± 14.6	96 ±10.5	93 ±18.3	42 ± 4.7
Salivary cAMP (pmoles/ml)	6.1 ± 3.3	3.8 ± 0.7	7.0 ± 2.3	4.6 ± 0.7	6.8 ± 2.4	4.4 ± 0.8	5.0 ± 0.45	9,17 ± 2.4	6.4 ± 2.7
Heart rate (min⁻¹)	78 ± 5	78 ± 4	72 ± 6	73 ± 7	73 ± 1	68 ± 4	70 ± 3	73 ± 6	71 ± 5

Table 2: Changes of concentrations of plasma cAMP and salivary cAMP ($\bar{x}$ ± *SEM*) after *i. v.* injection of 0.04 mg/kg cAMP in 3 healthy volunteers. — Despite a 35-fold increase in plasma cAMP there occurred no increase in concentration of salivary cAMP.—Heart rate remains unaltered after injection of cAMP (−3→0 min).

	Time (min)	−15	−5	0	+3	+6	+10	+20	+30	+60
Salivary cAMP (pmoles/ml)	Controls	3.3 ± 1.0	2.7 ± 0.5	6.6 ± 1.2	10.0 ± 2.9	5.5 ± 1.2	4.6 ± 1.2	3.0 ± 0.4	3.6 ± 0.9	2.7 ± 0.4
	Patients	3.5 ± 0.3	3.0 ± 0.5	8.4 ± 2.3	12.5 ± 4.6	8.6 ± 2.5	6.9 ± 2.0	4.8 ± 1.5	5.2 ± 1.3	4.7 ± 0.8
Salivary Protein (mg/ml)	Control	0.99 ± 0.24	0.86 ± 0.2	4.12 ± 1.0	4.37 ± 1.0	2.97 ± 0.64	1.99 ± 0.42	1.87 ± 0.27	1.55 ± 0.27	1.44 ± 0.19
	Patients	1.46 ± 0.25	1.18 ± 0.18	2.77 ± 0.62	4.58 ± 1.40	3.49 ± 0.74	2.34 ± 0.51	1.88 ±0.37	1.62 ± 0.23	1.45 ± 0.39
Plasma cAMP (pmoles/ml)	Controls	14.0 ± 0.9	13.5 ± 0.4	17.5 ± 1.2	20.9 ± 1.7	20.1 ± 2.1	21.8 ± 1.5	19.9 ± 1.3	17.4 ± 1.3	16.0 ± 1.3
	Patients	13.4 ± 0.7	13.9 ± 0.6	16.8 ± 0.8	21.0 ± 0.9	22.5 ± 1.5	25.2 ± 2.8	21.3 ± 1.5	19.7 ± 1.7	17.3 ± 1.1
Heart rate (min^{-1})	Controls	68 ± 2	71 ± 4	76 ± 3	74 ± 4	73 ± 4	72 ± 4	69 ± 3	71 ± 3	67 ± 4
	Patients	78 ± 6	75 ± 5	88 ± 7	84 ± 5	81 ± 5	80 ± 4	75 ± 5	74 ± 6	72 ± 6

Table 1: Changes of concentrations of cAMP and protein in parotid saliva and cAMP in plasma $\bar{x} \pm$ *SEM*) in asthmatic patients ($n = 6$) and healthy volunteers (controls; $n = 6$) after *i. v.* injection of 0.01 mg/m^2 fenoterol ($-3 \rightarrow 0$ min).

Discussion

It has been shown by numerous authors that in response to a β-adrenergic agonist cAMP concentrations in plasma are increased. This might be due to an efflux of cAMP from several organs, especially from the liver. According to the results described above, it is now possible to measure the biochemical consequence of the stimulation of β-adrenoceptors in an organ-specific compartment in man: Increase of the concentrations of cAMP in the parotid saliva is due to an organ-specific stimulation of β-adrenoceptors in the parotid gland. This increase of salivary cAMP concentrations is not the consequence of a preceding increase of cAMP concentrations in plasma: Inspite of a 35 fold increase of cAMP in plasma after *i. v.* injection of cAMP, there is obviously no filtration into the saliva. Our results obtained in man are obviously in contrast to those obtained in dogs (KANAMORI *et al.*, 1975): These authors suggested that salivary cAMP is mainly filtrated from the blood.
According to our results, increase in salivary cAMP concentrations after application of fenoterol should be an indicator for the reponsiveness of β-adrenoceptors in this organ. Until now, however, we have not been able to detect any differences between the sensitivity of β-adrenoceptors in healthy volunteers and in asthmatic patients.
Hence, these results do not support the general assumption of Szentivanyi (1968). Szentivanyi's assumption, however, may still hold for lung tissue and may not be applicable to the β-adrenoceptors in the parotid gland. Some authors have recently questioned SZENTIVANYI's assumption by showing that chronic treatment of, *e. g.* asthmatic, patients with β-adrenoceptor agonists leads to a diminished adrenergic response indicating a desensitization phenomenon (*c. f.* CONOLLY and GREENACRE, 1976). The model used in our studies may be useful to characterize in the parotid gland a probably organ-specific capability to respond to chronic β-sympathometic stimuli by a desensitization phenomenon; such investigations in man are now in progress.

References

Conolly, M. E., Greenacre, J. K.: J. Clin. Invest. *58*, 1307—1316 (1976).

Galant, S. P., Duriseti, L., Underwood, S., Insel, P. A.: New Engl. J. Med. *299*, 933—936 (1978).

Kanamori, T., Nagatsu, T., Matsumoto, S.: J. Dent. Res. *54*, 535—539 (1975).

Lowry, O. H., Rosebrough, N. J., Farr, A. L.: J. biol. Chem. *193*, 265—275 (1951).

Schmid, G., Hempel, K., Fricke, L., Wernze, H., Heidland, A.: Dtsch. med. Wschr. *100*, 1435—1437 (1975)

Steiner, A. L., Parker, C. W., Kipnis, D. M.: J. biol. Chem. *247*, 1106—1113 (1972).

Szentivanyi, A.: J. Allergy *42*, 203—232 (1968).

Correlation of pharmacodynamic activity and pharmacokinetics of Molsidomine

J. Ostrowski, K. Resag, D. Voegele
Pharmaforschung Cassella AG (Direktor: Dr. R.-E. Nitz), Frankfurt/Main.

K. Lehmann, D. Röhl
Kreiskrankenhaus Main-Taunus (Chefarzt: Dr. J. Schmidt-Voigt), Bad Soden/Ts.
Akademisches Lehrkrankenhaus der Universität Frankfurt/Main

Abstract: With Molsidomine (M.) [Corvaton®] a double blind cross-over study in patients with coronary heart disease was performed. 2 mg M. (*s. l.*) reduced the ST-segment-depression and increased workload capacity over five hours. There is a good correlation to the M. plasma concentration. An inverse relationship between pharmacodynamic activity and pharmacokinetics can be obtained by plotting the mean transit times of M. in the body (v. HATTINGBERG [2]) *v.* the mean transit times of clinical response of each patient. This indicates that M. belongs to the group of so-called "prodrugs."

The antianginal effect of Molsidomine* (N-carboxy-3-morpholinosydnonimin-ethylester) was established by a double blind cross-over study *v.* placebo [1]. Object of the following analysis was to correlate this clinical effect of the drug with its pharmacokinetics.

Methods

Nine patients with coronary heart disease, effort angina (since at least 8 weeks), and ST-segment depression of at least 1 mm *i. e.* 0.1 mV, were selected for the clinical trial.
The patients did not show congestive heart failure or insufficiency of liver and kidney. The chosen patients were informed about type and objective of the study.
The following measurements were made: workload capacity with maximal physical exercise in bicycle ergometry, ST-segment depression under identical workload, heart rate, systemic blood pressure, Molsidomine plasma concentration by HPLC. For methodical details see ref. [1].
Statistical analysis was done by the standard operating procedure in statistics of Hoechst AG**.
Mean transit times ($\bar{T}$ (sys)) were estimated by the following routine [2] (see scheme):
1) Generate the time course of cumulative loss

* INN (Corvaton®); manufacturer: Cassella-Riedel Pharma GmbH, D-6000 Frankfurt/Main 61
** We thank Dr. PASSING, AMP Hoechst AG, for cooperation and discussion.

$$Z(n) = \sum_{i=1}^{n} \left((P(i) + P(i+1))\right)/2)^{*} \left(T(i+1) - T(i)\right)$$

$i = 1, 2, \ldots, n, n+1, \ldots, N$; $P(N)$ must be zero or almost zero again.

2) Estimate ABC, AUC and $\bar{T}$ (SYS). (The time course of the Molsidomine plasma concentration was to be extrapolated to the detection limit for this purpose).
3) Do this for the kinetic *and* clinical parameters of each patient.

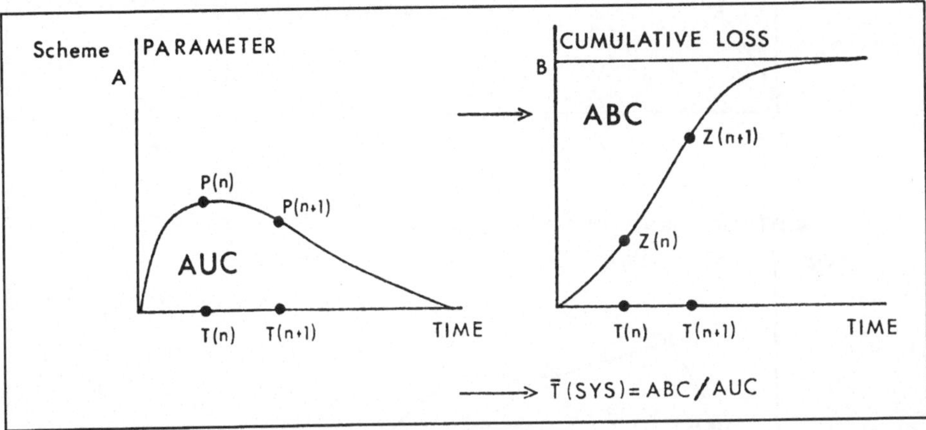

Results

Molsidomine, 2 mg administered sublingually reduced the ST-segment depression and increased workload capacity over five hours ($p < 0.05$) with maximal effects after 1 hour. The mean plasma concentration of Molsidomine shows a similar time course (Figure 1, Table 1). Heart rate and arterial blood pressure were not changed significantly. There is a good correlation between increase of workload capacity and plasma concentration of Molsidomine, *but* the slopes of the regression lines are different for each patient (Figure 2).

Using the method of v. HATTINGBERG [2] for calculation of mean transit times, a relationship between pharmacodynamic activity and plasma concentration of Molsidomine can be abtained by the inverse correlation of (Figure 3, Table 2).

$\bar{T}$ (SYS) clin. *v. s.* $\bar{T}$ (SYS), kin.

$\bar{T}$ (SYS), clin. = mean transit time of the clinical response
$\bar{T}$ (SYS), kin. = mean transit time of Molsidomine

Discussion points

1. The reciprocal relationship (Figure 3) indicates that Molsidomine is a so-called prodrug.
2. The plasma concentration of Molsidomine *itself* is an adequate parameter to correlate kinetic and clinical effect.
3. The only *kinetic* information you need for this estimation is:
plasma concentration values (or urinary excretion data) of the drug
and the area between the cumulative loss and its asymptote.

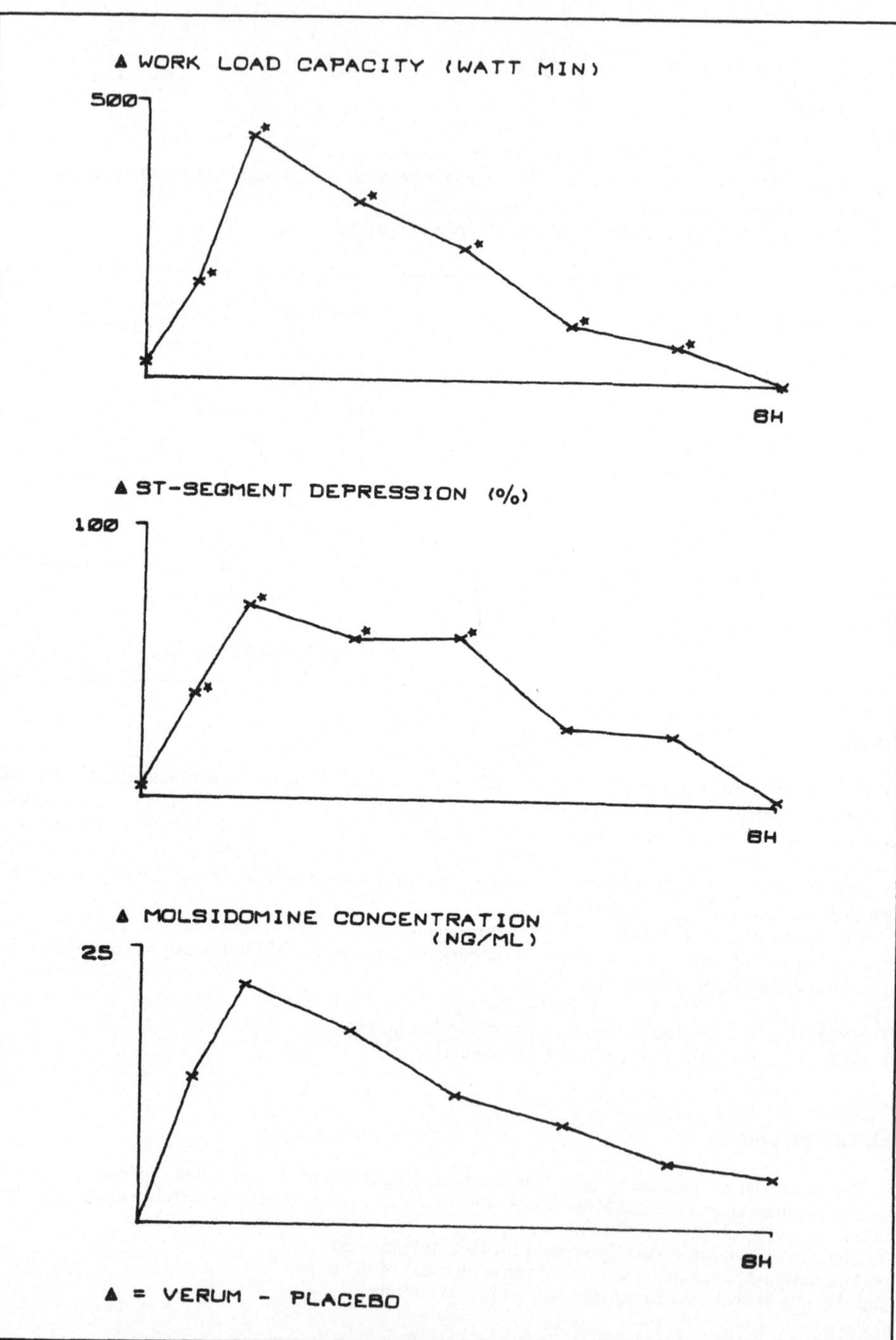

Figure 1: Clinical response and time-course of Molsidomine plasma concentration in patients after sublingual administration of 2 mg of the drug.

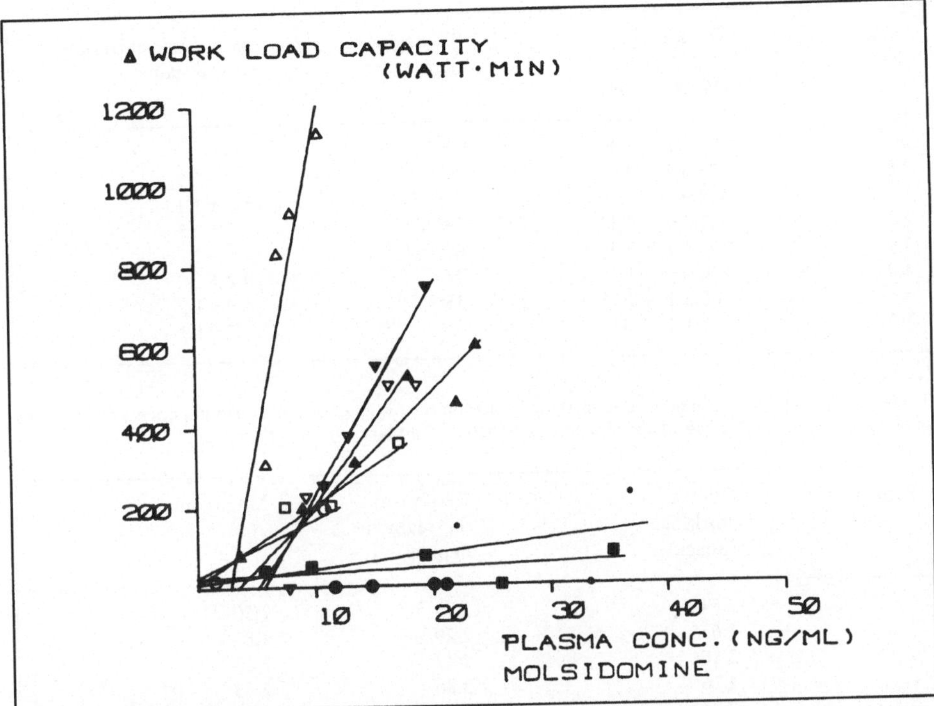

Figure 2: Correlation between workload capacity and Molsidomine plasma concentration of each patient after sublingual administration of 2 mg of the drug.

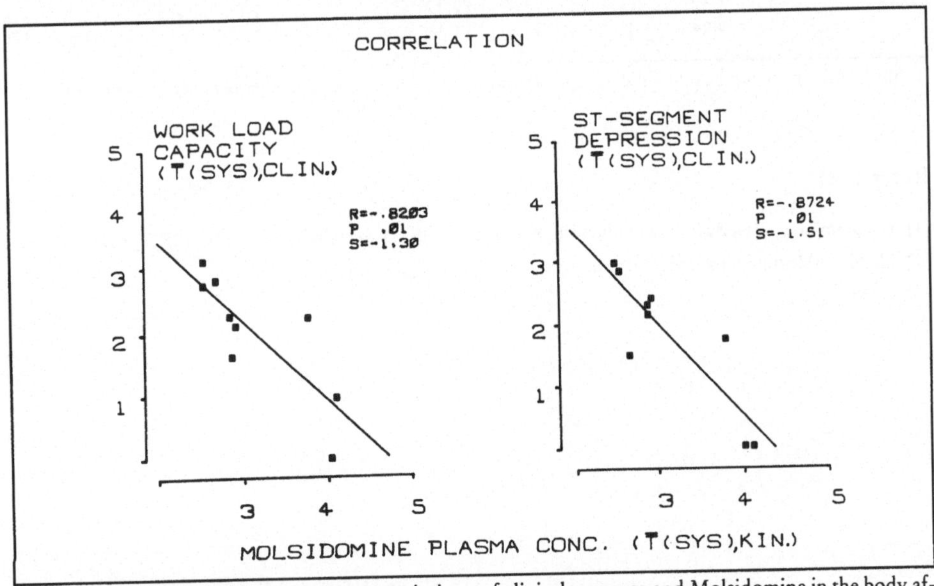

Figure 3: Correlation between the mean transit times of clinical response and Molsidomine in the body after sublingual administration of 2 mg of the drug.

Time (h)	Workload capacity (Watt × min)	ST-Segment depression (%)	Plasma concentration Molsidomine ($ng \cdot ml^{-1}$)
0	27.8 ± 21.4	4	0
0.5	173.3 ± 73.4*	39*	13.2 ± 2.9
1.0	438.9 ± 126.5*	71*	21.6 ± 3.1
2.0	321.0 ± 107.0*	59*	17.5 ± 2.8
3.0	237.4 ± 93.9*	60*	11.8 ± 2.2
4.0	100.0 ± 44.5*	27	9.2 ± 2.0
5.0	65.6 ± 22.0*	25	5.9 ± 1.2
6.0	1.1 ± 0.37	1.7	4.7 ± 1.1

* $p < 0.05$

Table 1: Clinical response and time-course of Molsidomine plasma concentration in patients after sublingual administration of 2 mg of the drug (Comparison with placebo).

Patient	Clinical workload capacity	Response ST-segment depression	Molsidomine
1	2.84	2.99	2.50
2	1.63	2.29	2.87
3	2.10	2.42	2.93
4	3.16	2.86	2.55
5	0.93	0	4.11
6	2.24	1.75	3.79
7	0	0	4.03
8	2.32	2.17	2.86
9	2.94	1.50	2.68

Table 2: Mean transit times of clinical response and of Molsidomine in the body for each patient (hours).

References

[1] K. Lehmann, Dissertation, Fakultät für Klinische Medizin der Universität Ulm, BRD, 1979.

[2] H. M. v. Hattingberg, Infection, in press.

Evaluation of long-acting diuretics; investigations on tizolemide, a new diuretic: Part 1 Methodological approach

Edmundo E. Dagrosa, Fritz Sörgel, Rainer M. Zapf, Reinhard Bender, and Thomas Royen
Hoechst AG, Frankfurt/Main

A standardized electrolyte and fluid intake is one of the most important conditions to be observed in trials with diuretics on healthy volunteers [1]. It is especially relevant in investigations on long-acting drugs, if dose-response curves are to be established. In this case intra- and interindividual variations have to be reduced as much as possible to obtain accurate results.

The coefficient of variation $\left(\text{C.V.\%} = \frac{\text{Standard deviation}}{\text{Mean}} \times 100\right)$ of the main urine variables respresents a good indicator, in addition to the mean, of the interindividual variations, (the C.V.% declining gradually) during the standardization (Figure 1).

A suitable time for drug administration can be achieved as early as 48 hours after commencement of standardization [2]. It is also necessary for subjects to abstain from drugs, foods and drink, other than those included in the standardization, and also from smoking. Strenuous excercise is not allowed and wash-out periods of at least 6 days between two consecutive drug administrations are required. Each study period lasts for 4 days. On the first day of the trial the subjects take breakfast in the Clinical Pharmacology Department at about 7 *a. m.* after emptying their bladders and being weighed. They are given the amount of fluids for this day with careful instructions regarding its intake and told when urine should be collected in the specially provided bottles. Then they carry on with their normal working routine. A standard lunch is taken in the Clinical Pharmacology Dept. and the subjects are then given a standard evening meal and return to their work. This process is repeated on all days of the trial. However, the day on which the substance is taken (3rd day) is spent lying in the Clinical Pharmacology Unit, in an air-conditioned room.

For dose-response studies on tizolemide, a new long-acting diuretic, the conditions already mentioned were used, and in addition the subjects were requested to drink a constant amount of fluid at intervals of exactly one hour over 16 hours, in order to diminish the incidence of acute changes in antidiuretic hormone and aldosterone release. In order to secure better standardization regarding possible water and electrolyte loss through sweating, as well as to minimise excretion due to different physical activities, subjects spent 12 hours of the second day (06:00 – 18:00 approx.) lying in the Clinical Pharmacology Dept. The selected fluid and electrolyte intake remained unchanged (±5%) during the 4 days of each trial period (Table 1).

Eight single-dose double-blind trials were performed with this model. Placebo was used as control for the saluretic effect as well as to determine the duration of action of tizolemide. Since placebo responses often vary it was included twice in the drug administration plan to obtain values as reliable

FLUID, SODIUM, POTASSIUM AND CHLORIDE INTAKE

	TIME	FLUID ml/24 h	SODIUM INTAKE mmol/24 h	POTASSIUM INTAKE mmol/24 h	SODIUM / POTASSIUM INTAKE RATIO/24 h	CHLORIDE INTAKE mmol/24 h
MONDAY	-48 to -24 hours	2475	238	82	2.90	223
TUESDAY	-24 h to 0	2475	225	84	2.68	214
DOSING →						
WEDNESDAY	0 to 24 h p. Appl.	2475	225	84	2.68	214
THURSDAY	24 to 48 h p. Appl.	2475	234	81	2.89	223

Table 1: Fluid and electrolyte intake during standardization

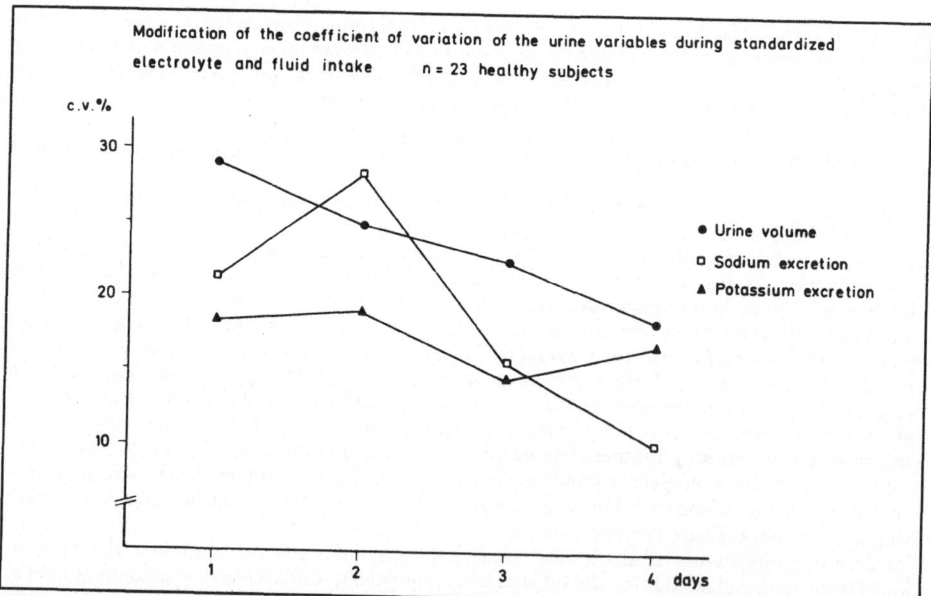

Figure 1: Coefficient of variation under standardization

as possible. Figure 2 shows the reproducibility in the hourly profile of the cumulative sodium excretion in urine after placebo. The placebo treatment which produced in the subject the highest sodium excretion in 24 hours, was used for the calculations. The duration of action of each tizolemide dose was determined individually by comparing the placebo excretion of sodium with the amount excreted after tizolemide during the observation period. The saluretic effect was considered to last until net excretion became smaller. As Figure 3 shows, the duration of tizolemide's saluretic effect was found to be dose-dependent, varying from about 6 hours for 3.1 mg tizolemide to more than 16 hours for doses higher than 25 mg.

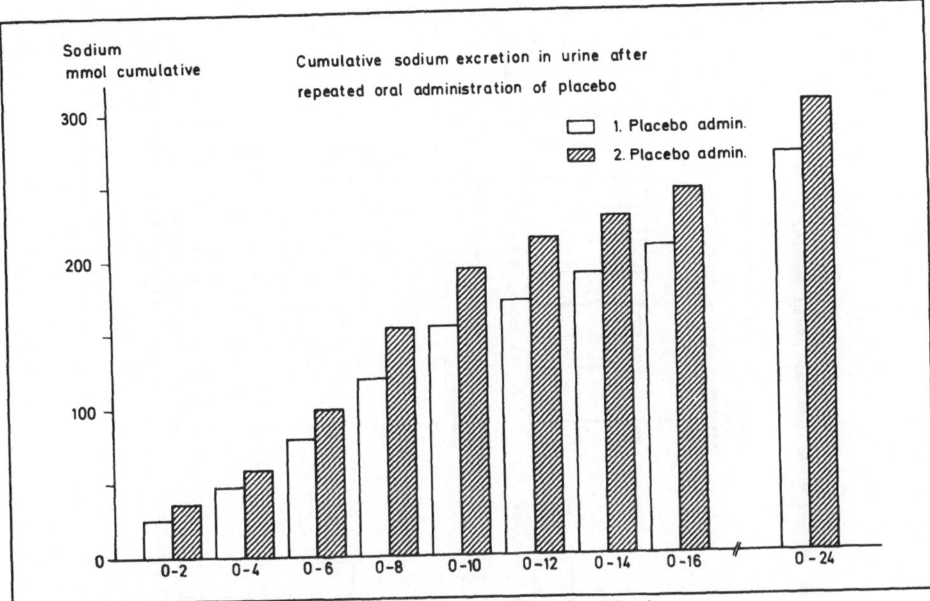

Figure 2: Accumulated sodium excretion in a normal subject after placebo

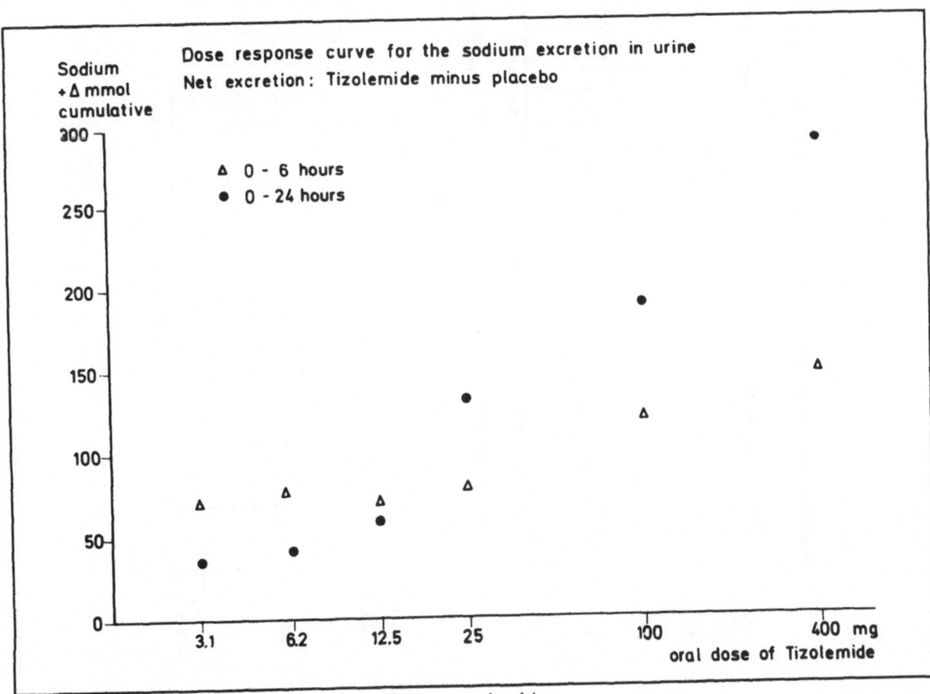

Figure 4: Tizolemide dose-response curve in a normal subject

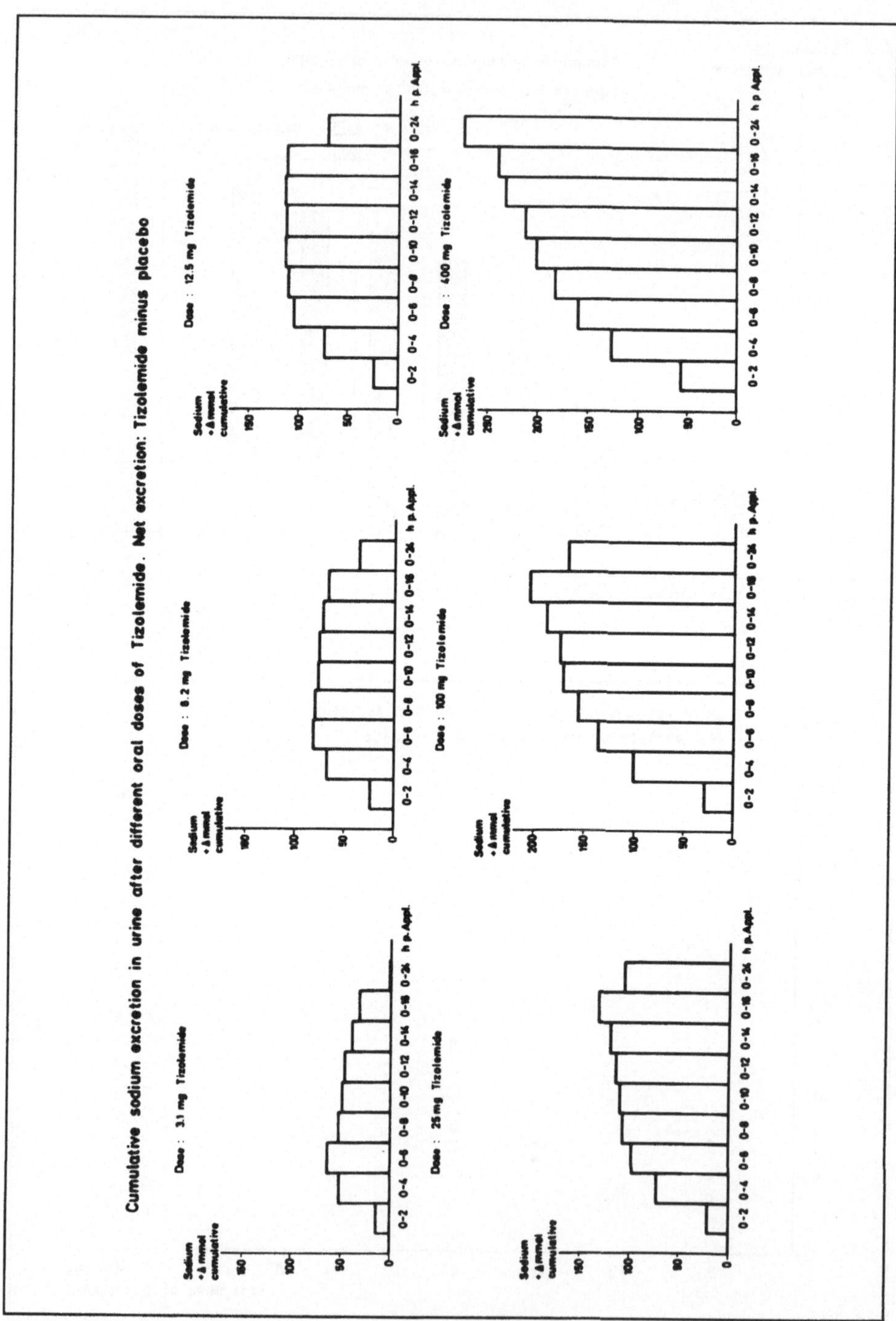

Figure 3: Net sodium excretion in a normal subject after tizolemide

Dose-response curves for tizolemide were constructed based on differences between drug effect and that of placebo, the dose-reponse curves being examined for different cumulative periods. Figure 4 shows the relationships for the 0—6 h and 0—24 h periods. A dose-dependent effect was observed between 3.1 mg and 400 mg tizolemide, and the slope varied depending upon the length of the observation period.

References

[1] Rupp, W.: Praktische Beispiele zur Dosisfindung bei Diuretika. — Arzneim.-Forsch./Drug Res. *27*, 2a, 289—295 (1977)

[2] Dagrosa E. E., Rupp W., Bender R., Schirmer M.: Stabilization of renal electrolyte excretion during standardized diet. — Upsala J. Med. Sci., Suppl. 26, 12 (1979). Abstracts from the III European Colloqium on Renal Physiology.

Evaluation of long-acting diuretics; investigations on tizolemide, a new diuretic: Part 2 Comparison with hydrochlorothiazide

F. Sörgel*, E. E. Dagrosa**, T. Royen**, and R. Bender**

* Institut für Gerontologie der Universität Erlangen-Nürnberg
** Hoechst AG, Frankfurt/Main

Introduction

In recently published data from the laboratories of Lang *et. al.* [1], the action of the new diuretic tizolemide [HOE 740] were evaluated in animals. Tizolemide is a sulfonamide diuretic with basic physicochemical properties, which makes it different from most other diuretics, which are mainly organic acids. The main site of action of tizolemide, like the thiazides [2], is the distal tubule.

Aims of these studies

The studies were carried out to evaluate the action of tizolemide in man. The drug hydrochlorothiazide (HCT) was chosen for comparison.

Methods

Electrolytes, osmolarity and pH-measurements were measured by standard procedures.

Subjects

Only healthy male volunteers participated in the studies. They were subjected to a thorough medical examination including clinical chemistry, hematology, and urine analysis.

Diet, fluid intake and drug administration (Figure 1)

In all studies involving oral administration of the drug, medication was administered to the subject during breakfast.

Total Fluid Intake	(24 h):	2475 ml
Total Sodium Intake	(24 h):	229 m mol
Total Potassium Intake	(24 h):	78 m mol
Total Chloride Intake	(24 h):	228 m mol

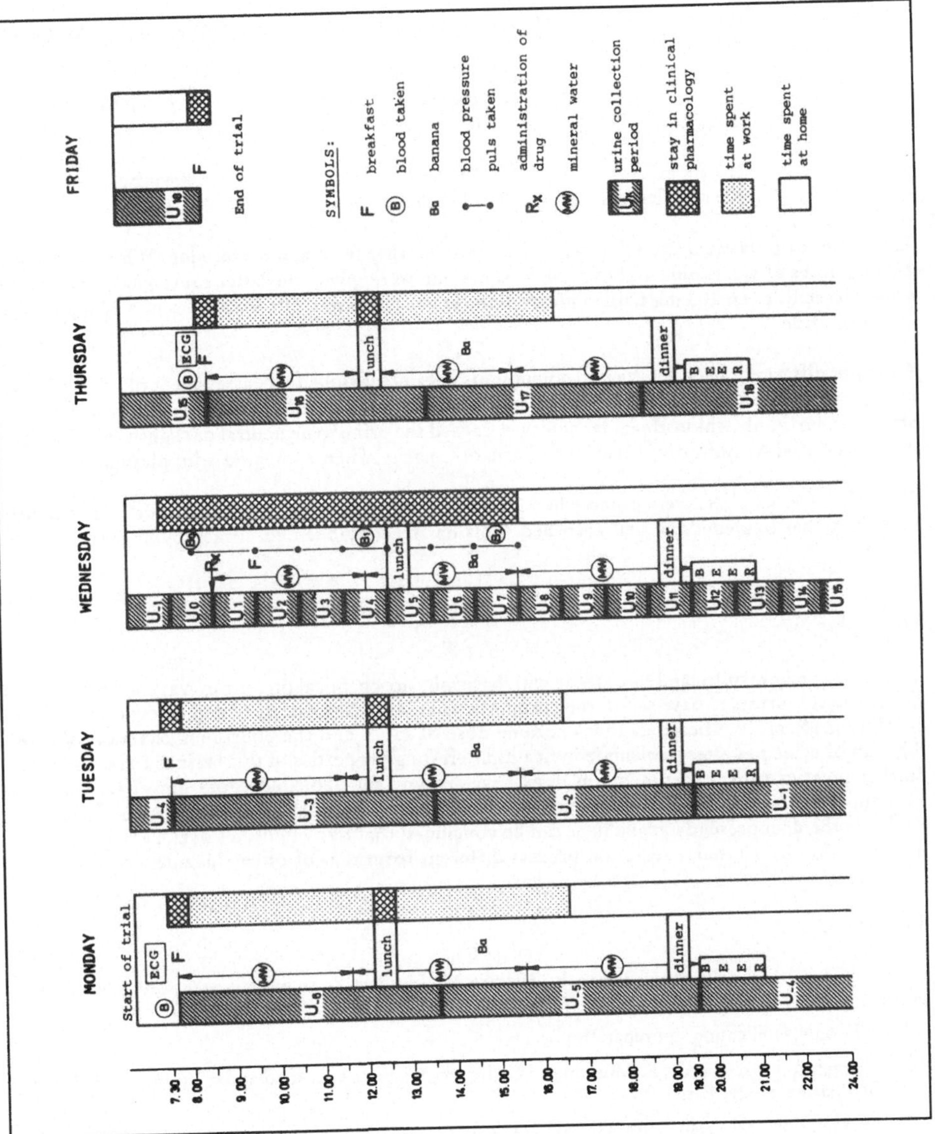

Figure 1: Protocol of the studies

Results

Diuresis and natriuresis following 50 mg HCT were significantly lower ($p \leqq 0.05$) (variance analysis, intra-individual comparison) than those following 50 mg tizolemide ($\bar{x}$, $n = 10$).

Dose (p. o.)	Increased diuresis (0—24 hrs.)	Increased natriuresis (0—24 hrs.)
50 mg HCT	832 ml	130.6 mEq
50 mg Tizolemide	1088 ml	201.8 mEq

No significant differences were observed in increased urine and sodium excretion following 200 mg of either drug ($\bar{x}$, $n = 10$).

Dose (p.o.)	Increased diuresis (0—24 hrs.)	Increased natriuresis (0—24 hrs.)
200 mg HCT	1318 ml	208.3 mEq
200 mg Tizolemide	1151 ml	228.2 mEq

The curve for potassium excretion was different from that for sodium excretion. When 50 mg and 200 mg doses of tizolemide and hydrochlorothiazide were given, the latter caused more potassium to be excreted. Even 200 mg tizolemide brought about less potassium excretion than 50 mg hydrochlorothiazide.

A further difference between the two compounds became obvious from assessment of urine pH. After treatment with tizolemide the urine was acidic in comparison with the initial pH levels and those after placebo. Hydrochlorothiazide, however, caused the urine to be neutral or slightly alkaline. The urine produced by both drugs had hyperbaric osmolarity when compared with plasma.

No differences of effect were noted when 25 mg of tizolemide were given orally and intravenously indicating that tizolemide is well absorbed. This has recently been confirmed by pharmacokinetic studies.

Discussion

Tizolemide, a new sulfonamide-diuretic with basic physicochemical properties was shown in studies in healthy volunteers to have salidiuretic properties similar to those of thiazides. 50 mg of tizolemide is saluretically more efficacious that the same dose of HCT and the potassium excretion is lower. The fall of urine pH after tizolemide indicates interesting properties of this basic diuretic and needs further investigation. Experiments in dogs have shown that tizolemide does not effect the renal clearance of furosemide which is secreted by the anionic transport system in the proximal tubule [3, 4]. From the data presently available it can be concluded that tizolemide, a thiazide—like drug, exerts its action by a tubular secretion process different from that of other thiazides.

Literature:

[1] Lang, H.-J., Knabe, B., Muschaweck, R., Hropot, M., Lindner, E., In diuretic agents, ACS Symp. series No. 83, p. 24—37, Washington DC (1978)

[2] M. Hropot publication in preparation

[3] F. Sörgel, R. Muschaweck, E. Mutschler, M. Hropot, Abstract presented at the 7th International Congress of Pharmacology, Paris (1978)

[4] F. Sörgel, doctoral thesis, University of Frankfurt/Main (1978)

Pharmacokinetics of cyclophosphamide (Endoxan): The balance of cyclophosphamide metabolites in the mouse

G. Voelcker, R. Haeglsperger, H.-J. Hohorst
Gustav-Embden-Zentrum der Biologischen Chemie, Abteilung Zellchemie,
Theodor-Stern-Kai 7, D-6000 Frankfurt/Main

Introduction and description of study

With regard to the mechanism of action of cyclophosphamide some controversy exists whether 4-hydroxycyclophosphamide ("activated cyclophosphamide") or phosphoramide mustard, a metabolite formed from it by β-elimination of acrolein, is the therapeutically effective metabolite. In the following report, pharmacokinetic measurements after intravenous injection into the mouse show that 90% of cyclophosphamide administered is activated to 4-hydroxycyclophosphamide and that 80% thereof is detoxified to 4-ketocyclophosphamide and carboxyphosphamide. From therapy tests on heterotransplanted human breast cancers only 4-hydroxycyclophosphamide (liberated *in vivo* from cyclophosphamide) but not phosphoramide mustard, can imitate the therapeutic effects of cyclophosphamide. These results exlude the extracellular formation of phosphoramide mustard having a significant role in the therapeutic effects of cyclophosphamide.

Materials and Methods:

^{3}H-cyclophosphamide (specific activity 5940 Bq/nmol) was purified by TLC on 1,3-propandiol impregnated cellulose plates using ethyl acetate as a mobile phase [1]. 4-hydroxycyclophosphamide and ^{3}H-4-ketocyclophosphamide (specific activity 6200 Bq/nmol) were prepared by the method of Peter *et al.* [2].
Pharmacokinetic measurements were carried out on female NMRI mice (bodyweight 27—30 g). Blood samples for determination of cyclophospamide and cyclophosphamide metabolites were drawn from the retrobulbar plexus by means of 20 µl heparinised glass capillaries (capilette, Labora/Mannheim).
4-hydroxycyclophosphamide in blood samples was determined fluorometrically [3]. After intravenous administration of ^{3}H-cyclophosphamide, carboxyphosphamide was determined by TLC on 1,3-propandiol impregnated cellulose plates and 4-ketocyclophosphamide by TLC on precoated silicagel plates with ethyl acetate as a mobile phase. As cyclophosphamide and one 4-hydroxycyclophosphamide diastereomer have nearly the same Rf-values on 1,3 propandiol impregnated cellulose plates the concentration of cyclophosphamide in the blood samples was calculated from the difference of the sum of cyclophosphamide, both the 4-hydroxydiastereomers and aldophosphamide de-

termined by TLC [1] and the fluorometrically determined concentration of 4-hydroxycyclophosphamide-diastereomers and aldophosphamide. After intravenous administration of carboxyphosphamide and ^{3}H-4-ketocyclophosphamide, carboxyphosphamide in blood was determined by NBP-test [4] and 4-ketocyclophosphamide by radioactivity measurements.
Therapy tests with cyclophosphamide, 4-hydroxycyclophosphamide and phosphoramide mustard were carried out on human breast cancers in nu/nu-mice (for breeding, keeping, and heterotransplantation of tumors see [5]). The drugs were administered on day 1, 7, and 14. The animals were killed on day 21 and the results expressed as:

$$\frac{C}{T} = \frac{\text{mean tumor weight of excised tumors from control group}}{\text{mean tumor weight of excised tumors from test group}}$$

The tumor weights were approximately 0.2 g at the beginning of the therapy test and in the range of 1.0—1.5 g (control groups) when animals were killed for tumor excision.

Results:

The aim was to determine the *in vivo* yield (bioavailability) of 4-hydroxycyclophosphamide and phosphoramide mustard after administration of a therapeutically, effective dose of cyclophosphamide and to examine the therapeutic effects of equivalent dosages of each on human breast cancers in nu/nu-mice.
There was no method available which permitted quantitative determination of phosphoramide mustard *in vivo* and therefore the highest amount of phosphoramide mustard was estimated from the difference between the sum of 4-hydroxycyclophosphamide and its tautomeric form, aldophosphamide, and the sum of detoxification products, 4-ketocyclophosphamide and carboxyphosphamide (see Scheme 1).

cyclophosphamide → 4-hydroxycyclophosphamide → 4-ketocyclophosphamide
↓ ↑
aldophosphamide → carboxyphosphamide
↓
phosphoramide mustard + acrolein

Scheme 1: Metabolism of cyclophosphamide.

Figure 1 shows the blood concentration curves of cyclophosphamide and cyclophosphamide-metabolites after intravenous administration of 100 mg/kg ^{3}H-labelled cyclophosphamide into female mice.

In order to calculate the bioavailability of 4-hydroxycyclophosphamide, 4-ketocyclophosphamide and carboxyphosphamide after cyclophosphamide administration from these curves, references tests were required. In these references tests the total body clearances of these metabolites were calculated from the intravenous dose administered and the corresponding area under the curve (auc). The intravenous administered dosages were: 4-hydroxycyclophosphamide 10, 31.6, 43.3, 65.1 mg/kg; 4-ketocyclophosphamide 56 mg/kg; carboxyphosphamide 200 mg/kg.

The total body clearances and the corresponding auc of Figure 1 permit the determination of the bioavailability from the equation

$$D = Cl_{tot} \cdot \text{auc} \ [6]$$

where: $Cl_{tot} = \frac{D_{iv}}{\text{auc}_{iv}}$ (total body clearance)

D = bioavailability
D_{iv} = intravenous administered dose of the metabolite in the reference test.
auc_{iv} = area under curve calculated from the blood concentration curve of the metabolite in the reference test.
auc = area under curve calculated from the blood concentration curve of the metabolite after cyclophosphamide administration (Figure 1).

Using this equation we assume a linear relationship between the dose of metabolite administered and auc. This was proven to be true for 4-hydroxycyclophosphamide in the range of 10 to 65 mg/kg *i.v.* and assumed to be true for 4-ketocyclophosphamide and carboxyphosphamide.

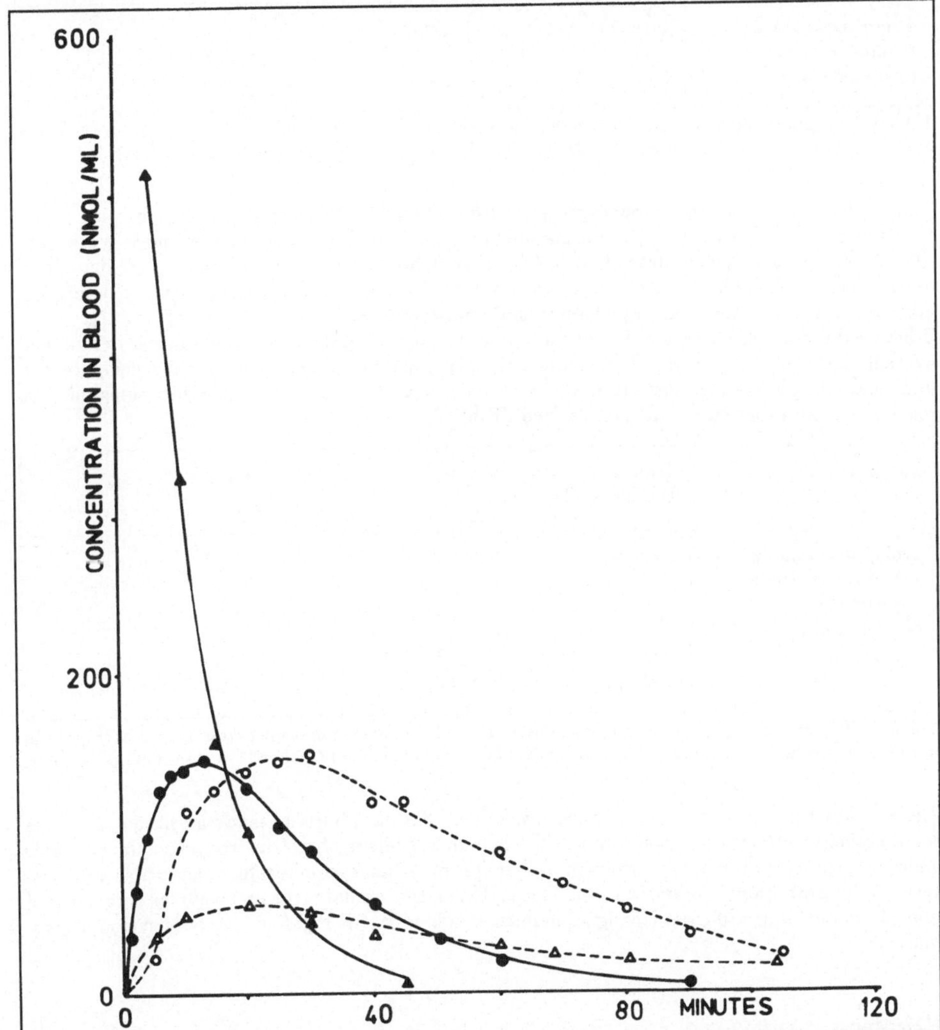

Figure 1: Blood concentration vs. time of cyclophosphamide (▲———▲), 4-hydroxycyclophosphamide (●———●), 4-ketocyclophosphamide (Δ— — — —Δ) and carboxyphosphamide (O— — — —O) following intravenous administration of ^{3}H labelled cyclophosphamide into female mice. Mean of 5—8 animals.

The results of these measurements are summarized (Table 1).

Substance	Apparent first order rate const. of formation (min^{-1})	Total body clearance $\left(\frac{ml}{min \cdot g}\right)$	Bioavailability $\left(\frac{nmol}{g}\right)$
cyclophosphamide	—	0.046	358
4-hydroxycycloph. 4-ketocycloph. carboxyphosph.	0.14 0.12 0.06	0.059 0.011 0.031	322 47 217

Table 1: Formation, total body clearance and bioavailability of cyclophosphamide metabolites after intravenous administration of cyclophosphamide into female mice (mean of 5—8 individual values).

From Table 1, 322 nmol/g cyclophosphamide are activated to 4-hydroxycyclophosphamide corresponding to 90% of cyclophosphamide administered (358 nmol/g). 47 nmol/g of the 4-hydroxycyclophosphamide formed are detoxified to 4-ketocyclophosphamide and 217 nmol/g are detoxified to carboxyphosphamide. From this it appears that the highest amount of 4-hydroxycyclophosphamide which can be converted to phosphoramide mustard is $322-(217+47) = 58$ nmol/g. Whether this amount is converted to phosphoramide mustard in the blood could not be determined by analytical methods, but the therapeutic effects of cyclophosphamide, 4-hydroxycyclophosphamide and phosphoramide mustard on human breast cancers in nu/nu-mice can be compared. The results of these experiments are summarized (Table 2).

Substance	Dose ($nmol \cdot g^{-1}$)	n	$\frac{C}{T}$
cyclophosphamide	358 i.p.	6	7.1
4-hydroxycyclophos-phamide	245 i.p	6	11.1
phosphoramide mustard	208 i.v. 208 i.p.	12 11	1.0 1.2

Table 2: Therapeutic efficacy of cyclophosphamide, 4-hydroxycyclophosphamide and phosphoramide mustard on human breast cancers. For further details see "Material and Methods". n = number of animals.

Table 2 shows that only 4-hydroxycyclophosphamide but not phosphoramide mustard can imitate the therapeutic effects of cyclophosphamide. It is thus evident, that 4-hydroxycyclophosphamide which is not detoxificated to carboxyphosphamide or 4-ketocyclophosphamide, is also not converted to phosphoramide mustard in the blood. This result excludes the extracellular formation of phosphoramide mustard from having an important role in the therapeutic effects of cyclophosphamide.

References:

[1] Voelcker, G., Draeger, U., Peter, G., Hohorst, H. J., Studies on the spontanous decomposition of 4-hydroxycyclophosphamide and 4-hydroperoxycyclophosphamide by means of thin layer chromatography, Arzneim. Forsch. 24, 1172—1176 (1974).

[2] Peter, G., Wagner, T., Hohorst, H.-J., Studies on 4-hydroperoxycyclophosphamide (NSC-181815): A simple preparation method and its application for the synthesis of a new class of "activated" sulfur containing cyclophosphamide (NSC 26271) derivatives, Cancer Treatment Reports 60, 427—435 (1976)

[3] Voelcker, G., Haeglsperger, R., Hohorst H.-J., Fluorometric determination of "activated" cyclophosphamide and ifosfamide in blood. J. Cancer Res. Clin. Oncol. 93, 232—240 (1979)

[4] Friedman, O. M., Boger, E., Colorometric estimation of nitrogen mustard in aqueous media Anal. Chem. 33, 906—910 (1961)

[5] Bastert, G., Fortmeyer, H. P., Schmidt-Matthiesen, H., Thymusaplastic nude mice and rats in clinical oncology, G. Fischer, D-7000 Stuttgart (in press)

[6] Dost, F. H., Grundlagen der Pharmakokinetik, Georg Thieme Verlag, D-7000 Stuttgart (1968)

Measurement of activity of immunosuppresive drugs *in vitro*

F. L. Shand,
Department of Experimental Immunobiology,
The Wellcome Research Laboratories, Beckenham, Kent, UK.

Our interest in the pharmacological aspects of immunosuppressive drugs originated from observations which indicated that the alkylating agent cyclophosphamide (CY), induced lesions in lymphocyte populations of mouse spleen that were not attributable directly to inhibiton of cellular proliferation. It was established that B lymphocytes from the spleens of mice injected 24 hours previously with 150 mg/kg of CY were unable to regenerate their surface immunoglobulin receptors following treatment with anti-immunoglobulin serum and subsequent incubation. This lesion was identified by means of an immunofluorescence assay utilizing rhodamine-labelled rabbit anti-mouse immunoglobulin for the initial capping treatment. Newly regenerated receptors were detected after incubation with an indirect immunofluorescence test using the (Fab')$_2$ fragment of rabbit anti-mouse immunoglobulin serum in conjunction with a fluoroscein-labelled sheep anti-rabbit conjugate. The use of a (Fab')$_2$ fragment excluded the possibility of detecting Fc receptors on B lymphocytes in this model.

Since the impairment of B cell receptor regeneration induced by a prior injection of CY could not be reproduced with various other immunosuppressive drugs (azathioprine, 6-mercaptopurine, chlorambucil or melphalan), it appeared that this activity was a selective attribute of CY which deserved further evaluation. Moreover, this inhibition of B cell regenerative capacity, linked to the fact that CY-injected mice were equisitely sensitive to tolerance induction by thymus-independent antigens implied a causal relationship between these two phenomena.

To explore the system further, it was deemed necessary to treat lymphoid cell suspensions *in vitro*. Unfortunately, CY in its native state is virtually devoid of activity *in vitro* since the drug requires microsomal activation within the liver before those metabolites which actively alkylate nuclear DNA are formed. Therefore, advantage was taken of the *in vitro* activation system described by workers in the tumour field in which CY was activated with isolated rat liver microsomes and a NADPH generating system. The procedure utilized is outlined below:

Washed rat liver microsomes	3 ml
$MgCl_2$ at 10 mg/ml	1 ml
Nicotinamide adenine dinucleotide phosphate (Sigma) at 2.1 mg/ml	1 ml
D-glucose-6-phosphate (Sigma) at 15.5 mg/ml	1 ml
Glucose-6-phosphate dehydrogenase (Sigma) at 10 units/ml	0.3 ml
Cyclophosphamide monohydrate (Koch-Light) at 5 mg/ml	1 ml
Tris buffer pH 7.4	2.7 ml

All reagents are prepared in Tris buffer pH 7.4 and mixtures incubated at 37° C for 30 minutes. The concentrations of the activated drug used to treat spleen cells *in vitro* were calculated from the 500

μg/ml level in the original activation mixture and no account was taken of possible differences in the efficiency of activation.
Preliminary experiments on the transfer of spleen cells pretreated with 20—50 μg/ml of microsomally-activated CY to lethally irradiated syngeneic recipients, indicated that such cells were unable to respond to antigen if challenged 24 hours after transfer. Furthermore, supplementation experiments revealed that both B and T lymphocytes were affected to an equal extent. However, if antigen challenge was delayed for approximately one week, then CY-treated cells responded normally to both thymus-dependent and -independent antigens. The use of congenic mouse strains differing in immunoglobulin allotype confirmed that the antibody response observed was of donor and not of host origin. This implies that immunosuppression induced by CY is a fully reversible event possibly mediated by an intracellular enzymatic repair mechanism of nuclear DNA. This recovery from immunosuppression is also paralleled by a similar recovery in the ability of CY-treated B cells to regenerate their surface immunoglobulin receptors after capping with anti-immunoglobulin serum.
We were fortunate in being able to acquire a number of defined metabolites and derivatives of CY which had been investigated previously for their cytotoxic, alkylating and anti-tumour activities. Those metabolites with proven activity (4-hydroxy-CY, phosphoramide mustard and nor-nitrogen mustard) were all capable of reproducing the immunosuppressive effects of microsomally-activated CY when used to pretreat spleen cells *in vitro*. A further derivative of CY, 4-hydroperoxy-CY, which undergoes spontaneous hydrolysis to form 4-hydroxy-CY, was also found to be effective. In contrast, the metabolites carboxyphosphamide, 4-keto-CY and acrolein, were devoid of activity, as was 5,5-dimethyl-CY, a derivative which is activated in a similar manner to CY but is unable to form active alkylating products. Thus, it appears that the alkyalting activity of CY metabolites is indissociable from the immunosuppressive activity and inhibition of B cell receptor regenerative capacity.
Mouse spleen cells which had been pretreated with microsomally-activated CY *in vitro* and transferred to lethally-irradiated syngeneic recipients were also found to be hypersensitive to tolerance induction with the polysaccharide antigens levan or dextran, providing that tolerogen was administered shortly after transfer. It seems likely therefore that alkylated B cells which are not subjected to antigenic stimulation are able to repair their DNA lesion in an few days and thereafter respond normally to challenge. This interpretation is substantiated to some extent, by the observation that transferred spleen cells pre-treated *in vitro* with activated-CY, recover their immunocompetence to both levan and dextran in a week or so. Since normal adult bone marrow cells take in excess of 50 days to become immunocompetent to these same antigens after transfer to lethally-irradiated recipients, it is probable that the early recovery of CY-treated cells results from a reversible event in mature B cells rather than maturation from stem cell precursors.
When the effect of microsomally-activated CY on T lymphocyte function was investigated a similar phenomenon was observed. The injection of CBA parental spleen cells into a lethally-irradiated (CBA × C57BL) F_1 hybrid recipient results in death from graft-versus-host disease within approximately 14 days. However, if the parental cells are pretreated with 20 μg/ml of activated-CY *in vitro* prior to injection, then death does not ensue and recipient animals become demonstrably chimaeric. More importantly, surviving chimaeras were able to produce a near normal plaque forming cell response against sheep erythrocytes, part of which was shown to originate from cells of donor origin. The practical implications of these observations to bone marrow transplantation in man without accompanying graft-versus-host disease, are obvious.
These experimental immunopharmacological approaches have an obvious practical application to the design and testing of immunosuppressive drugs. In particular, it becomes possible to explore potential modes of action by pretreating defined lymphocyte populations *in vitro*.

Chapter 3

Developmental aspects of pharmacodynamic and pharmacokinetic theory

Simultaneous modelling of pharmacokinetics and pharmacodynamics

Brian Whiting, M.D., F.R.C.P.
Department of Materia Medica, University of Glasgow
Andrew Kelman, B.Sc., Ph.D.
Department of Clinical Physics and Bio-Engineering, West of Scotland Health Boards

Introduction

An ability to derive a concentration-time profile which accurately reflects the pharmacokinetic characteristics of a drug is now undisputed. The generation of an analogous effect-time profile, however, is still a challenge which involves repeated measurement of drug effect over extended periods of time. The demands on subjects and observers alike may be somewhat eased by the application of non-invasive methods but these will not always be appropriate. If, however, kinetic and dynamic data can be obtained simultaneously, the opportunity arises to analyse the corresponding concentration-effect relationship in both qualitative and quantitative terms.

The simplest approach is to pose the question—is observed effect related to *plasma concentration*? Or indeed, having determined the pharmacokinetic characteristics of the drug—is observed effect related to drug levels in *any particular compartment*? Galeazzi *et al.* [3] showed how this approach could be realised in graphical terms by plotting observed effect against plasma concentration or predicted amount of drug in a peripheral compartment and linking the points in time order. Any obvious loop contained within the figure so formed (*i. e.* a significant degree of *hysteresis*) would indicate lag of effect behind changes in concentration or in amount of drug in a peripheral compartment. Bryson *et al.* [1] used this approach to examine the relationship between plasma concentrations of disopyramide after *oral* administration and prolongation of the electrocardiographic QT interval. An absence of hysteresis in the plasma concentration-QT prolongation plot indicated that changes in concentration were essentially mirrored by changes in effect and it was easy to propose a simple linear relationship between concentration and effect, where the slope expressed sensitivity to the drug. In these circumstances, kinetic considerations (principally absorption) dictated "parallelism" between all compartmental and effect changes (Figure 1b).

After *intravenous* administration, however, the situation was different (Figure 1a). An intravenous bolus of disopyramide was followed by a period of disequilibrium and it is in this kind of setting when plasma and peripheral compartment levels are rapidly changing that we have to model changes in effect. It is perhaps obvious from Figure 1a that once pseudodistribution equilibrium was attained (at approximately 24 minutes), equilibrium was also established with effect, but these relationships are not so clear when a more complex model, such as that associated with digoxin, is considered. Sumner *et al.* [6] have shown that plasma concentration kinetics after intravenous digoxin are consistent with a three-compartment open model. Changes in effect (*e. g.* shortening of the left ventricu-

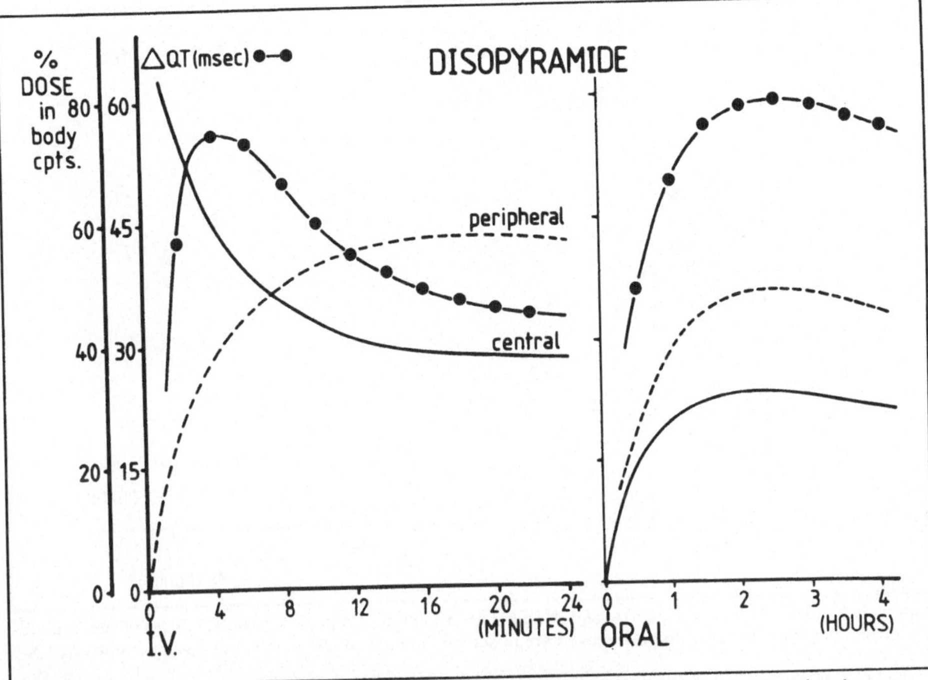

Figure 1: Theoretical amounts of disopyramide (% dose) in the central (plasma) and peripheral compartments after intravenous (a) and oral (b) administration. Superimposed are points (●—●) which represent typical changes in the electrocardiographic *QT* interval (ΔQT msec).

lar ejection time, ΔLVET) after *i. v.* digoxin must be seen in relation to changes in the level of digoxin in the three compartments of this model, viz the central (plasma), shallow and deep compartments (Figure 2). KRAMER *et al.* [4] have demonstrated a close correlation between predicted digoxin levels in the *deep* compartment and another non-invasive measure of cardiac function, viz changes in the QS_2 index, but their analysis was based on *averaged* serum digoxin concentration-time and response-time data, and they were unable to comment on *individual* subjects.
With individual *patient* response in mind, it is essential that we should now address ourselves to the development of measurement techniques and mathematical models which will adequately discriminate between individuals. Moreover, there may be no obvious correlation between response and drug level changes (measured and/or predicted) in any of the compartments of a pharmacokinetic model (Figure 3). Following 1 mg of digoxin intravenously (data corresponding to Figure 2), all plots in this individual showed a marked degree of hysteresis.

Multiple regression effect model

Having recognised that it may be impossible to correlate response with drug level changes in any *particular* compartment, it seems sensible to ask—can response be seen in terms of the changes in drug level in *more than one* compartment? In other words, is it possible to assess the contribution made by each compartment to the overall response? If so, effect can then be seen as a function of drug level changes in any chosen comparments and the data can be applied to the following first-order model with two independent variables

$$E = \theta_0 + \theta_1 X_1 + \theta_2 X_2$$

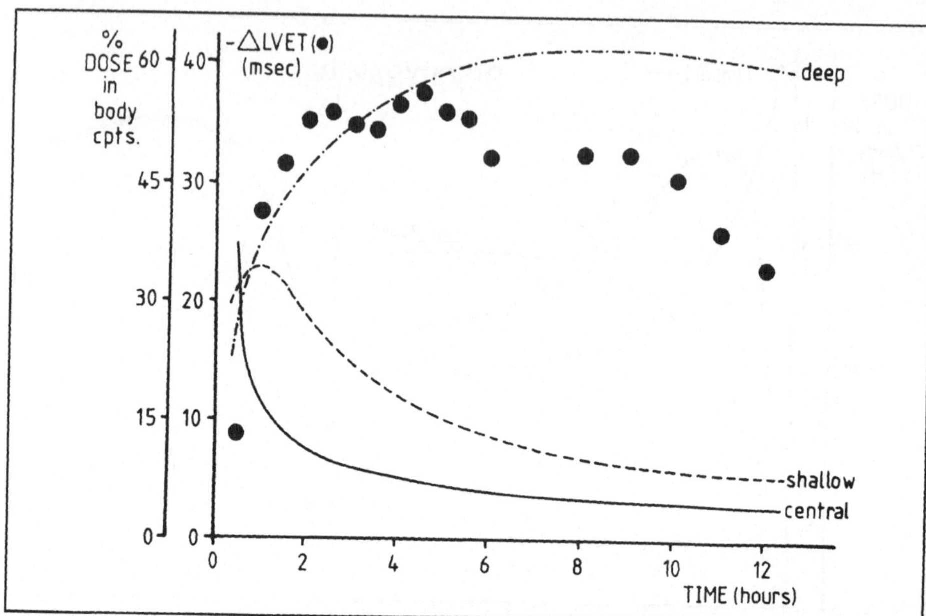

Figure 2: Central (plasma), shallow—and deep compartment amounts of digoxin (% dose) in one individual after 1 mg intravenously. Superimposed are observed changes in left ventricular ejection time (ΔLVET msec).

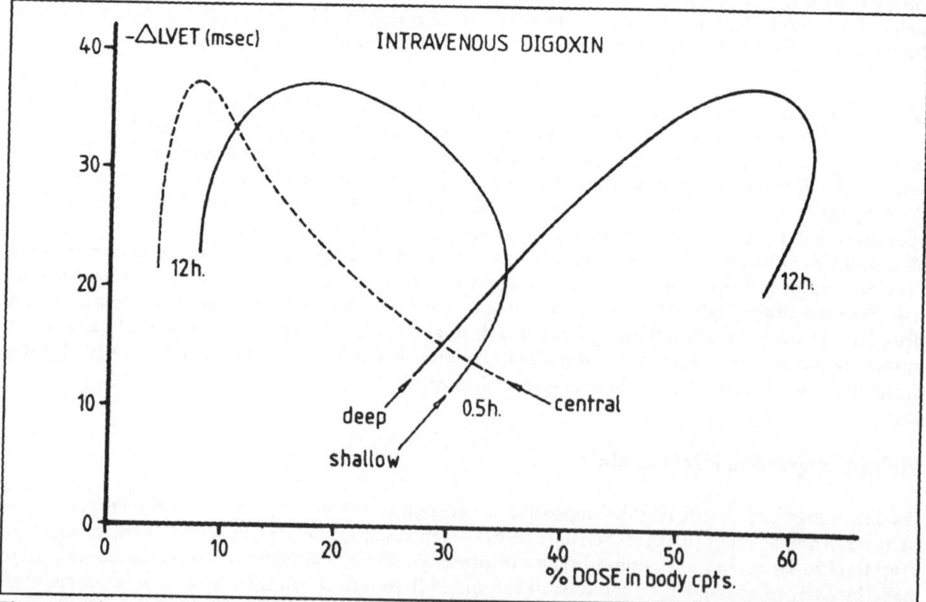

Figure 3: Change in LVET after digoxin plotted against calculated amounts of digoxin in the central, shallow—and deep compartments based on the data presented in Figure 2. The obvious hysteresis in each case indicates that ΔLVET cannot be considered as a function of changes in the amount of digoxin in any *particular* compartment.

where, in terms of a pharmacodynamic model, E is observed effect, X_1 and X_2 are functions of the amounts of drug in two body comparments and θ_0, θ_1 and θ_2 are the parameters of the model. θ_1 and θ_2 are the partial regression coefficients; θ_0 is the Y intercept of the regression plane. This, then, gives us the basis for a generalised empirical effect model which can be analysed by multiple regression. Taking digoxin as an example, the appropriate equation would be

$$E = i + A \cdot f_1(Q_S) + B \cdot f_2(Q_D)$$

where Q_S and Q_D are the calculated time-dependent amounts of digoxin in the shallow and deep compartments respectively, i is the Y intercept and E is the effect (ΔLVET) observed at times corresponding to the calculated drug amounts. Input to the multiple regression programme therefore, consists of the dependent variable, E, and the two independent variables, Q_S and Q_D. Three parameters are then estimated, i, A and B. Figure 4 shows the observed changes in LVET in one subject after 1 mg digoxin intravenously with the predicted form of the effect-time relationship generated from the following final parameter estimates ($\pm$ SD), $i = -206.5$ ($\pm$ 138.9); $A = 15.6$ ($\pm$ 1.0); $B = 49.1$ ($\pm$ 5.7) ($r = 0.96$). (This particular analysis was based on independent variables which had undergone logarithmic transformation, *i. e.* $f_1(Q_S) = ln(Q_S)$ and $f_2(Q_D) = ln(Q_D)$ but we subsequently decided that such a transformation was not necessary as it did not improve the fit.)

When this approach was applied to QT prolongation following intravenous disopyramide, estimation of the three parameters i, A and B, led to predicted effect changes which again were wholly consistent with the data. Individual effect-time profiles were modelled from calculated amounts of drug in the central (Q_C) and peripheral (Q_P) compartments of the two compartment kinetic model thus,

$$E = i + A(Q_C) + B(Q_P)$$

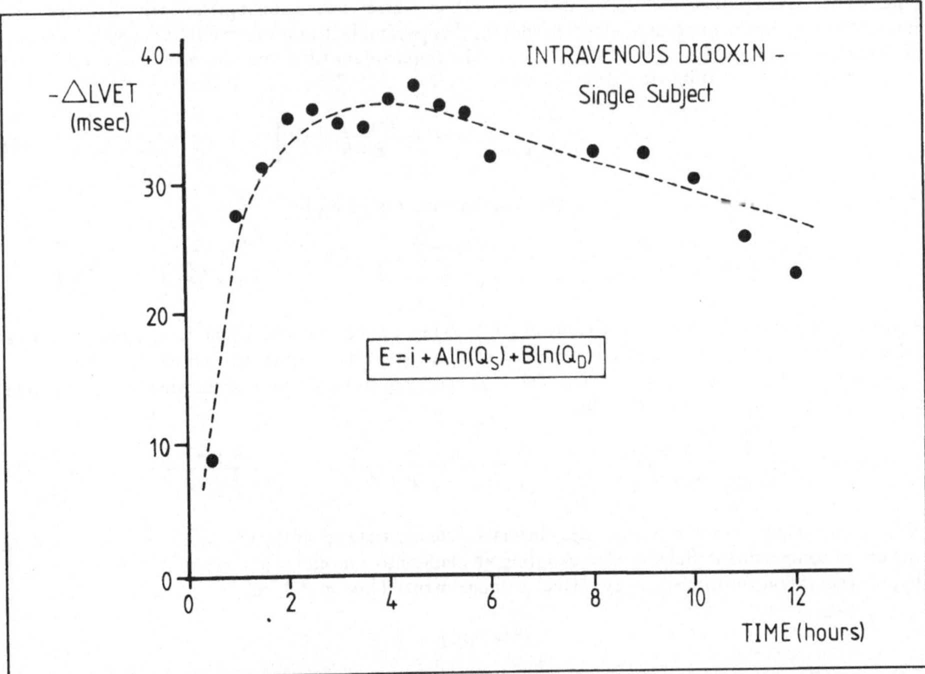

Figure 4: Observed (•) and predicated (- - -) changes in LVET in one individual after 1 mg digoxin intravenously. The data, as shown in Figure 2, was analysed by multiple linear regression. The dotted line represents the best fit of the multiple regression model to the data.

Without any transformation of variables a typical individual set of parameter values was $i = -5.6$ ($\pm$ 11.4); $A = 0.417$ ($\pm$ 0.001); $B = 0.272$ ($\pm$ 0.001). Intercept units are the units of effect (in this case, msec) and regression coefficient units are effect/unit of drug amount (in this case, msec/% dose in relevant compartment).

Integrated effect model

Another interesting approach has been proposed by SHEINER *et al.* [5] who postulate that changes in pharmacological effect can be related to plasma concentrations by a first order process. The classical pharmacokinetic model (Figure 5, with compartments 1, 2, 3, ..., N) is extended by a hypothetical effect compartment, E, whose input and output functions have no influence on the formal kinetc solution for mass of drug in the body. Effect is then considered to be some function of (hypothesised) changes in effect compartment concentration and k_{eq} is the first order rate constant which expresses any discrepancy between changes in plasma concentration and changes in pharmacological effect. As all the information about this discrepancy is available *before any equilibrium is established*, the model allows simultaneous fitting of plasma concentration and effect data obtained during the initial disequilibrium phase following drug administration, or from any other non-equilibrium phase. DAHLSTROM *et al.* [2] have also put forward a similar concept, applied to the analysis of the analgesic response to morphine in rats.
To illustrate the use of this model, consider again the problem of analysing the disopyramide concentration-effect data. BRYSON *et al.* [1] showed that after oral administration, effect (QT prolongation) could be thought of as a simple linear function of plasma concentration. After intravenous administration, however, WHITING *et al.* [7] have subsequently shown that the form of the plasma concentration-effect relationship cannot be modelled satisfactorily without accommodating the diseqilibrium between plasma concentration and effect which occurs during the early distributional phase. In terms of the integrated effect model for disopyramide, therefore, we first derive the expression for the amount of drug (Q_C) in the central compartment of a two compartment model after intravenous administration of a dose, D, thus

$$Q_C = D\left[\frac{k_{21}-\alpha}{\beta-\alpha}e^{-\alpha t} + \frac{k_{21}-\beta}{\alpha-\beta}e^{-\beta t}\right] \tag{1}$$

The corresponding solution for the effect compartment is given by

$$Q_E = k_{1e}D\left[\frac{k_{21}-\alpha}{(\beta-\alpha)(k_{eq}-\alpha)}e^{-\alpha t} + \frac{k_{21}-\beta}{(k_{eq}-\beta)(\alpha-\beta)}e^{-\beta t} + \frac{k_{21}-k_{eq}}{(\alpha-k_{eq})(\beta-k_{eq})}e^{-k_{eq}t}\right] \tag{2}$$

Assuming as usual a partition coefficient of 1.0 between the central and effect compartments, and a value of k_{1e} which is extremely small compared with k_{eq} or with any other rate constant in the model, the concentration in the effect compartment (C_E) can be derived in terms of the steady state volume of the central compartment (V_C), thus

$$C_E = k_{eq}\frac{D}{V_C}\left[\frac{k_{21}-\alpha}{(\beta-\alpha)(k_{eq}-\alpha)}e^{-\alpha t} + \frac{k_{21}-\beta}{(k_{eq}-\beta)(\alpha-\beta)}e^{-\beta t} + \frac{k_{21}-k_{eq}}{(\alpha-k_{eq})(\beta-k_{eq})}e^{-k_{eq}t}\right] \tag{3}$$

Where C_E can now be referenced to the plasma as "steady state equivalent" concentrations of drug in the effect compartment. Substitution can then be made into a model which relates observed effect to hypothesised concentrations in the effect compartment. This model can be of the linear form

$$E = mC_E + i \tag{4}$$

(where E is the effect corresponding to a concentration C_E, m is the slope and i the intercept; WHITING *et al.* [7]) or of a sigmoid form, allowed, for example, by an equation such as the Hill equation

$$E = \frac{(C_E)^\gamma}{(C_E)^\gamma + (C_E(50))^\gamma} \quad (5)$$

(where E is the intensity of pharmacological effect expressed as a fraction of the maximal effect, C_E is as defined above, $C_E(50)$ is a constant giving the value of C_E at 50% effect and γ is a parameter that allows sigmoidicity in the relationship; SHEINER *et al.* [5]).

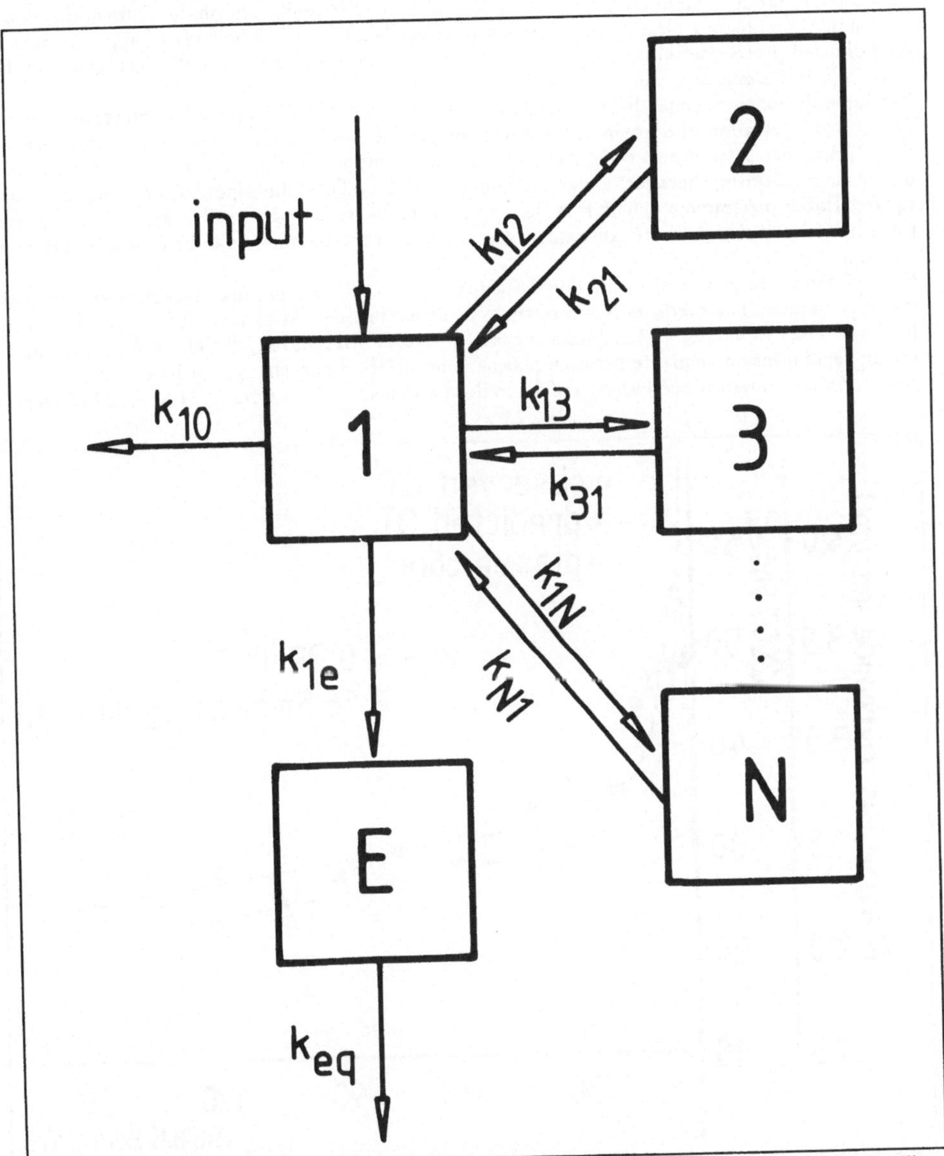

Figure 5: Diagrammatic representation of the integrated effect model. The *N*-compartment mamillary pharmacokinetic model is extended by an "effect" compartment (*E*) whose input and output functions have no influence on the formal pharmacokinetic solution for mass of drug in the body.

As the range of QT prolongation following disopyramide is considered to be relatively small—without any approach to a maximum—the linear model (Eqn. 4) is appropriate. Three parameters, therefore, have to be estimated, m, i and k_{eq}, and because equation 3 is not linear in k_{eq}, nonlinear least squares data fitting is used for parameter estimation. All other constants (V_C, k_{21}, α and β) are assigned values based on previous pharmacokinetic analysis.

Figure 6 shows the results of fitting one individual's QT-plasma concentration data with the integrated effect model—highlighting the early (0—20 min) disequilibrium phase. Estimation of k_{eq} (0.39 min^{-1}, implying a plasma concentration to effect "equilibration" half-life of approximately 2 min) allowed precise definition of the sensitivity relationship between C_E and effect, given by the slope (m), 16.5 msec/mcg/ml.

The same approach can equally be applied to the digoxin data already referred to. Here, the expression for concentration of digoxin in the effect compartment will contain *four* exponentials because the effect model is based on a three compartment kinetic model. Again, the data only permits a simple linear relationship between C_E and changes in LVET. Thus the input to the nonlinear least squares fitting programme is LVET vs time, the constants are DOSE, V_C, k_{21}, k_{31}, α, β and γ (the three hybrid dispositional rate constants for digoxin) and the parameters to be estimated are m, i, and k_{eq}.

Figure 7 shows the results of fitting one individual's LVET-digoxin plasma concentration data with the effect model. The predicted form of the effect-time profile was generated from the following final parameter estimates, m, 32.27 msec/ng/ml; i, -20.41 msec and k_{eq}, 0.15 h^{-1}, the latter implying an "equilibration" half-life between plasma concentration and changes in LVET of 4.6 h. Rate constant values assigned to k_{21} and k_{31} in this particular analysis were 0.761 h^{-1} and 0.074 h^{-1}

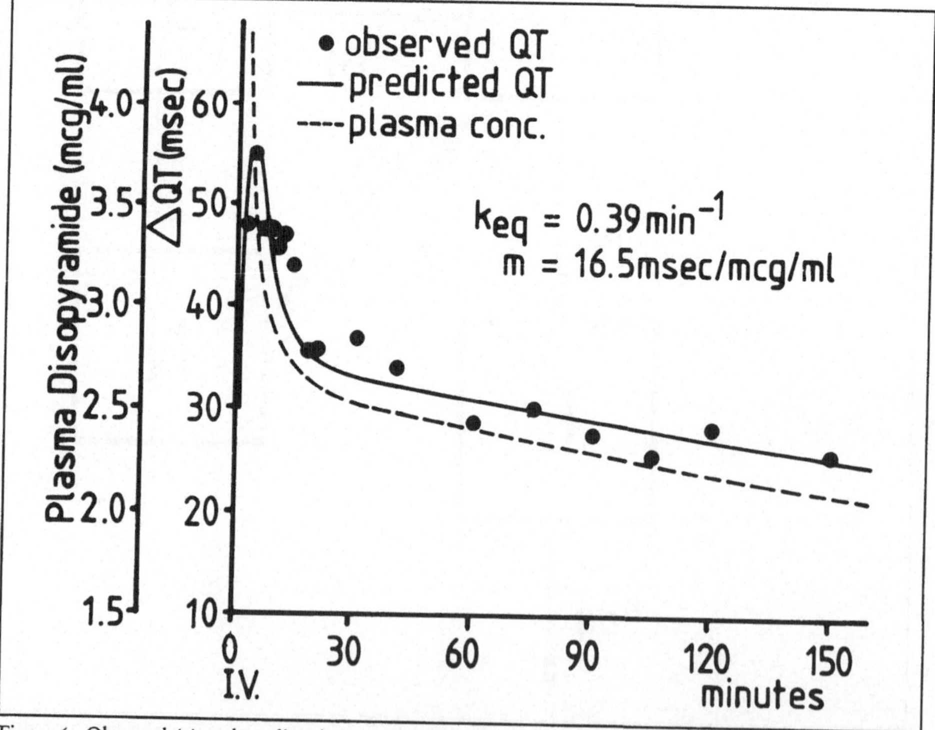

Figure 6: Observed (•) and predicted (——) changes in the QT interval in one individual after 150 mg disopyramide intravenously. Also shown is the form of the plasma concentration-time profile (---). The solid line represents the best fit of the effect model to the data.

respectively. k_{eq} was therefore intermediate in value between k_{21} and k_{31}, implying that changes in concentration responsible for LVET shortening are *not* directly related to either the shallow or deep compartment as has been previously suggested [4]. The value of k_{eq} relative to the other microscopic rate constants is useful in "placing" effect relative to the established kinetic compartments. If k_{eq} assumes a very large value, effect kinetics will be indistinguishable from those of the central compartment—*i. e.* the two will be in parallel. If k_{eq} assumes a value equal to the value of a rate constant linking a peripheral compartment to the central compartment, effect kinetics will parallel the kinetics of drug in that compartment.

Summary

This paper has outlined four possible approaches to the analysis of concentration-effect data.
1. Initial exploratory data analysis with the construction of hysteresis plots.
2. Modelling of effect as a function of drug level changes in a *particular* kinetic compartment.
3. Modelling of effect using multiple regression analysis: parameters reflect the contribution of each defined kinetic compartment to overall effect.
4. Modelling of effect using the integrated effect model: parameters define (a) the proportionality constant, *m*, relating equilibrium plasma concentrations to effect and (b) the first order rate constant, k_{eq} which expresses the discrepancy between plasma concentration and effect which is manifest during periods of disequilibrium.

References

[1] Bryson, S. M., Whiting, B., Lawrence, J. R.: Disopyramide serum and pharmacologic effect kinetics applied to the assessment of bioavailability. B. J. Clin. Pharmac. 6, 409—419 (1978).

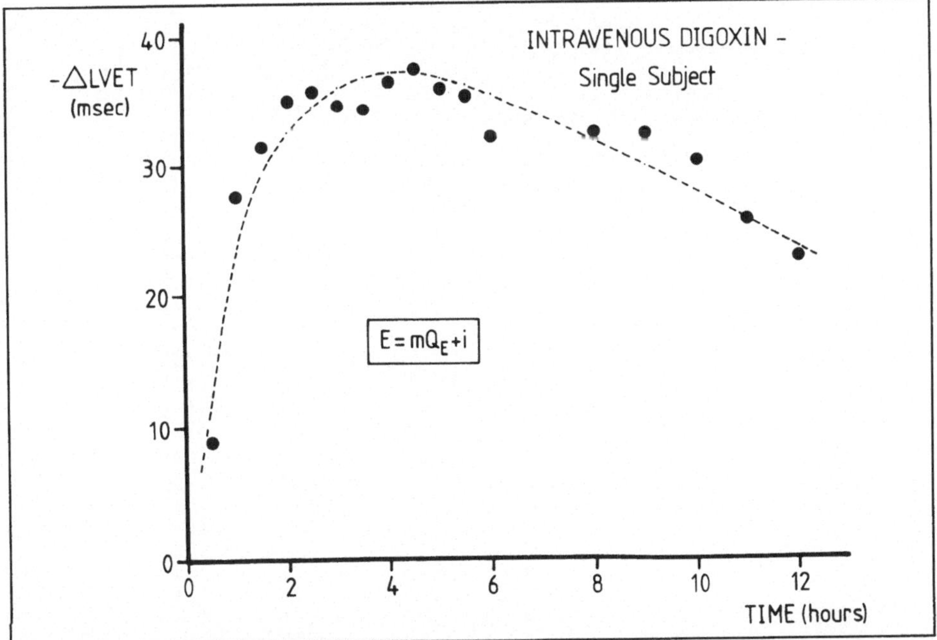

Figure 7: Observed (•) and predicted (---) changes in LVET in one individual after 1 mg digoxin intravenously (data as in Figure 2). The broken line represents the best fit of the effect model to the data.

[2] Dahlstrom, B. E., Paalzow, L. K., Segre, G., Ågren, A. J.: Relation between morphine pharmacokinetics and analgesia. J. Pharmacokinet. Biopharm. 6, 41—53 (1978).

[3] Galeazzi, R. Benet, L. Z., Sheiner, L. B.: Relationship between the pharmacokinetics and pharmacodynamics of procainamide. Clin. Pharmacol. Ther. 20, 278—289 (1976).

[4] Kramer, W. G., Kolibash, A. J., Lewis, R. P., Mohinder, B. S., Visconti, J. A., Reuning, R. H.: Pharmacokinetics of digoxin: relationship between response intensity and predicted compartmental drug levels in man. J. Pharmacokinet. Biopharm. 7, 47—61 (1979).

[5] Sheiner, L. B., Stanski, D. R., Vozeh, S., Miller, R. D., Ham, J.: Simultaneous modelling of pharmacokinetics and pharmacodynamics: Application to d-tubocurarine. Clin. Pharmacol. Ther. 25, 358—371 (1979).

[6] Sumner, D. J., Russell, A. J., Whiting, B.: Digoxin kinetics: Multicompartmental analysis and its clinical implications. Br. J. Clin. Pharmac. 3, 221—229 (1967).

[7] Whiting, B., Holford, N. H. G., Sheiner, L. B.: Quantitative analysis of the disopyramide concentration-effect relationship. Br. J. Clin. Pharmac. 9, 67—75 (1980).

Volume terms in pharmacokinetics

Renato L. Galeazzi
University of Berne, Department of Medicine, Inselspital, 3010 Bern

Although every kineticist calculates and reports volumes of distribution, there is a great deal of misunderstanding and discussion about the meaning of this term, the methods of calculation and its practical applications.
In this communication I shall try to define the meaning of this "volume", to explain why there are and have to be different volume terms, and to discuss the different methods to calculate the "volume" (with special reference to the non-compartmental methods).

Definition

The reason for a "volume of distribution" is the fact that we cannot measure the amount of drug in the body. We *know* the dose, which is an amont, but we *measure* a concentration. In order to transform concentrations into amounts and *vice versa* we need a volume term. This term is mathematically speaking a proportionality constant and has no physiologic meaning. We therefore define "volume of distribution" in pharmacokinetics *as the number with the dimension of VOLUME, with which the concentration of a drug has to be multiplied to get the amount of drug in the body.*
If the concentration in plasma is measured, it gives the volume with respect to the total plasma-concentration. If only the free fraction is considered, then the volume of distribution may be different and relates to the "free plasma-concentration."
In this definition no physiological space which could correspond to the volume is mentioned, because there is no such space. This "volume" is a proportion between amount of drug in the body and its plasma-concentration, it is no real volume.

One compartment model

If the elimination of a drug follows first order kinetics and can be described with a one compartment body model, the determination of the Vd is easy. Drawn on semilogpaper the data points can be extrapolated back to the time $t = 0$. This Cp_0 is the hypothetical concentration which would occur if the dose were instantaneously and homogeneously distributed throughout the distribution space. Therefore

$$Vd = \frac{\text{Dose}}{Cp_0} \tag{1}$$

Multi-compartment model

However, if the distribution phase is important, there is no straight line at the beginning of the plasma-concentration *vs.* time curve. The drug is not instantaneously distributed in the space of final distribution. During a certain time there is distribution in the body *and* elimination from the body. Redistribution from the plasma (plasma-compartment) to the tissues (peripheral compartment) takes place. This again means that the ratio "Amount in plasma *vs.* Amount in the body" varies with time. Vd, therefore, is not a constant value.
At the beginning all the drug given (the dose) is in the central compartment. Back extrapolation of the real data point at the beginning of the curve will reveal the initial Vd or V_1, the volume of the central compartment.

$$V_1 = \frac{\text{Dose}}{\text{“}Cp_o\text{”}} \tag{2}$$

V_1 is a very important parameter if Cp data are fitted to equations explicitly describing more-compartment models. In this case it is a "scaling" parameter. Moreover it is used to calculate Vd_{ss}; see Equation 12.
After a certain time distribution will be finished and the ratio of drug in plasma to drug in body will remain constant. At this point the log-linear-portion of the curve starts. Back extrapolation of this straight line (on "semilog" paper) to time $t = 0$ will give a hypothetical initial concentration as if the dose were homogeneously distributed with the final plasma to body ratio. If B is the intercept of this line at $t = 0$ then

$$Vd_{\text{extrap}} = \frac{\text{Dose}}{B} \tag{3}$$

However, during the distribution phase drug is not only distributed, but also eliminated. Therefore using the actual dose to calculate Vd_{extrap} will give a high value for this volume of distribution. This value is artificially high and will never correspond to a true Vd unless the drug follows one-compartmental kinetics.

$$Vd_{\text{extrap}} > V_1$$

A formula to calculate the Vd at any point in time was given by NIAZI [1]. The amount of drug at time t, A_t, is equal to the dose times the fraction of the dose remaining in the body. According to DOST's law of corresponding areas [2]:

$$A_t = \text{Dose} \frac{\int_0^\infty Cp\,dt}{\int_t^\infty Cp\,dt} \tag{4}$$

$$Vd_t = \frac{A_t}{Cp_t} \tag{5}$$

$$Vd_t = \frac{D \cdot \int_t^\infty Cp\,dt}{\int_0^\infty Cp\,dt \cdot Cp} \tag{6}$$

but

$$\frac{D}{\int_0^\infty Cp\,dt} = \text{Clearance} \tag{7}$$

therefore

$$Vd_t = \text{Clearance} \cdot \frac{\int_t^\infty Cp\,dt}{Cp} \tag{8}$$

The volume of distribution at pseudo-equilibrium

Vd_t will become constant if $\int_t^\infty Cp\,dt/Cp$ is constant. This will be the case in the monoexponential (log-linear) phase, after completion of distribution. Then

$$\frac{Cp}{\int_t^\infty Cp\,dt} = \beta \tag{9}$$

where β is the slope of the log-linear line.
Therefore the constant Vd after completion of distribution in the phase of the pseudo-equilibrium will be [3]

$$Vd_\beta = \text{Clearance} \cdot \frac{1}{\beta} \tag{10}$$

This Vd_β must be larger than V_1 (the smallest of the volume terms) and smaller than Vd_{extrap} (the false and largest one)

$$Vd_{extrap} > Vd > V_1$$

Vd_β is the volume with which the plasma-concentration has to be multiplied to get the amount of drug in the body in the log linear phase (*e.g.* the phase of pseudo-equilibrium).
This volume term is "non-compartmental." This means, that no explicit compartmental model has to be solved for. Clearance is model independent and can be calculated by different area methods and β can be determined from the terminal slope of the concentration *vs.* time curve alone.
This advantage however is balanced by the fact that Vd_β is dependent on the elimination process [4]. If elimination is fast the difference between the concentration in the plasma compartment (out of which the elimination occurs) and the concentration in the peripheral compartments becomes bigger, therefore Vd_β becomes larger. If elimination is slow, the concentrations are less different, Vd_β becomes smaller.
Vd_β therefore is not suitable for the comparison of the distribution of different drugs or of the same drug in different diseases affecting the elimination of the drug.

The volume of distribution at steady-state

Another stable state, where the ratio plasma-concentration to drug in the body does not change is the "steady state." Here, by definition, the concentrations in all compartments (of the model, not in the real body) are equal. Therefore the inter-compartmental clearances have to be equal, too:

$$V_1 \cdot k_{12} = V_2 \cdot k_{21} \tag{11}$$

$$Vd_{ss} = V_1 + V_2 = V_1 \left(1 + \frac{k_{12}}{k_{21}}\right) \tag{12}$$

This volume term is larger than V_1 but it is smaller than Vd_β,

$$Vd_{extrap} > Vd_\beta > Vd_{ss} > V_1$$

because, for equal plasma-concentrations there is less drug in the body at the steady state than at the pseudo-equilibrium. This is due to the fact that in the pseudo-equilibrium the concentration in the peripheral compartments will always be larger than in the central compartment. This volume, as it can be seen in Equation 12, is independent of the elimination, but a full compartmental model has to be solved.
The same is true for the formula given by VAN ROSSUM [5] and later by WAGNER [6].

$$Vd_{ss} = \frac{D \cdot \sum_{i=1}^{n} \frac{A_i}{\lambda_i^2}}{\left(\sum_{i=1}^{n} \frac{A_i}{\lambda_i} \right)^2} \tag{13}$$

where A_i are the intercepts and λ_i are the exponents of an n-exponential equation (that is an n-compartment model).
However,

$$\sum_{i=1}^{n} \frac{A_i}{\lambda^2} = \int_0^\infty t \cdot Cp \, dt \tag{14}$$

and

$$\sum_{i=1}^{n} \frac{A_i}{\lambda} = \quad Cp \, dt = \text{AREA under the curve} \tag{15}$$

and

$$\frac{\int_0^\infty t \, Cp \, dt}{\int_0^\infty Cp \, dt} = \text{MTT} \tag{16}$$

MTT is the "Mean Transit Time" of the physiologists [7]. It is also identical to the "first moment about zero" of the Cp *vs.* time curve [8]. In physical terms it is the x-axis of the center of gravity of the Cp *vs.* time curve [9]. Using these terms in equation 13 we can say that

$$\begin{aligned} Vd_{ss} &= \text{Clearance} \cdot \text{Mean Transit Time} \\ &= \frac{D \int_0 d \, Cp \, dt}{\left(\int_0^\infty Cp \, dt \right)^2} \end{aligned} \tag{17}$$

The two integrals in Equation 17 can be solved in different ways, *e. g.* using spline functions and their integral. They can also be calculated by numerical approximations using the trapezoidal rule either in its normal form

$$AUC_{Cp_1 - Cp_2} = (Cp_1 + Cp_2) \cdot (t_2 - t_1) \cdot \frac{1}{2} \tag{18}$$

or, for the log-linear descending portion [10],

$$AUC_{Cp_1 - Cp_2} = \frac{(Cp_1 - Cp_2) \cdot (t_2 - t_1)}{ln\ Cp_1 - ln\ Cp_2} \quad (19)$$

The integral from the last data point Cp_L, to infinity has to be extrapolated by the following equations:
For the integral in the numerator

$$AUC_{Cp_L \to \infty} = \frac{t_L \cdot Cp_L}{\beta} + \frac{Cp_L}{\beta^2} \quad (20)$$

For the integral in the denominator

$$AUC_{Cp_L \to \infty} = \frac{Cp_L}{\beta} \quad (21)$$

This Vd_{ss} calculated according to Equation 17 is the non-compartmental volume of distribution at steady state. It is also independent of elimination.
This *Vd*, which can be calculated also after bolus doses, can be used [1] to calculate amounts of drug in the body at steady state *(it is the volume with which the plasma-concentration has to be multiplied to get the amount of drug in the body at steady state)* and [2] to compare the distribution characteristics of a drug in different diseases affecting the elimination of the drug.
We have calculated $Vd\beta$ and Vd_{ss} for cefamandol in normals and in patients with end stage renal failure, using published data [11]. $Vd\beta$ is markedly different in the two groups, because elimination of cefamandol is very slow in renal failure. This result could lead to the conclusion that not only the elimination process is altered but also the distribution characteristics. However, *Vd_{ss} is identical in the two groups, clearly showing the fact that the difference in $Vd\beta$* is not due to changes in the distribution but rather due to the altered elimination. The error in calculating Vd_{ss} according to Equation 17 can be substantial. Errors may occur due to the numerical approximation of the integrals with the trapezoidal rules. This has been described in details by CHIOU [12]. The use of Equation 19 [10] in the descending portion of the *Cp vs.* time curve and/or more data points per time can be of help and the error can be minimised. Another error which is difficult to assess is the error due to extrapolation using Equations 20 and 21. Slight errors in β or in the value of the last data point can lead to markedly erroneous extrapolations. Therefore it is very important to sample as long as possible in order to maximize the reliability of our β and to minimise the portion of the integrals which has to be extrapolated.

Conclusion

The volume term in pharmacokinetics is a proportionality constant used to relate concentration of drugs in plasma to amount in the body. As this proportion is different at different times after the dose, more than one volume term must exist. Each has its meaning and its value. Each should only be used in the context in which it is defined; *e. g.*, Vd_{ss} should not be used to calculate amounts of drug in the body at pseudo-equilibrium.
Because of the lack of correlation with physiological spaces, *Vd* terms have little meaning for the clinician. They are, however, primary parameters for the kineticist.

References

[1] Niazi, S.: Volume of distribution as a function of time. J. Pharm. Sci. 65, 452—454 (1976).

[2] Dost, F. H.: Grundlagen der Pharmakokinetik. Georg Thieme, Stuttgart, 1968.

[3] Gibaldi, M., Nagashima, R., Levy, G.: Relationship between drug concentration in plasma or serum and amount of drug in the body. J. Pharm. Sci. 58, 193—197 (1969).

[4] Jusko, W. J., Gibaldi, M.: Effects of change in elimination on various parameters of the two-compartment open model. J. Pharm. Sci. 61, 1270—1273 (1972).

[5] van Rossum, J. M.: Significance of pharmacokinetics for drug design and the planning of dosage regimens. In: Drug Design (Ed. E. J. Ariens), pp. 469—521. Academic Press, New York and London, 1971.

[6] Wagner, J. G.: Linear pharmacokinetic equations allowing direct calculations of many needed pharmacokinetic parameters from coefficients and exponents of poly exponential equations which have been fitted to the data. J. Pharmacokin. Biopharm. 4, 443—467 (1967).

[7] Perl, W., Samuel, P.: Input-output analysis for total input rate and total traced mass of body cholesterol in man. Circ. Res. 25, 191—199 (1969).

[8] Yamaoka, K., Nakagawa, T., Uno, T.: Statistical moments in pharmacokinetics. J. Pharmacokin. Biopharm. 6, 547—558 (1978).

[9] Meier, J., Nuesch, E., Schmid, R.: Pharmacokinetic criteria for the evaluation of retard formulations. Europ. J. Clin. Pharmacol. 7, 429—432 (1974).

[10] Yeh, K. C., Kwan, K. C.: A comparison of numerical integrating algorithms by trapezoidal, lagrange, and spline approximation. J. Pharmacokin. Biopharm. 6, 79—98 (1978).

[11] Aziz, N. S., Gambertoglio, J. G., Grausz, H., Benet, L. Z.: Pharmacokinetics of cefamandole using HPLC-assay. J. Pharmacokin. Biopharm. 6, 152—164 (1978).

[12] Chiou, W. L.: Critical evaluation of the potential error in pharmacokinetic studies of using the linear trapezoidal rule method for the calculation of the area under the plasma level-time curve. J. Pharmacokin. Biopharm. 6, 539—546 (1978).

A method for *in vivo-in vitro* correlation using the additivity of Mean Times in biopharmaceutical models

H. M. von Hattingberg, D. Brockmeier
Zentrum für Kinderheilkunde, D-6300 Giessen
D. Voegele
Cassella, D-6000 Frankfurt/Main

Supported by "Bundesminister für Forschung und Technologie der Bundesrepublik Deutschland", Bioverfügbarkeit von Arzneimitteln (BAM 02).

Summary

The Mean Time—mittlere Verweildauer—as defined by Dost [3] is the statistical mean of all particular times any individual molecule of a dose is held up within a pharmacokinetic system prior to being eliminated from it. It is demonstrated that this mean time is as model independent as Dost's rule of areas. Operational algorithms for its assessment are presented. It can be used to characterize the time dependencies of a drugs "*in vivo* dissolution" from *in vitro* measurements. This is possible, since in a model consisting of a chain of, although undefined, subsystems, the mean Time in the model is the algebraic sum of all mean Times attributable to such subsystems. This linear relationship between *in vitro* and *in vivo* mean Times is found valid for different pharmaceutical formulations of carbocromene-HCl.

Introduction

In vitro dissolution tests on pharmaceutical formulations are necessary tools in quality control, and they can provide valuable information to explain observations from *in vivo* studies. They have, however, no predictive value, unless significant correlation to *in vivo* situations have been established. For certain dissolution test equipment such a correlation between amount dissolved *in vitro* and amount absorbed *in vivo* has been demonstrated for a few drugs, and sometimes the relationship was found invalid for some of their formulations (Frömming [5], Ritschel [8]).
The use of the mean Time, discussed here, may help to add to the list of drugs and formulations, for which *in vitro* tests allow predictions on the time course of drug concentrations *in vivo*. It is a mathematically defined, overall time parameter which summarizes all time dependencies in complex systems, and it is easy to assess experimentally.

Definition and method for assessment

DOST [3] defined the mean Time T ("mittlere Verweildauer") as the arithmetic mean of all times during which any particular molecule of an amount of drug remains within *i. e.*, is not eliminated from, a system in which it did reside at the time zero.

From the statistical definition it follows, irrespective of any model, that the mean of all(!) lifetimes is

$$T = \frac{\int t \cdot dM(t)}{\int dM(t)} \tag{1}$$

(VAN DER WAERDEN [11]).

Which, by partial integration and rearranging, becomes (VON HATTINGBERG and BROCKMEIER [6, 7])

$$T = \frac{\int_0^\tau [M(\tau) - M(t)]\, dt}{\int_0^\tau dM(t)} \tag{2}$$

Here the integrand is the time course of the amount of drug (number of drug molecules) within an as yet undefined system, $M(\tau)$ its value at the end of the integration interval, and $\int dM(t)$ the total amount under considerations.

The numerator in Equation 2 is the Area Between a Curve, ABC, and a constant value (horizontal line), and it can be obtained by pragmatic methods. Thus the algorithm is reduced to

$$T = \frac{\text{ABC}}{\text{total amount}} \tag{3}$$

If $M(t)$ is defined as the amount within a total pharmacokinetic system, *i. e.*, "not excreted", ABC is identical with the area under that curve, since $M(\tau)$ for infinity is zero.

If, however, M(t) describes cumulative loss, $M(\tau)$ is the amount finally eliminated, and identical with the total amount observed. ABC is then the Area Between Cumulative appearance at the output and its asymptote.

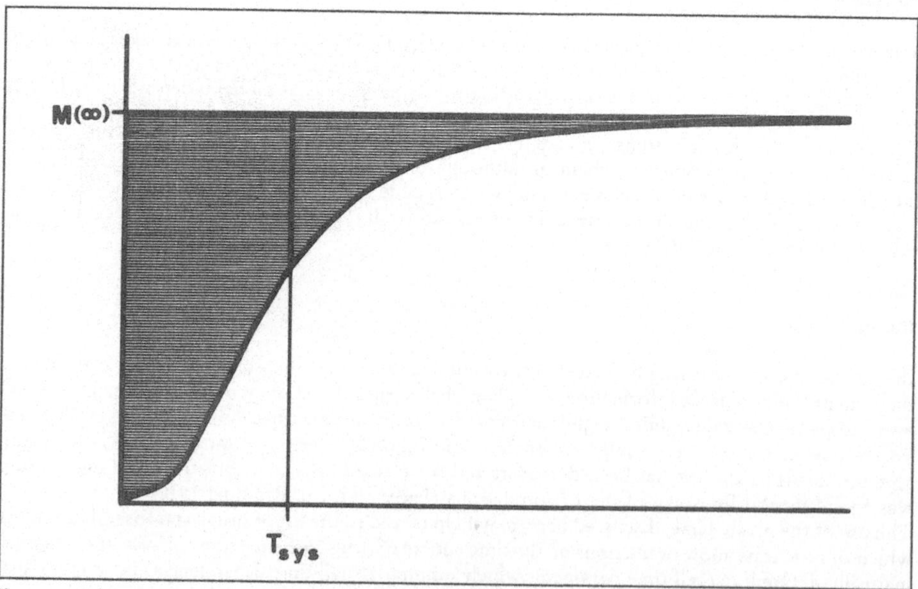

Figure 1: Schematic presentation of the cumulative output from a pharmacokinetic system, *e. g.* by cumulative urinary excretion: In the hatched area each horizontal line represents the actual persistence Time of one fraction of the dose within the—unknown—system. ABC/asymptote thus yields their mean.

This is visualized in Figure 1, where cumulative urinary excretion is shown, and where three important aspects become apparent:
1. *T-sys* may be regarded as the mean of all horizontal lines, each representing the actual life time of a subfraction of the total amount.
2. *T-sys* encompasses all time dependencies attributable to all processes possibly involved after zero time, which includes, *e. g.*, the influence of a pharmaceutical formulation and absorptive processes. This is indicated by the subscript "*sys*". After *iv.* administration *T-vss* for the body model *i. e.* the "mean transit time", is obtained.
3. Estimates of *T-sys* from urinary excretion date are unaffected by parallel metabolic degradation of the drug. This would only change the scale of the ordinate, but not the ratio ABC/asymptote. They are independent of incomplete bioavailability since only drug amounts which actually reach the system investigated are considered.
From a multiexponential equation describing the theoretical time course in the central compartment, *Vc*, from which irreversible elimination takes place at a relative rate of *k-el*, the timecourse of amounts not excreted can be predicted, *e. g.* for an *i. v.* bolus administration. Substituting such predictions in either of Equation 1 through 3, we then obtain the mean transit time, *T-vss*, for the body model

$$T\text{-}vss = \frac{\Sigma Cj/y_j^2}{\Sigma Cj/y_j} \qquad (4)$$

and we find (von HATTINGBERG *et al.* [6], VAN ROSSUM [10],

$$T\text{-}vss = Vss/Cl\text{-}tot \qquad (5)$$

and

$$V\text{-}vss/T\text{-}vss = Vc \cdot ke \qquad (6)$$

If there are no interactions of the rates between subsystems connected in a chain, *i. e.* if there are no saturable procecces, or compartmentally interacting forces, *e. g.* as in reversibly exchanging side compartments involved, the statistical rules of additivity of means apply.

Mean Time in mathematically defined subsystems

In Figure 2 four different models together with their cumulative outputs and the Areas Between Curves and final values are shown. The mean Times obtained from these are listed in the last column.
a) For an infusion device delivering an amount D at a constant rate $\dot{D}$, the mean Time is one half of the infusion time. This trivial result is obtained by division of the triangular area above the cumulative delivery function by $\dot{D} \cdot \tau$.
b) The area above the cumulative disposition curve from a first order compartment is equal to the dose, divided by the rate constant, and it is identical to the area under the curve of amounts within that compartment. It has been shown by DOST [3] that the "mean life time" then is $1/k$.

Additivity

c) If these two models are combined to, *e. g.*, a one compartment model with zero order administration, the concentration time course "within" the compartment is described by different equations before and after the total dose is infused. The sum of the two respective areas "within", again, *is* $\dot{D}\tau/k$ (DOST [3]). The Area Between Cumulative disposition, however, is the sum of the two areas obtained from the two models taken separately. Thus the mean Time for the entire system, *i. e.* infusion pump and pharmacokinetic model together, is the sum of both individual mean Times.
d) Combining two first order compartments in series leads to the Bateman function, where the rule

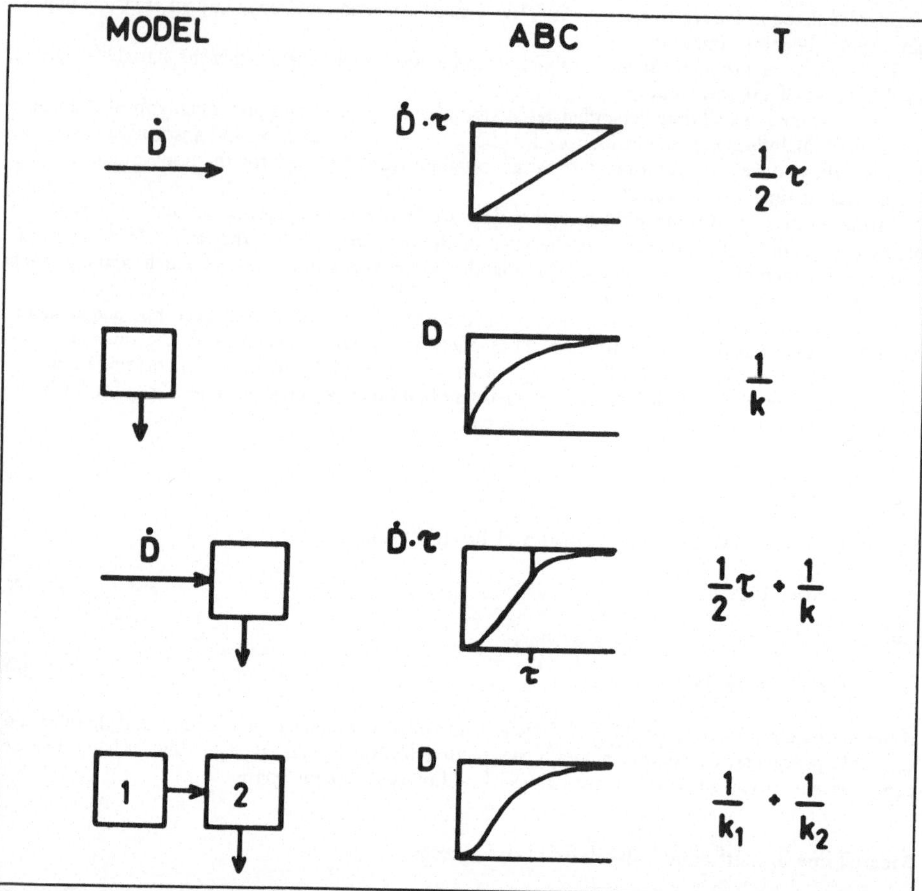

Figure 2: Different models (first column), the graphical presentation ot their outputs (second column) and the corresponding mean system Times as obtained by division of the Area Between Curves—or by Equation 1 through 3—(last column).
First row: zero order output; second row: first order output; third row: first order and second order in series; fourth row: two second order compartments in series. In sequential systems the mean Times of the system is the sum of the mean Times of the components.

of areas defines the rate constant *k-el*, and its reciprocal, *T-vc*, for the body model. The numerical result if Equation 3 is the sum of the mean Times from each compartment.
The output ot these last two examples are very similar in shape, and the correct mean Time can be obtained numerically from ABC without identification of the model.

Parallel processes

If parallel processes act on a total dose, the mean system time *T-sys* is the weighted sum of mean Times describing the particular components. The weights are the fractions of dose undergoing the different processes: If, *e. g.*, a drug is administered in part (D1) by an *i. v. bolus* (priming dose), and in part (D2) by constant infusion over the time, τ (Figure 3), the entire dose will be subject to the mean Time for the body model, whereas the additional one half of the infusion time applies only for the fraction administered at a constant rate.

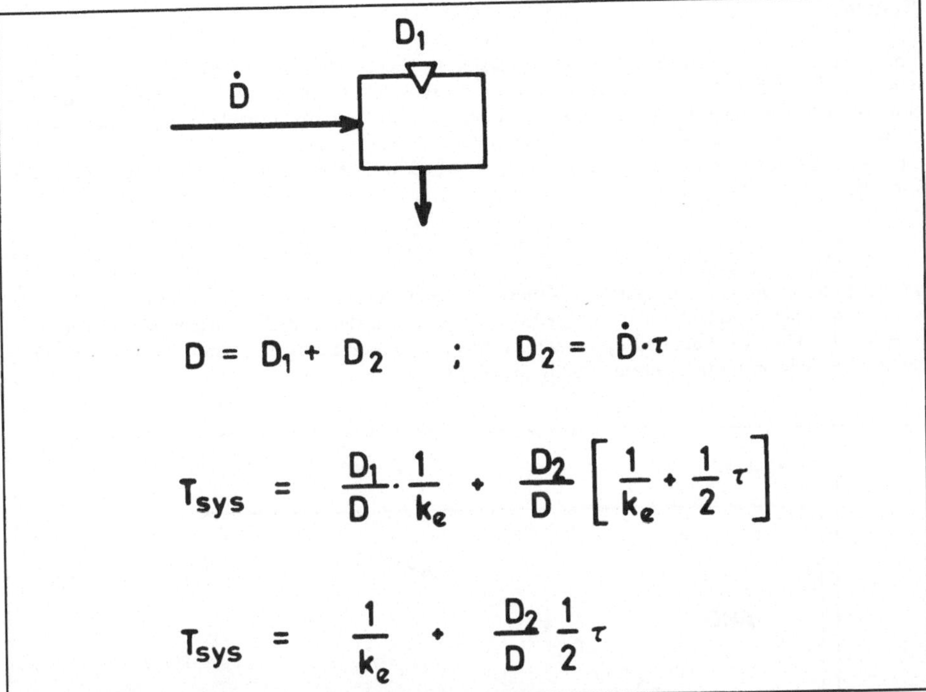

Figure 3: Two different inputs acting in parallel on a first order compartment: The mean Time attributable to the compartment pertains to the total dose, whereas the additional mean infusion Time pertains only to the fraction administered at a constant rate.

In vitro dissolution Time

The similarity of the curves just discussed to *in vitro* dissolution curves is obvious.
We therefore expect a "mean *in vitro* dissolution time," *T-diss,* obtained by the same method as before, to encompass the time dependencies attributable to all conceivable, although undefined, elementary subsystems involved in the solubility of a pharmaceutical formulation.
The significance of this parameter could possibly exceed that of the time required for a certain percentage, *e. g.* 60% or 90%, to dissolve.
If this is true, *T-diss* for a given formulation, obtained in an *in vitro* apparatus providing appropriate physical and chemical conditions, must prove to be additive to the *in vivo* mean system Time, if the time scales *in vivo* and *in vitro* are the same, or, if a constant factor, *f,* exists, relating the time scale *in vitro* to *in vivo* time.

This postulate can be expressed by a linear equation:

$$T\text{-}sys = T\text{-}biol + f \cdot T\text{-}diss \tag{7}$$

where *T-biol* is the mean transit time for the body model, *T-vss* [12], plus the mean Time of all biological processes affecting absorption, and

$$f \cdot T\text{-}diss = T\text{-}diss\text{-}vivo$$

Results

The validity of this thesis (Equation 7) was tested by linear regression of mean dissolution Times determined in a Sartorius® apparatus versus *T-sys* assessed in volunteers. Four different formulations of carbocromene-HCl (Intensain®) were tested: A soft gelatine capsule, a sugar-coated tablet, a film-coated tablet and the core of a retard tablet.
The Weibull function (RRSB distribution [4]) modified to contain a linear component and allowing for a lag time of dissolution

$$y = A + Bt + C \cdot \exp(G \cdot t \uparrow P) \quad (8)$$

was fitted to the *in vitro* observations, without linearizing transforms, on a desk top computer. The modification provided better least square fits for all formulations tested. An example is shown in Figure 4. The ABC was obtained by numerical integration of the function, and *T-diss* was obtained from it by division by the amount finally dissolved.

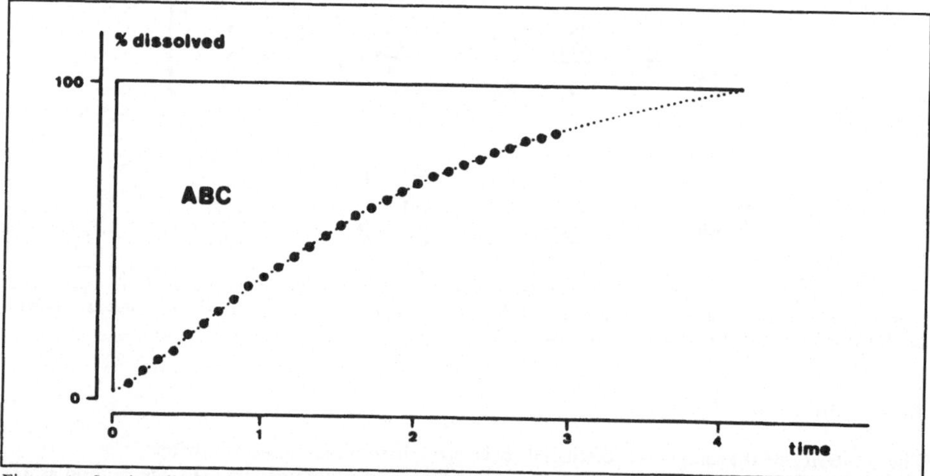

Figure 4: *In vitro* dissolution of carbocrome-HCl. Heavy points signify dissolution observed in a Sartorius® apparatus using a pH-gradient. Small points demonstrate the mathematical prediction of dissolution against time as obtained from non linear curve fitting of Equation 8 to the dissolution data. ABC is the area between the predicted curve and 100% dissolved. Ordinate: Dissolution (%); abscissa: Time in hours.

For the *in vivo* results (Figure 5), experimentally obtained plasma levels were integrated by stepwise parabolic interpolation to yield a function proportional to cumulative disposition. The difference of this function and its asymptote (AUC) was again integrated by the same method. A monoexponential fit to the last data was used to extrapolate integrals to infinity and to define the asymptote. The determination of the mean system Time from experimental plasma levels requires two subsequent integrations and *T-sys* then simply is

$$T\text{-}sys = \frac{ABC}{AUC} \quad (9)$$

In Figure 6 the regression of *in vivo versus in vitro* is shown: The coefficient of correlation is 0.9996. The time converting factor, f, is 1.4 with a relative standard deviation of 2%. The intercept defining *T-biol* is 1.77 h with the same relative standard deviation. There is no reason to reject our postulate as improbable ($P < 0.01$).

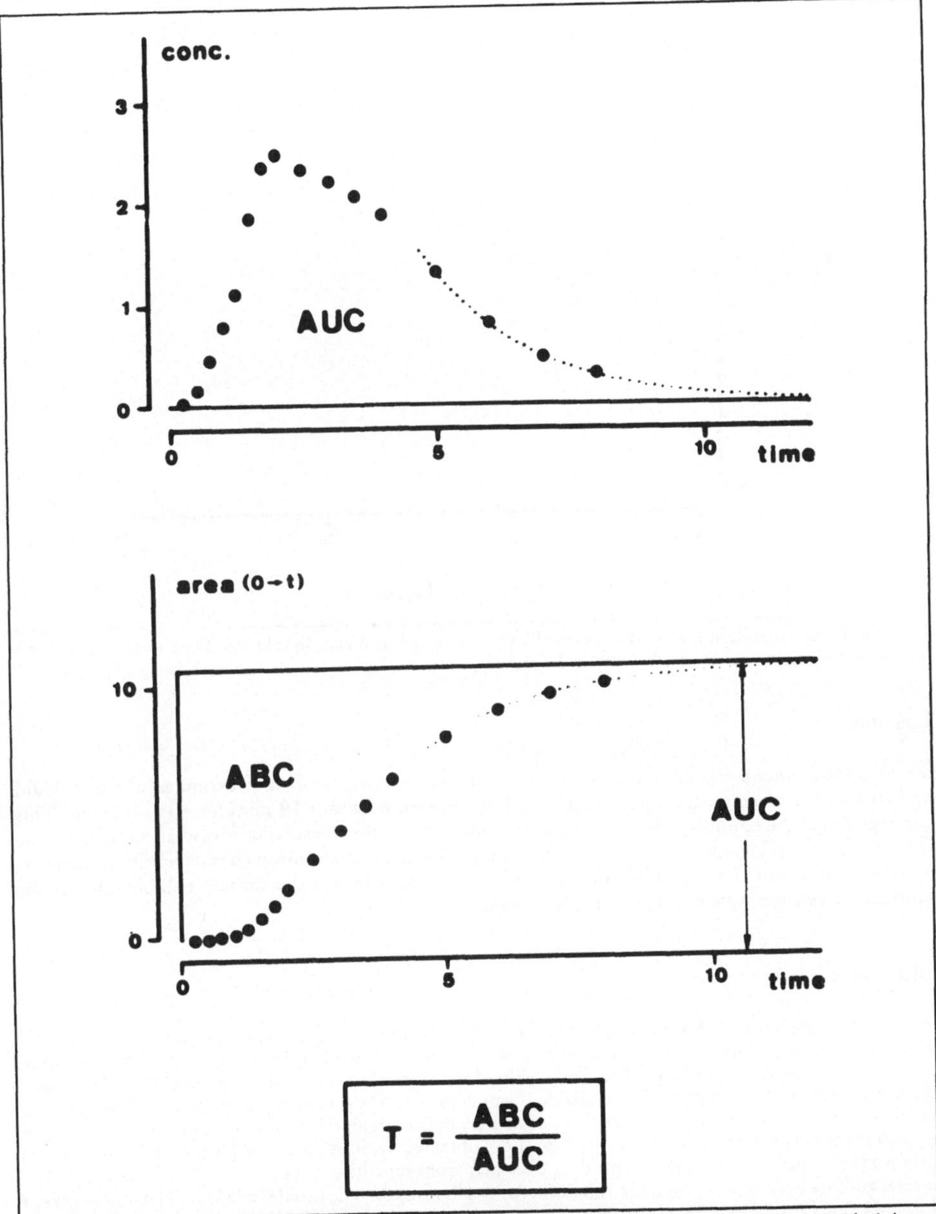

Figure 5: Mean plasma concentrations (heavy points) of carbocromenic acid in plasma upon administration of carbocromene-HCl to volunteers. Small dotted curve: Monoexponential fit to the data indicated. AUC and ABC can be estimated by numerical, parabolic interpolation and extrapolation to infinity using the monoexponential fit. Ordinate: Concentrations in nmol/ml; abscissa: Time in hours.

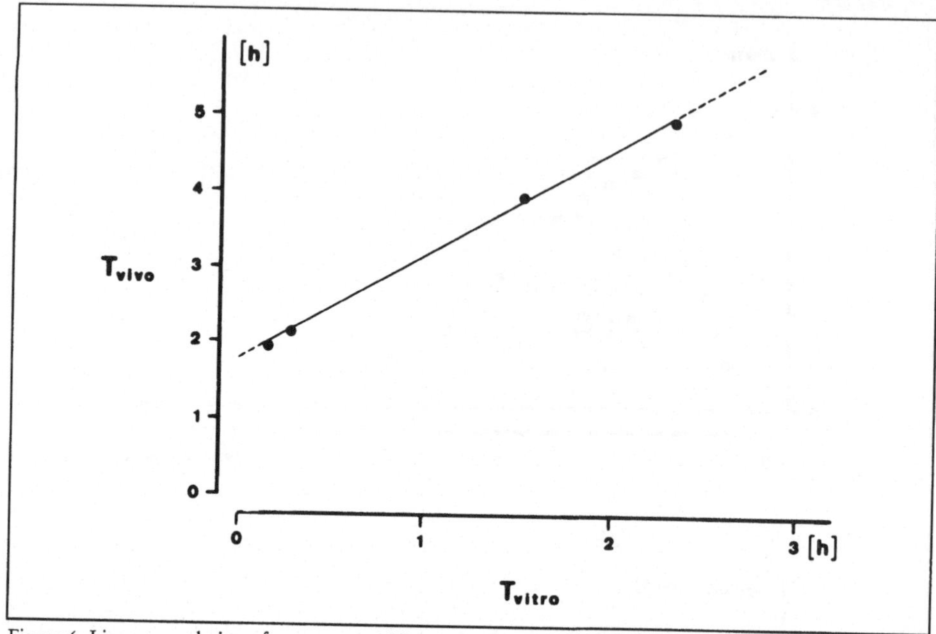

Figure 6: Linear correlation of mean system Time *in vivo* versus mean dissolution Time *in vitro* for carbocromene. Ordinate and abscissa: Time in hours.

Lagtime

When carbocromene was administered orally as an aqueous solution, a bi-exponential curve could be fitted to the plasma data, and a lagtime of absorption of about 19 minutes was obtained. This corresponds to 14 minutes *in vitro* dissolution time. The fastest dissolving formulation, namely the soft gelatine capsule had liberated 95% at that time. Hence the dissolution characteristics of this formulation exert only a small effect on the profile of plasma levels; the capsule exhibits almost the same mean *in vivo* system Time as the solution.

Discussion

Provided that the Sartorius® apparatus and carbocromene were not an unusually lucky choice, we have demonstrated that the concept of mean Times provides tools for efficient biopharmaceutical work. The 'mean *in vivo* dissolution time' can be used to predict blood concentration curves from *in vitro* data, if the basic pharmacokinetics of the most readily available formulation are known (VOEGELE *et al.* [13]). The principle has also been used successfully in the analysis of urinary data of gentamicin where 'model fitting' has failed [7], and the results where strictly comparable to those obtained by SCHENTAG *et al.* [10], who had performed a rigorous pharmacokinetic analysis on data obtained from repetitive dosing.
Several authors have applied the mean time concept to pharmacokinetic problems. DOST [3] defined $1/ke$ as the mean time for the central compartment by a statistical approach; from this he derived the rule of areas. VAN ROSSUM [12] characterizes a multicompartment body model by the mean time assessed after *i. v. bolus* administration. BENET and GALEAZZI [1] proposed it as a means to estimate total volumes of distribution independently of pharmacokinetic models. YAMAOKA *et al.* [14] discuss statistical moments as an approach to assess variability in blood levels. MEIER *et al.* [8] rejected the time coordinate of the gravity centre of plasma level curves as a measure for slow release formulations on the grounds of low sensitivity.
All authors used the statistical algorithm following from Equation. 1 for linear pharmacokinetic systems, where $y(t)$ represents plasma levels:

$$T\text{-}sys = \frac{\int t\,y(t)\,dt}{\int y(t)\,dt} \tag{11}$$

which recently was proposed again by CUTLER [2] who presented the theory of a mean absorption time. Pragmatic integration of experimentally obtained concentration x time products is difficult and likely to carry considerable numerical error.
The more operational algorithm given in Equation 3 (VON HATTINGBERG and BROCKMEIER [6 and 7] or Equation 9, presented here, has to our knowledge, not been used before.

References

[1] Benet, L. Z.: Galeazzi, R. L.: Non compartmental determination of the volume of distribution in steady state. Abstracts of papers, Acad. Pharm. Sci. 7, 162 (1977).

[2] Cutler, D. J.: Theory of the mean absorption time, an adjunct to conventional bioavailability studies. J. Pharm. Pharmac. 30, 476—478 (1978).

[3] Dost, F. H.: Über ein einfaches statistisches Dosis-Umsatzgesetz. Klin. Wschr. 36, 655—657 (1958).

[4] DIN 66145: "RRSB-Netz". Deutscher Normenausschuß, Januar 1970.

[5 Frömming, K.-H.: *In vitro* experiments as information of bioavailability. In: Titisee conference October 1978: Pharmacokinetics during drug development: Data analysis and evaluation technisques, van Rossum, J. M. (ed.) in press.

[6] von Hattingberg, H. M., Brockmeier, D.: A concept for the assessment of bioavailability in complex systems in terms of amounts and rates. In: Titisee conference October 1978: Pharmacokinetics during drug development: Data analysis and evaluation techniques, van Rossum, J. M. (ed.) in press.

[7] von Hattingberg, H. M., Brockmeier, D.: Pharmacokinetic basis for an optimum dose of antibiotics. Infection 8, Suppl. 1, 21—24 (1980).

[8] Meier, J., Nüsch, E., Schmidt, R.: Pharmacokinetic criteria for the evaluation of retard formulations. Europ. J. clin. Pharmacol. 7, 429—432 (1974).

[9] Ritschel, W. A.: Grundlagen der Biopharmazie und Bioverfügbarkeit. In: Kümmerle, H. P. (ed.): Methoden der klinischen Pharmakologie. Urban-Schwarzenberg, München 1978.

[10] Schentag, J. J., Jusko, W. J., Vance, J. W., Cumbo, T. J., Abrutyn, E., de Lattre, M., Gerbracht, L. M.: Gentamicin disposition and tissue accumulation on multiple dosing. J. Pharmacokin. Biopharm. 5, 559—577 (1977).

[11] van der Waerden, B. L.: Mathematische Statistik. Springer, Berlin, 3. Auflage 1971.

[12] van Rossum, J. M.: Basic parameters in pharmacokinetics. In: Titisee Conference October 1978: Pharmacokinetics during drug development: Data analysis and evaluation techniques, van Rossum, J. M. (ed.), in press.

[13] Voegele, D., Brockmeier, D., van Hattingberg, H. M.: The mean transit time as an aid in the development of galenical dosage forms. International Symposium on Methods in Clinical Pharmacology, Frankfurt, 6.—8. May 1979.

[14] Yamaoka, K., Nakagawa, T. Uno, T.: Statistical moments in pharmacokinetics. J. Pharmacokin. Biopharm. 6, 547—558 (1978).

The mean-transit-time as an aid in the development of galenical dosage forms

D. Voegele, D. Brockmeier, H. M. von Hattingberg
Pharmaforschung Cassella AG, Frankfurt/Main and Zentrum für Kinderheilkunde, Giessen

It is often said that *in vitro* dissolution cannot reflect *in vivo* dissolution conditions at all, because the human body is no "beaker with stirrer".
The contrary statement is that *in vitro* dissolution measurements may include basic properties of the *in vivo* dissolution process.
To confirm the second thesis a correlation between *in-vivo* and *in-vitro* dissolution must be demonstrated.

The additivity of mean-times in a series of biopharmaceutical subsystems defines a linear relationship between the mean-time of *in vitro* dissolution and the mean-transit-time of the drug in the total *in vivo* system for a given pharmaceutical formulation [1]. Thus T-Diss-vivo can be obtained experimentally; see Figures 1 and 2.
Under the preliminary assumption of first order *in vivo* dissolution at a rate of k = 1/T-Diss-vivo rough predictions of blood concentration curves can be computed for different dosage forms if the basic pharmacokinetics of the most bioavailable preparation are known; see Figures 3 and 4.
The method is applied to Carbocromene HCL* administered to humans in various Intensain®-dosage forms that exhibit differing dissolution characteristics in an *in vitro* model [5]; see Figure 6, soft gelatine capsules, sugar-coated tablets, film-coated tablets/retarded and uncoated tablet cores/retarded.
The shapes of the predicted curves compare favourably with observations [4, 3]; see Figures 5 and 7.
Bioavailability was accounted for under the thesis that loss of drug is due to intraluminal first order degradation in parallel to absorption [2]; see Figure 4.
The predictions may serve as guides in the search for a pharmaceutical drug design based on the drugs pharmacokinetic properties.

Acknowledgements

The authors gratefully thank Dr. R. E. Nitz, Dr. J. Ostrowski, Dr. K. Resag, and Dr. E. Schraven for providing blood concentration data.

* INN (Intensain®; Manufacturer: Cassella-Riedel Pharma GmbH, D-6000 Frankfurt/Main 61).

[1] von Hattingberg, M. H., Brockmeier, D., Voegele, D., A method for *in vivo-in vitro* correlation using the additivity of mean-times in biopharmaceutical models. International symposium on methods in clinical pharmacology, Frankfurt/Main, May 1979.

[2] von Hattingberg, H. M., Brockmeier, D., Standardisierung von Rechenmodellen zur Prüfung der Bioverfügbarkeit von Arzneimitteln. Rietbrock, N., Schnieders, B. (ed.), Bioverfügbarkeit von Arzneimitteln. Gustav Fischer, Stuttgart 1979.

[3] Internal report, Pharmaforschung Cassella.

[4] Schraven, E., Nitz, R. E., Klarwein, M., Arzneim. Forsch. 20, 1905 (1970).

[5] Stricker, H., Pharm, Ind. 33, 446 (1971.)

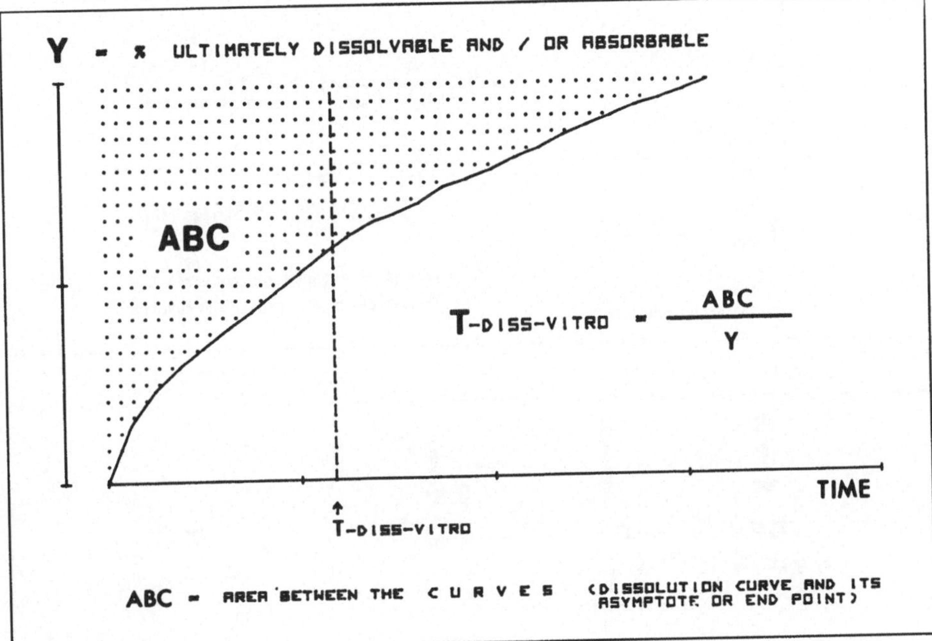

Figure 1.

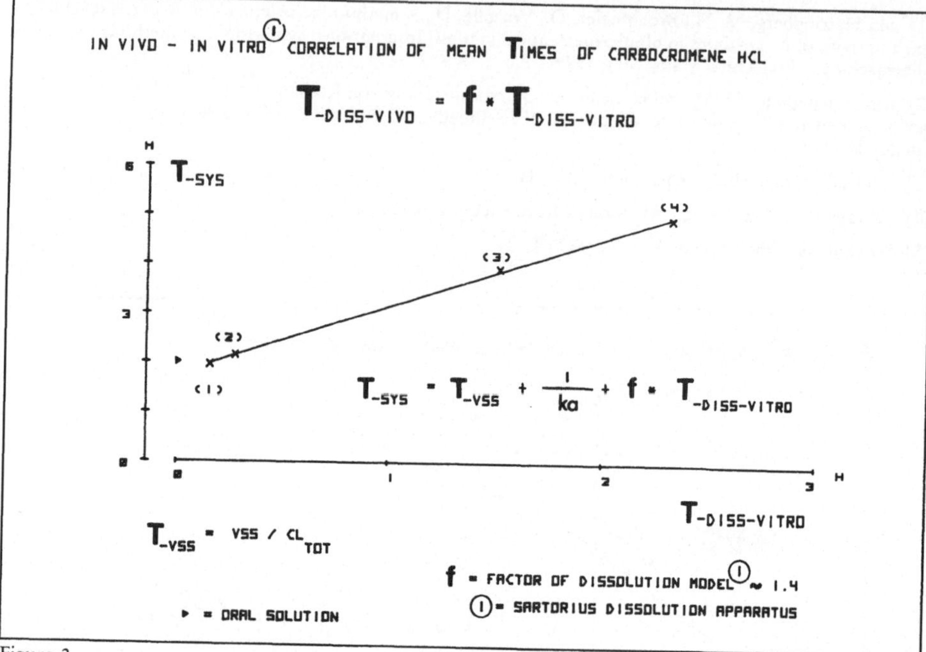

Figure 2.

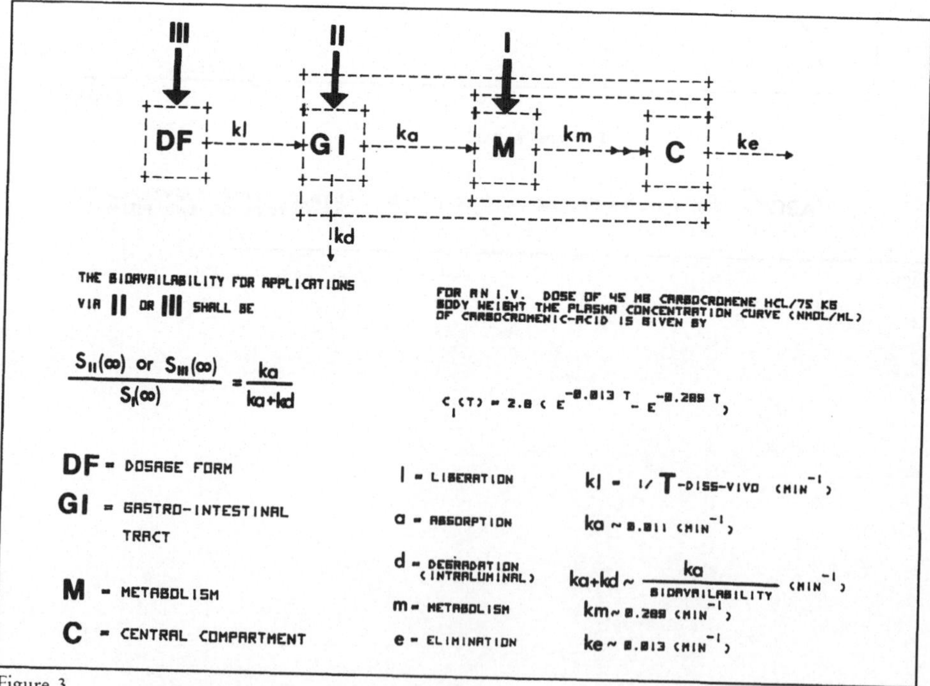

Figure 3.

$$c_{I}(t) = \sum_{1}^{n} C_j \, e^{-\gamma_j t}$$

$$c_{II}(t) = \sum_{1}^{n} C_j \, \frac{ka}{\gamma_j - (ka + kd)} \left(e^{-(ka+kd)t} - e^{-\gamma_j t} \right)$$

$$c_{II}(t) = \sum_{1}^{n+1} \hat{C}_j \, e^{-\gamma_j t} \qquad \gamma_{n+1} = ka + kd$$

$$c_{III}(t) = \sum_{1}^{n+1} \hat{C}_j \, \frac{kl}{\gamma_j - kl} \left(e^{-kl\,t} - e^{-\gamma_j t} \right)$$

$$c_{III}(t) = \sum_{1}^{n+2} \hat{\hat{C}}_j \, e^{-\gamma_j t} \qquad \gamma_{n+2} = kl$$

Figure 4.

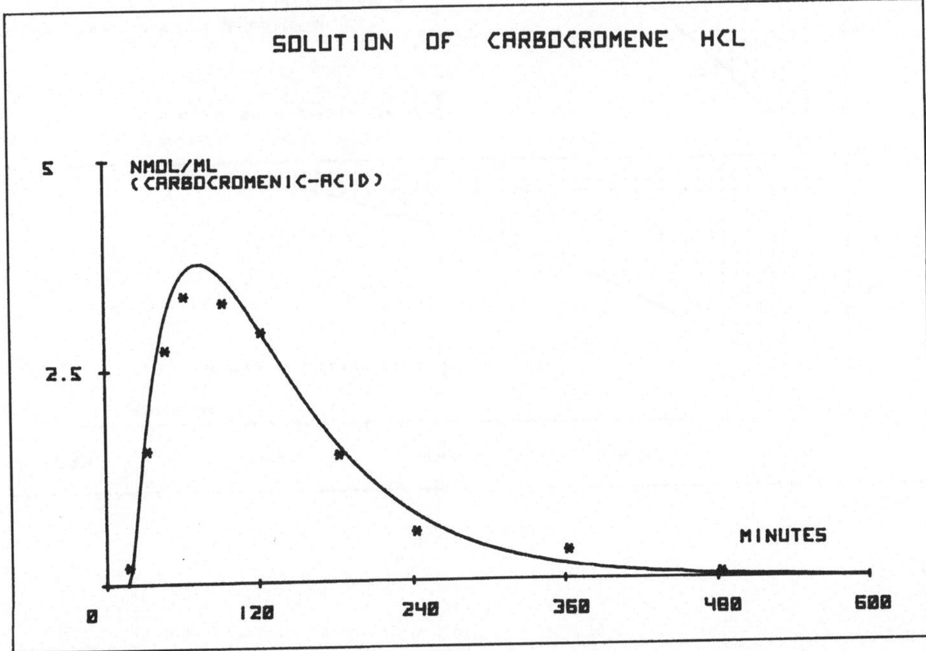

Figure 5.

IN-VITRO DISSOLUTION
% - DISSOLVED
100
50
0
- = • SARTORIUS DISSOLUTION APPARATUS •
T-DISS-VITRO = 8.24 MIN.
T-DISS-VITRO = 10.58 MIN.
□ = DESINTEGRATION TEST
PH EUR III
(22 MM LIFT / WITH DISKS)
T-DISS-VITRO = 88.84 MIN.
T-DISS-VITRO = 130.88 MIN.
MINUTES
0
120
240
360
480

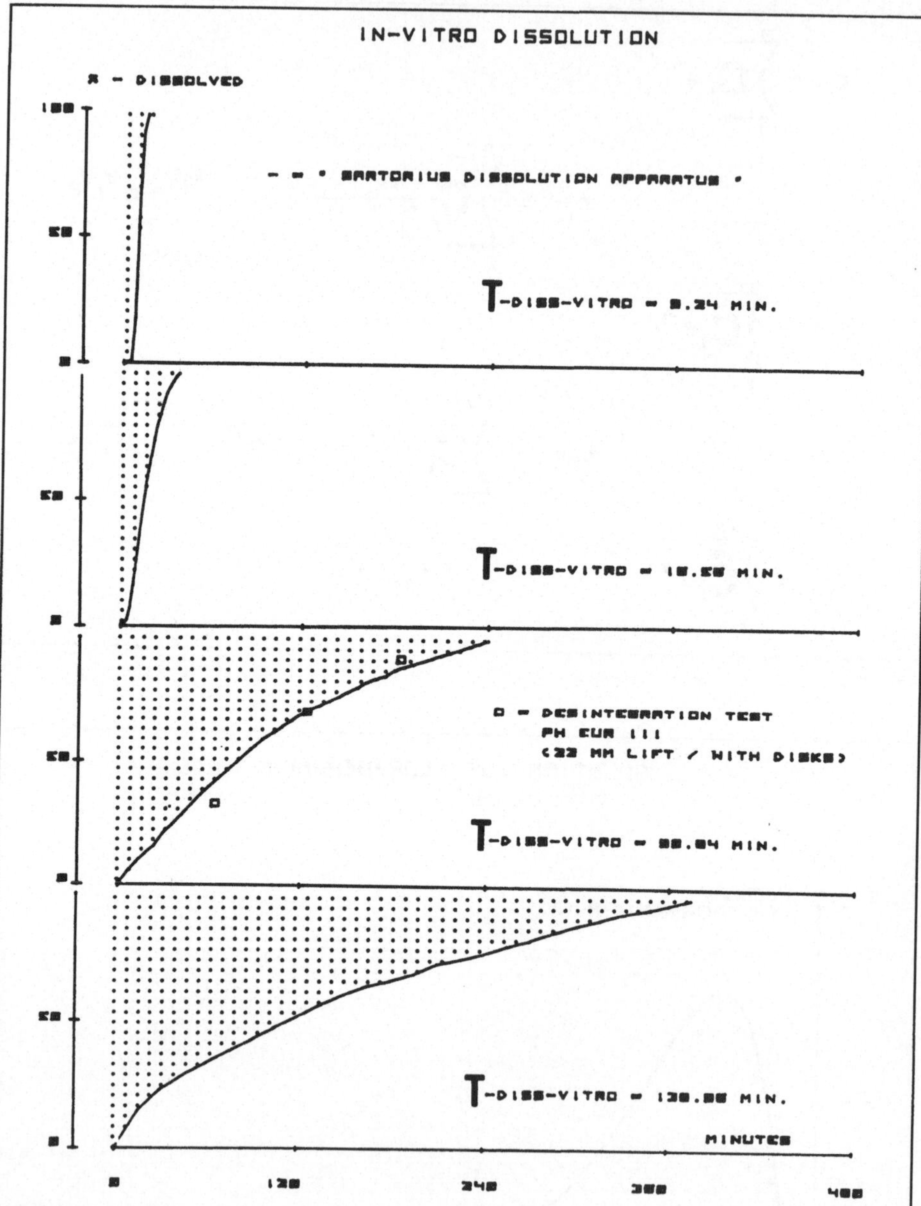

Figure 6.

PREDICTED BLOOD CONCENTRATION CURVES
NMOL/ML
(CARBOCROMENIC-ACID)
INTENSAIN - LANITOP
SOFT-GELATINE CAPSULES (1)
SUGARCOATED TABLETS (2)
INTENSAIN RETARD
FILMCOATED TABLETS (3)
INTENSAIN RETARD
TABLETS (4)
1
120
240
MINUTES

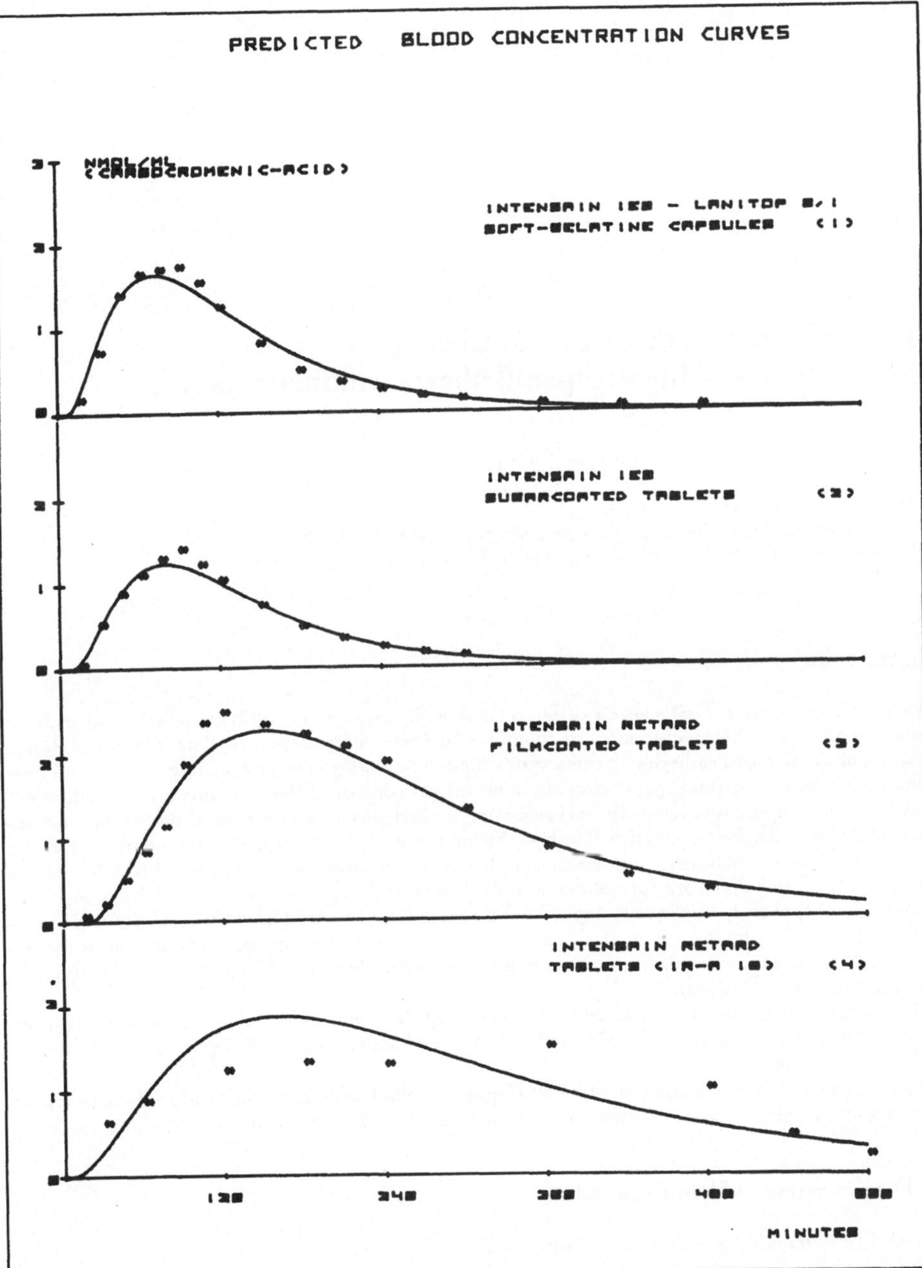

Figure 7.

Two different methods for calculating constants describing verapamil pharmacokinetics in man

A. Laßmann*, G. Lazarus**, and Ingrid Rietbrock**

* Department of Clinical Pharmacology,
Klinikum der Johann Wolfgang Goethe-Universität Frankfurt/Main
** Institut of Anaethesiology, Klinikum der Julius Maximilians-Universität Würzburg

Introduction

Two different ways for calculation of pharmacokinetic parameters will be demonstrated with an analog-computer. Their requirement of computer facilities will be described. The Method of Residuals ("Subtraction or Feathering"), done with a *digital-* or *analog-computer* (analog circuit 1), or graphically on semilogarithmic paper provides a means for control of the mathematical procedure because of the stepwise way in which the calculation is carried out and because of the visual tests one has available. With the Subtraction-Method the important pharmacokinetic parameters such as the β-constant can be obtained, from which the physician can calculate the biological half-life of the drug in blood and therefore formulate multiple dosage regimes.
These visual approaches have been applied to verapamil kinetics and describe plasma concentration-time curves as the sum of *e*-functions. This can be accomplished by iterative adjustment of the *hybrid-constants* until the calculated curves best aproximate the observed plasma concentrations (Gauß-Newton Iteration Method).
Pharmacokinetic parameters obtained by the *Method of Residuals*, will be compared with *analog-computer simulation* and the iteration programm *SAAM 25*, which allow *curve fitting* by direct adjustment of the *rate-constants.*
Plasma verapamil concentration-time curves (Figure 1) following *i. v.* administration in four subjects (3 patients, 1 control) were selected so as to provide a broad range of plasma clearance values.

I. Determination of Hybrid-Constants

Method of Residuals ("Subtraction or Feathering")
The calculation of pharmacokinetic parameters using the Subtraction Method is described by Gladtke and von Hattingberg [1]. In the case of most drug elimination curves a β-constant can be obtained from the data points in the monoexponential elimination phase. Subtraction of this *e*-function from the area under the plasma concentration-time curve leads to another semilogarithmic interpretable α-phase. The two hybrid constants, α and β and the intercepts with the ordinate are listed in Table 1.

Subject	$A_{1\,corr}$*	$A_{2\,corr}$*	α	β
C	19.6	9.6	0.0201	0.0055
L_d	19.4	8.1	0.0262	0.0008
ICP_1	29.6	20.2	0.0247	0.0038
ICP_2	5.1	10.7	0.0695	0.0071

Table 1: Estimation of the hybrid-constants for verapamil elimination of a healthy volunteer and 3 patients by the subtraction method [1]. Same subjects as Figure 1.

* In the case of slow drug administration the hypothetical concentration intercepts of the exponential terms with the ordinate

$$(A_{1\,\text{post inf.}} \text{ and } A_{2\,\text{post inf.}})$$

are corrected for an intravenous bolus-injection of the same amount of drug according to Loo and RIEGELMANN [2].

$$A_{1\,\text{corr.}} = \frac{A_{1\,\text{post inf.}} \cdot \alpha \cdot T}{(1 - e^{-\beta \cdot T})} \qquad A_{2\,\text{corr.}} = \frac{A_{2\,\text{post inf.}} \cdot \beta \cdot T}{(1 - e^{-\alpha \cdot T})}$$

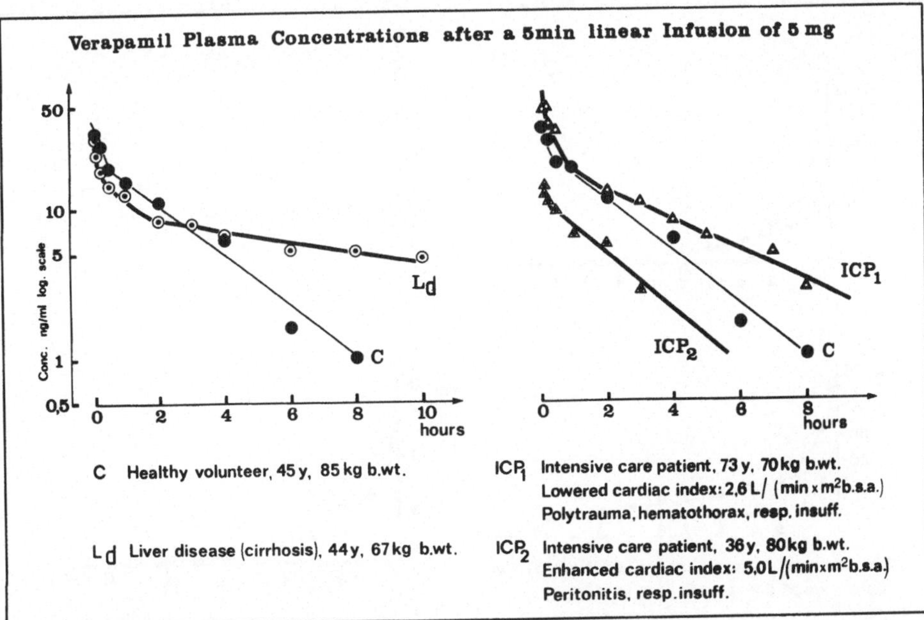

Figure 1: Verapamil plasma concentration-time curves of three patients and one healthy volunteer.

Analog computer drawn curves:
Parameters obtained directly with the Method of Residuals are suitable for simulation of four different verapamil elimination curves (Figure 3). These curves and their corresponding α- and β-phases are drawn by an analog-computer. The chosen potentiometer settings, proportional to the values of Table 1, are indicated in the analog circuit 1 (Figure 2). Each integrator delivers the voltage equivalent (= analog) for drug elimination from the compartment.
The analog-computer drawings, when compared to the original data, demonstrate that verapamil elimination can be described satisfactorily with an open two compartment model (Figure 4).

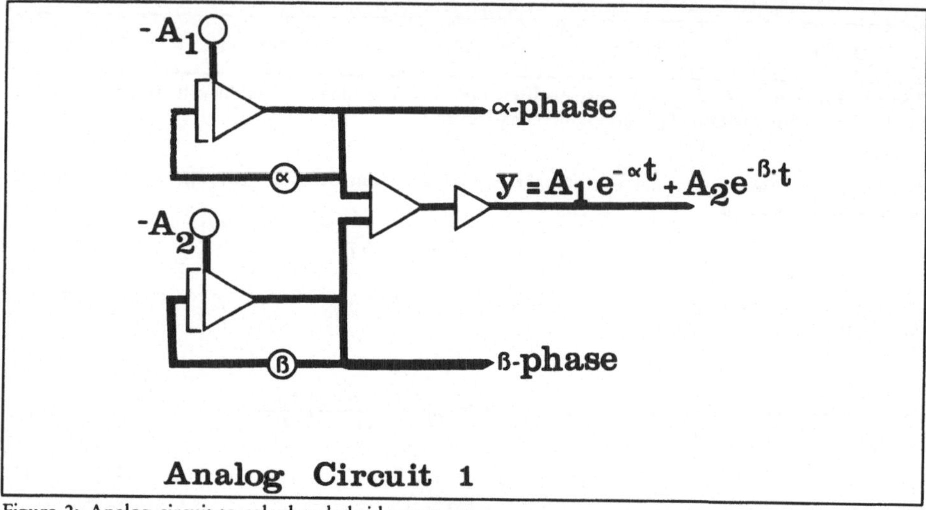

Figure 2: Analog circuit to calculate hybrid-constants.

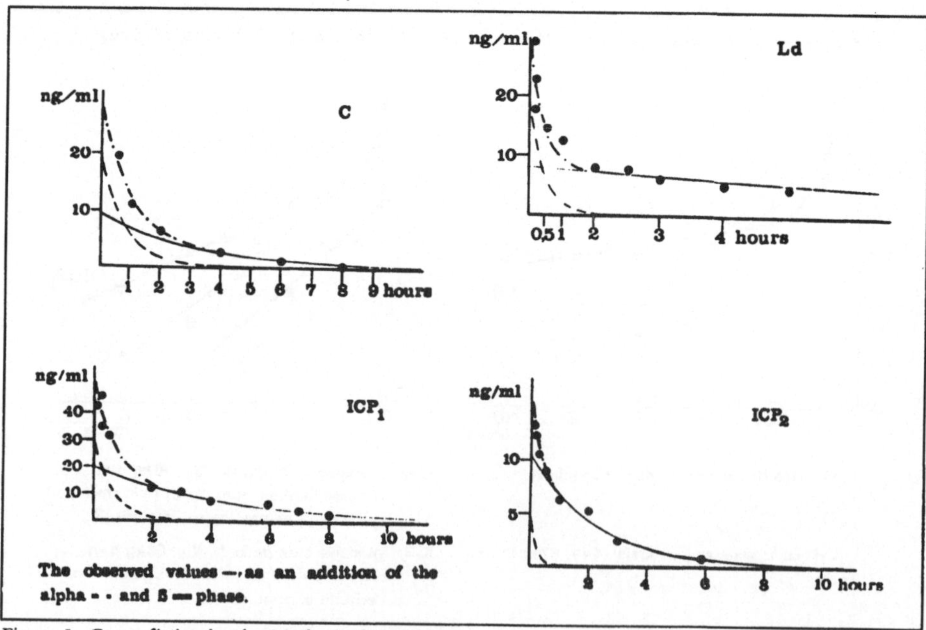

Figure 3: Curve fitting by the Method of Residuals.

II. Determination of Rate-Constants

a) Analog-Computer Simulation

With an analog-computer it is possible to estimate directly the rate constants of distribution ($k_{1,2}$, $k_{2,1}$) and the elimination rate constant (k_{el}) from the central compartment (analog circuit 2, Figure 5). This is demonstrated with the verapamil plasma concentration data of a patient with liver disease (Figure 6).

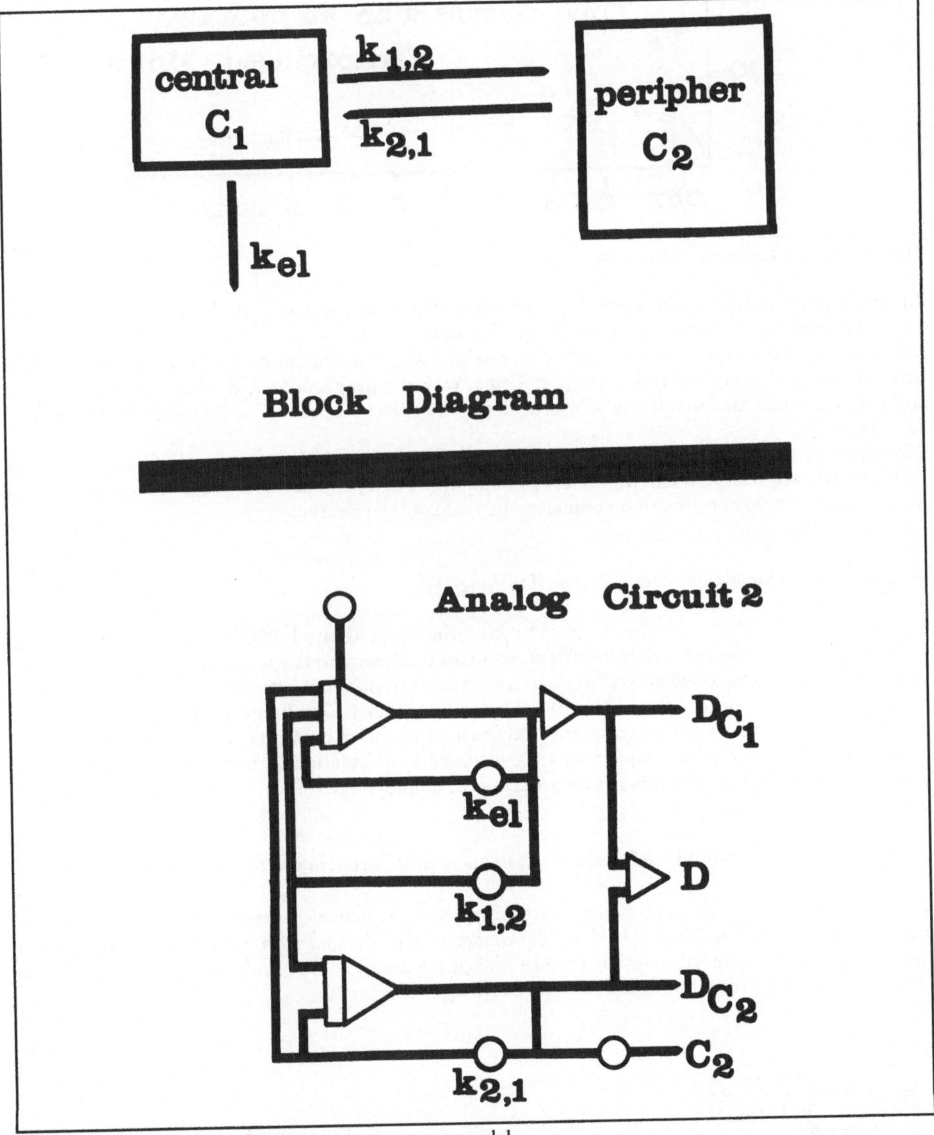

Figure 4 (Upper figure): Open two compartment model.
Figure 5 (Lower figure): Analog circuit to calculate rate-constants.

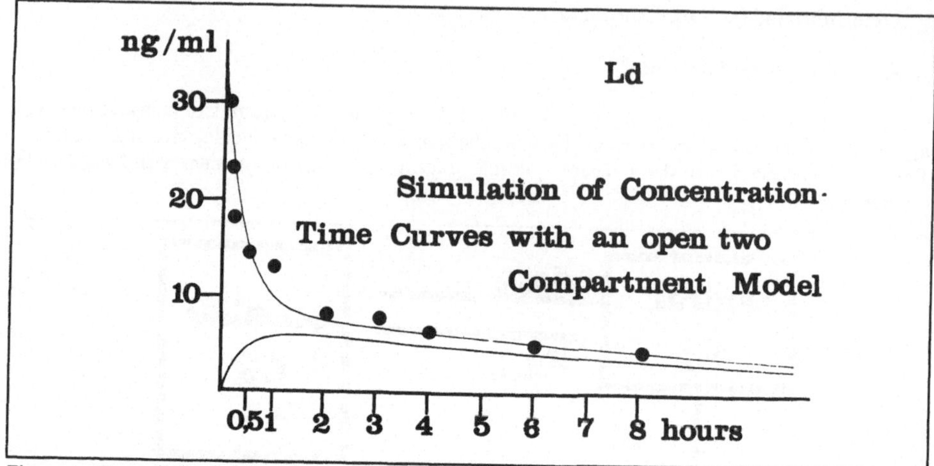

Figure 6: Curve fitting by the adjustment of rate-constants.

In the program SAAM 25 there are the same adjustable parameters as in the analog circuit 2. These rate constants are indicated in Figure 5 and Figure 6.
Comparison of the rate constants derived by analog computer simulation with the calculated values after an iterative adjustment of these parameters with the program SAAM 25 shows that the analog-computer data are outside the 95% confidence intervals (*i. e.* $\pm$ 1.96 $\times$ S.D.) for SAAM 25 data (see Table 2).
However, the advantage and usefulness of the analog-computer is that one can visualize directly the influence of each compartment on the drug elimination curve, and in this way the correct pharmacokinetic model (one, two or three compartment *etc.*) can be selected.

b) SAAM 25 *(Simulation Analysis and Modelling* [3])

The program SAAM 25 contains over 150 subroutines and about 10000 Fortran statements. The complexity of the program makes it difficult to adapt it to computers without a 32 K word memory. In the same way as described above for analog-computer simulation, curve fitting with the SAAM 25 program is possible without the estimation of hybrid-constants. Simultaneous differential equations describe mathematically the concentration-time curve in the chosen pharmacokinetic model. The primary parameters, *e. g.* rate constants are calculated by simulation of the measured data, and in general a nonlinear least squares fitting procedure is employed to adjust the primary parameters by iteration.

Comparison of the Method of Residuals *("Subtraction of Feathering with the Program SAAM 25")*

The rate constants $k_{1,2}$; $k_{2,1}$; and k_{el} are related directly to the hybrid-constants α and β and the intercepts A_1 and A_2 listed in Table 1*. If these parameters are adjusted with a short iteration program routine, the rate constants derived by the Method of Residuals are in good agreement with the data obtained from the program SAAM 25 (see Table 2).

$$^{*}\ k_{2,1} = \frac{A_1 \cdot \beta + A_2 \cdot \alpha}{A_1 + A_2};$$

$$k_{el} = \frac{\alpha \cdot \beta}{k_{2,1}}; \quad k_{1,2} = \alpha + \beta - k_{2,1} - k_{el};$$

Comparison of Rate Constants Obtained by three different Methods to calculate Verapamil Elimination

Subject	Method	Rate Constant (min^{-1})		
		$k_{1/2}$	$k_{2/1}$	k_{el}
	analog	.0256	.0113	.0048
Ld	subtract.	.0161	.0083	.0026
	SAAM 25	.0154	.0075	.0025
	S. D.	.0050	.0019	.0004
	subtract.	.0086	.0123	.0078
ICP_1	SAAM 25	.0133	.0153	.0080
	S. D.	.0105	.0076	.0013
	subtract.	.0173	.0493	.0102
ICP_2	SAAM 25	.0273	.0678	.0105
	S. D.	.0007	.0007	.0010
	subtract.	.0046	.0103	.0108
C	SAAM 25	.0068	.0115	.0117
	S. D.	.0030	.0019	.0017

Table 2

References

[1] Gladtke, E., von Hattingberg, H. M., Pharmakokinetik, Springer, Berlin (1977).

[2] Loo, J. C. K., Riegelmann, S., J. Pharm. Sci. *59*, 53—55 (1970).

[3] Berman, M., Ann. N. Y. Acad. Sci. *108*, 182—194 (1963).

Chapter 4

The clinical pharmacokinetic study in man—design and outcome

Cardiac glycosides in atrial fibrillation

George E. Mawer

Department of Pharmacology, Materia Medica and Therapeutics, University of Manchester.

I would like to emphasize three aspects of the clinical evaluation of a new drug intended for the treatment of chronic disease. Work on methyldigoxin will be quoted for illustration but the principles apply more widely.

1. Clinical evaluation of a new drug should include **direct comparison with a standard** reference drug. Ideally this should be a within-subject comparison. Otherwise we confound differences between drugs with differences between subjects.

The absorption of methyldigoxin and digoxin was compared in two healthy subjects (Table 1). Each drug was given on one occasion as an intravenous injection and on another occasion as tablets after a light breakfast. The cumulative 6 day urinary excretion of glycoside was used as an index of glycoside absorption. The area under the serum concentration time curve (AUC) could not be used because the sensitivity of the radio-immunoassay was not sufficient to measure accurately the prolonged tail of the curve. Subject GM was a poor absorber of digoxin but improved with methyldigoxin. In contrast subject GK absorbed both digoxin and methyldigoxin equally well. The need to compare both drugs in each subject is clearly shown. If we had measured digoxin absorption in GK and medigoxin in GM, we would have concluded that digoxin was better absorbed.

Sometimes circumstances prevent direct comparison with the standard reference drug in the same subject. It is nevertheless desirable to compare the two drugs in the same laboratory by the same methods. Otherwise we confound differences between drugs with differences between laboratories and methods.

subject	*digoxin 500 µg*			*methyldigoxin 300 µg*		
	iv sol	oral tab	absorption* %	iv sol	oral tab	absorption* %
GM	333	168	50	212	144	68
GK	369	304	82	241	183	76

Table 1: Cumulative 6 day urinary excretion of glycoside (µg) in healthy subjects

* proportion of oral dose absorbed calculated from the ratio = (excretion after oral dose/ excretion after intravenous dose)

Two independent research groups [6, 15] have studied the absorption of tritium-labelled cardiac glycosides from solutions taken by mouth (Table 2). Comparison of urinary excretion of radioactivity after oral and intravenous administration showed an unexpectedly large difference between methyldigoxin and digoxin. The digoxin absorption estimate was substantially lower than estimates obtained by other workers. This may be because different extraction methods were used before the measurement of urine radioactivity. Whatever the methodological explanation, the exaggeration of the absorption difference between methyldigoxin and digoxin emphasizes the need for direct comparison between the two drugs within one laboratory.

reference	*digoxin*			*methyldigoxin*		
	iv sol	oral sol	absorption* %	iv sol	oral sol	absorption* %
[6]	73.5	34	46			
[15]				62	55	89

Table 2: Cumulative 7 day urinary excretion of tritiated glycoside (% dose) reported by two groups of investigators

Methodological differences are less likely to occur when the same laboratory tests the two drugs at different times. BEERMANN and his colleagues [1, 2] reported about 50% absorption of digoxin and 83% absorption of methyldigoxin in separate papers (Table 3). Close inspection of the experimental results reveals however that once again we do not have comparable information about each drug. This is because an intravenous dose of digoxin was not given. Cumulative urinary excretion of glycoside after intravenous administration was therefore not available to provide the denominator of the absorption fraction.

reference	*digoxin*			*methyldigoxin*		
	iv sol	oral sol	absorption* %	iv sol	oral sol	absorption* %
[1]	—	—	—	82.3	74.6	91
[2]	?	50	?	—	—	—

Table 3: Cumulative 14 day excretion of tritiated glycoside (% dose) reported by one group of investigators

Subjects differ, investigators differ, even the same investigator does different things at different times. This is why I believe we should design our experiments from the start to include direct comparison of new drug with standard. There is a tendancy for this to be forgotten. Amongst 13 papers reporting estimates of methyldigoxin absorption only 4 or 5 included direct comparison with digoxin (Table 4).

2. Secondly I wish to emphasize the importance of **multiple dose studies** on drugs which are intended for prolonged therapeutic use.

Single dose studies are popular. Most of the papers I referred to earlier were based on single doses (Table 4). They take less time to complete, are amenable to conventional pharmacokinetic treatment and are more convenient for experimental subjects. They do however suffer from several drawbacks. Measurement of serum concentration half-time is liable to greater error. After the single dose the concentration even in the β phase falls as a consequence of redistribution as well as elimination. Thus the half-time is shortened and clearance is exaggerated. Predictions of maintenance dose requirements based on the estimates may therefore be excessive.

* proportion of oral dose absorbed, calculated as in Table 1

tablets/ solution		*measurement* response		concentration		patients/ volunteers		multiple/ single dose		estimate of absorption digoxin	methyldigoxin	cross-over	reference
T	S	HR	VP	RA	RIA	P	V	M	S	%	%		
+		+				+		+		67	91		17, 18
+			+			+		+			95		12
	+			+			+		+		ca 100		13
	+			+			+		+		94		3
	+			+		+			+	70	91		20
	+			+			+		+	?	91		1, 2
+					+	+		+		0.5 mg ≡	0.3 mg	+	19
+		+				+			+		ca 100		14
+			+			+		+			ca 100		5
+					+		+		+	0.5 mg ≡	0.3 mg	+	7
+					+		+		+	63	87		10, 11
	+			+			+		+		89		15
+					+		+		+	63	ca 100	+	8

Table 4: Availability of methyldigoxin given by mouth

HR heart rate
VP venous pressure
RA radioactivity
RIA radioimmunoassay

The concentration soon falls below the threshold for assay sensitivity. This reduces the time available for estimating the "terminal phase" half-time which in the interests of accuracy should extend over two or three half-times. Error in the estimation of slope leads to larger errors in the estimation of AUC by extrapolation.

The multiple dose study on the other hand allows drug to accumulate until a steady state is reached. The rate at which this is attained can be observed and used as a guide to the frequency of dosage adjustment in patients.

Because of the higher drug concentrations, the AUC during one dosage interval can be measured accurately. For a drug which obeys first order kinetics this equals the total AUC after the single dose which was so difficult to measure. After the last dose has been given the decay of drug concentration can be followed for a longer period giving more accurate half-time data. This half-time is also more relevant to the conditions of therapeutic use since sufficient time has elapsed for deep distribution compartments to be occupied.

The above argument was presented by RIETBROCK and coworkers [15, 16] who compared half-times of methyldigoxin after single and multiple doses (Table 5). The terminal phase half-time of 2.8 days, which is substantially longer than that usually quoted, (^{14}C-labelled methyldigoxin) was measured after the single dose at a time when the serum glycoside concentration was below the threshold for radioimmunoassay. After multiple dosage however the same phase could be measured by this method. Relying on radioimmunoassay after a single dose the terminal half-time would be falsely reported as 1.3 days.

phase of decay	*single dose* [15] period h	$t_{½}$ days	*multiple dose* [16] period h	$t_{½}$ days
2 or β	12—48/96	1.31	< 48	1.7
3 or γ	> 96	2.8*	> 48	2.8

Table 5: Serum glycoside concentration half-time ($t_{½}$) after single and multiple dose treatment with methyldigoxin

* concentration below threshold for radioimmunoassay

Single dose studies exaggerate the importance of *rate* of absorption. This may be relevant to the first dose of drug used in emergency treatment but it has little relevance to the more common situation of regular daily treatment of non-fasting patients. Often the clinical response appears to relate to the mean serum concentration over the dosage interval rather than to the height of the peak concentration. The kinetic equation which defines the mean concentration in the steady state ($\overline{C}_{pss}$ µg/l) is a simple one in which dosage rate (D/T µg/h), completeness of absorption (F) and clearance (CL l/h) are critical. The absorption rate constant (k_a h^{-1}) does not feature (Table 6).

drug input rate	=	drug output rate	
$F \cdot D/T$	=	$\overline{C}_{pss} \cdot CL$	---- (I)
$(D/T)/\overline{C}_{pss}$	=	CL/F	---- (II)

Table 6: Steady state pharmacokinetics

F fraction of dose D (µg) absorbed
T dosage interval (h)
$\overline{C}_{pss}$ mean plasma concentration (µg/l) in steady state
CL plasma clearance (total) (l/h)

Rearrangement of equation (I) gives the dosage rate for unit mean concentration in the steady state (II). Provided that the drug obeys first order kinetics—the mean serum concentration is proportional to dosage rate—this needs only to be multiplied by the desired mean serum concentration to give the therapeutic dosage rate.

In pharmacokinetic terms however the dosage rate for unit mean concentration is a hybrid. It only equals the clearance when absorption is complete ($F = 1$). An estimate of F itself can be obtained in the multiple dose study by comparing mean serum concentration during oral dosage with mean concentration during intravenous dosage. By this means RIETBROCK and coworkers [16] obtained a value for F with methyldigoxin of 0.75

A multiple dose study comparing methyldigoxin with digoxin was carried out in 6 healthy volunteers (Table 7). A crossover design was used in which the subjects received first either methyldigoxin 300 µg/day or digoxin 500 µg/day as tablets by mouth. Administration of each glycoside was continued for 12 days and on the final day the serum glycoside concentration profile was measured. The AUC was determined using the trapezoidal method and divided by the dosage interval (T) to give the mean glycoside concentration. The analysis of blood samples taken before each daily dose showed that 12 days were more than sufficient for the establishment of a steady state. After a "wash-out" period of not less than 9 days each subject received a second 12 day course of treatment with the other glycoside.

subject	*digoxin (500 µg/day)*	*medigoxin (300 µg/day)*
JV	1.58	1.54
GK	1.82	1.57
RF	1.53	1.53
BW	1.60	1.52
GM	1.05	1.43
JN	1.39	1.29
$n = 6$	1.49 ± 0.11	1.48 ± 0.04
$n = 7$	1.34 ± 0.10	1.40 ± 0.12
$n = 13$	1.41 ± 0.07	1.44 ± 0.07

Table 7: Mean serum glycoside concentrations (µg/l ± s. e. mean) in healthy volunteers on day 12 of treatment

The mean steady state serum glycoside concentrations are compared in Table 7. The mean values for the two drugs were equal but the variance was greater with digoxin (variance ratio = 6.1, $p = < 0.05$). This confirmed published statements about the equivalence of the two dosage schedules [7, 19] and suggested as hoped that the absorption of methyldigoxin was not only more complete but also less variable. This encouraged us to study more subjects and also to extend the study into patients. Close scrutiny of Table 7 however reveals that the smaller variance with methyldigoxin was attributable entirely to the poor digoxin absorption of one subject (GM) whose absorption characteristics were described earlier. When a further 7 subjects had been studied, extending the total number to 13, the mean serum glycoside concentrations became indistinguishable. The variance with methyldigoxin was no less than the variance with digoxin.

It soon became clear that the smaller dosage requirement for methyldigoxin could not be explained entirely on the basis of more complete absorption. It would be necessary to postulate 100% absorption of 300 µg methyldigoxin to equal the probable 60% absorption of glycoside from 500 µg digoxin tablets. Taking a broad view of the literature 80—90% seemed a more realistic estimate. Thus the smaller dosage requirement for methyldigoxin must be based partly on a lower clearance. Measurements of 24 hour glycoside excretion during the multiple dose study showed that the *renal* clearance of methyldigoxin was substantially less than that of digoxin.

Estimates of *total* glycoside clearance (CL) were obtained from the steady state pharmacokinetic equation (Table 6) by substituting published values for F and solving for CL. Values of F obtained for methyldigoxin tablets (0.87) [11] and digoxin tablets (0.63) [9, 10] were used. Estimates of *extra-renal* clearance were obtained by subtracting measured *renal* clearance from estimated *total* clearance (Table 8). Thus methyldigoxin appears to have a lower *total* clearance than digoxin and a greater

clearance ml/min	*digoxin*	*methyldigoxin*
total*	155	125
renal**	136	75
extra-renal***	19	51

Table 8: Renal clearance of glycoside and estimates of total and extra-renal clearance in healthy volunteers on day 12 of treatment [4]

* calculated from equation (II), Table 6, assuming published absorption fraction (*F*) for digoxin tablets of 0.63 [9, 10] and methyldigoxin tablets of 0.87 [11]

** (24 h urinary excretion) / (mean plasma/serum concentration)

*** total less renal

dependence on extra-renal mechanisms of elimination. The smaller dosage requirement for the same glycoside concentration appears to be associated with elimination differences as well as absorption differences.

During the process of absorption, to a small extent in the stomach but mainly in the liver, methyldigoxin undergoes partial demethylation [1]. Thus the resulting serum glycoside is a mixture of digoxin and methyldigoxin [15]. It is not sufficient therefore to show that the two dosage schedules give the same mean total glycoside concentration in serum.

3. Cross-over comparison using multiple dose studies must be extended to include patients in whom the **therapeutic responses** can be compared. Several of the early studies on methyldigoxin involved measurement of cardiac responses in patients receiving one or more doses of methyldigoxin (Table 4). Unfortunately however they were not continued long enough for a steady state to result nor was a direct comparison with digoxin made.

We opted to study patients with atrial fibrillation who were prescribed digoxin (Lanoxin, Wellcome Medical Division) at a dose of 500 µg/day but despite this had ventricular rates in excess of 100 beats per minute [4]. We believed that this selection might give a sample which was biased towards patients with poor absorption of digoxin.

Suitable patients were interviewed in the outpatient clinic and invited to participate. An electrocardiogram (ECG) was obtained and serum taken for digoxin assay about 6 hours after the prescribed morning dose of digoxin. The patients were then admitted to a six week study which consisted of two 14 day periods on digoxin 500 µg/day (digoxin 1 and 2) and one 14 day period on methyldigoxin 300 µg/day (medigoxin). On the 14th day of each treatment period each patient was admitted overnight for simultaneous blood sampling and ECG recording at 6, 12 and 24 hours after dosage. The first treatment period was digoxin 1 in each case. The patient was then allocated randomly to either digoxin 2 or medigoxin. The final treatment period was the alternative.

The results of the study were very clear. Admission to the study produced a dramatic rise in serum digoxin concentration and fall in ventricular rate; since there had been no change in prescribed dose this was attributed to improved compliance. By contrast, during the study compliance appeared to be good. There was no difference between digoxin periods 1 and 2 with respect to serum glycoside concentration, urine glycoside excretion, mean ventricular rate or the frequency of ventricular ectopic beats (Table 9). Similarly the change from digoxin to methyldigoxin produced no change in glycoside concentration or ventricular rate response. Methyldigoxin (300 µg/day) therefore proved to be therapeutically equivalent to digoxin (500 µg/day) under steady state conditions in patients with atrial fibrillation.

Conclusion

In this paper I have emphasized the importance of making a *direct, internal comparison* between new drug and standard reference drug. I have argued in favour of *multiple dose studies* when assessing

	digoxin 1	treatment period digoxin 2	methyldigoxin
serum glycoside concentration (μg/l ± s. e. mean)	2.2 ± 0.1	2.0 ± 0.1	2.1 ± 0.1
ventricular rate (beats/min ± s. e. mean)	89.0 ± 3.5	88.7 ± 3.3	90.9 ± 2.7
ventricular ectopic beats (beats/min, mean and range)	2 (0—7)	2 (0—7)	1.5 (0—7)

Table 9: Comparison of effects of maintenance treatment with methyldigoxin (300 μg/day) and digoxin (500 μg/day) in 12 patients with atrial fibrillation [4]

drugs used for long-term maintenance therapy and I have pointed out that such studies must be extended to involve patients in whom it is possible to measure a *therapeutic response.*
I have illustrated these points by reference to methyldigoxin and have reported with some disappointment that our comparative studies with methyldigoxin and digoxin in Manchester have shown no advantage for medigoxin in the treatment of patients with atrial fibrillation.

Acknowledgement

Comparative studies of methyldigoxin and digoxin in Manchester were assisted financially by Roussel Laboratories Ltd.

References

[1] Beermann, B.: The gastrointestinal uptake of methyldigoxin 12 α—^{3}H in man.—Eur. J. clin. Pharmac. 5, 28—33 (1972).

[2] Beermann, B., Hellström, K., and Rosén, A.: The absorption of orally administered 12α—^{3}H digoxin in man.—Clin. Sci. 43, 507—518 (1972).

[3] Carbonin, P. U., Zecchi, P., Bellocci, F., Ruffa, S., and Loperfido, F.: Turnover metabolico della metildigossina—^{3}H somministrata per via orale ed endovenosa nell'uomo normale.—Abstract from the 32nd Congress of the Italian Society of Cardiology (1971).

[4] Coburn, P., Kongola, G. M. W., and Mawer, G. E.: Comparison of medigoxin and digoxin in the control of atrial fibrillation.—Br. J. clin. Pharmac. 8, 53—58 (1979).

[5] Doering, W., König, E., Kronski, D., and Hall, D.: Bestimmung der Kenngrößen von β-methyldigoxin mit Einschwemmkatheterverfahren und nicht invasiven Methoden. Dt. med. Wschr. 98, 2274—2280 (1973).

[6] Doherty, J. E., Flanigan, W. J., Murphy, M. L., Bulloch, R. J., Dalrymple, J. W., Beard, O. W., and Perkins, W. H.: Tritiated digoxin. Enterohepatic circulation and excretion studies in human volunteers.—Circulation 42, 867—873 (1970).

[7] Hartel, G., Manninen, V., Melin, J., and Apajalahti, A.: Serum digoxin, concentrations with a new digoxin derivative, β-methyldigoxin.—Ann. clin. Res. 5, 87—90 (1973).

[8] Hayward, R. P., Greenwood, H., and Hamer, J.: Comparison of digoxin and medigoxin in normal subjects.—Brit. J. clin. Pharmac. 6, 81—86 (1978).

[9] Huffman, D. H., Manion, C. V., and Azarnoff, D. L.: Absorption of digoxin from different oral preparations in normal subjects during steady state. Clin. Pharmac. Ther. 16, 310—317 (1974).

[10] Johnson, B. F., and Bye, C. E.: Maximal intestinal absorption of digoxin, and its relation to steady state plasma concentration.—British Heart Journal, 37, 203—208 (1975).

[11] Johnson, B. F., Bye, C. E., Jones, G. E., and Sabey, G. A.: The pharmacokinetics of beta-methyldigoxin compared with digoxin tablets and capsules.—Eur. J. clin. Pharmac. 10, 231—236 (1976).

[12] König, E., and Ohly, A.: Quantitative Eigenschaften eines neuen Herzglycosids.—Medsche. Klin., 65, 296—299 (1970).

[13] Larbig, E., Scheler, F., Schmidt, H.-J, Betzien, G., and Kaufmann, B.: Untersuchungen zur enteralen Resorption von β-Methyl-Digoxin.—Klin. Wschr. 49, 604—607 (1971).

[14] Limbourg, P., Just, H., Fiegel, P., Michaelis, J., and Rosellen, E.: Untersuchungen zur Resorption und zum Wirkungseintritt von β-Methyl-Digoxin bei Patienten mit Vorhofflimmern.—Arzneimittel-Forsch. 23, 60—63 (1973).

[15] Rietbrock, N., Abshagen, U., Bergmann, K. V., and Rennekamp, H.: Disposition of β-methyldigoxin in man.—Eur. J. clin Pharmac. 9, 105—114 (1975).

[16] Rietbrock, N., Guggenmos, J., Kuhlmann, J., and Hess, U.: Bioavailability and Pharmacokinetics of β-Methyldigoxin after Multiple Oral and Intravenous Doses.—Eur. J. clin. Pharmac. 9, 373—379 (1976).

[17] Storz, H.: Zur Grundlage und Praxis einer Glykosidtherapie mit Digoxin.—Ärztl. Wschr. 10, 796—802 (1955).

[18] Storz, H.: Die quantitative wirksamkeit des herzglykosids β-methyldigoxin.—Medsche. Welt, Stuggt. 21, 2066—2070 (1970).

[19] Strobach, H., Greeff, K., Horster, F. A., and Wildmeister, W.: Radioimmunologische Glykosidbestimmungen nach Gabe von Digoxin und seinen Digoxinderivaten beim Menschen.—Naunyn—Schmiedebergs Arch. Pharmacol. 274, Suppl. R 113 (1972).

[20] Wirth, K., Bodem, G., and Dengler, H. J.: Kinetik und Stoffwechsel von Digoxin und verwandten Herzglycosiden beim Menschen.—Naunyn—Schmiedebergs Arch. Pharmacol. 269, 427—428 (1971).

Individual pharmacokinetic parameters in patients on long-term treatment

K.-O. Haustein
Section of Clinical Pharmacology, Institute of Pharmacology and Toxicology, Medical Academy Erfurt, Erfurt

Long-term treatment with drugs involves crucial but often neglected problems because in most cases the therapeutic effect has been assessed with purely clinical procedures. This judgement depends on criteria of different value, for example on changes in clinical symptoms or in laboratory data, in some other cases on changes in plasma drug concentrations. This is explained by the following examples:

1. Effective digitalization can be seen only with respect to improvement of clinical signs such as reduction of body weight and disappearance of oedema and of dyspnoea. The glycoside plasma level and shortening of systolic time intervals are uncertain criteria with respect to the restitution of compensation.
2. Prophylaxis of thrombo-embolic diseases with drugs is possible by laboratory control of the coagulation potential. The methods used for control of coagulation factors, however, lead to uncertain dosage regimen calculations. Nevertheless, control of medication will be better because it is oriented to more objective parameters than that of the first example.

Monitoring of most drugs such as antimicrobial drugs, antifibrillants, hormone preparations, cytostatics, antiepileptics, psychotropic drugs *etc.* follows the first example, while only some drugs such as hypoglycemics and antihypertensives follow example two.

The use of plasma level estimations for individualizing drug dosage is not always possible because of 1. expensive analytical methods such as radioimmunoassay, high pressure liquid chromatography and gas chromatography, and 2. uncertain correlations between plasma level and intensity of the therapeutic effect of many drugs [11]. In case of digitalis administration, the frequency of intoxications was reduced to 50 per cent in many hospitals after introduction of plasma level estimations [2].

The elimination half-life ($T_{\frac{1}{2}}\beta$) is the important parameter for calculation of effective doses and dose intervals. Therefore, it seems of special interest to measure this parameter under conditions of steady-state drug administration. Investigations were performed with the aim to test if there exist correlations between the elimination half-life and the administered dose during continous drug administration. Following the results of the radioimmunoassay technique, equilibrium between labelled and unlabelled drug bound to the corresponding antibody appears some minutes after starting the reaction [17, 23]. One can expect equilibrium between labelled and unlabelled drug under analogous conditions at the receptor protein and at all other structures which are biologically important for the drug action. Presupposed is that all the pharmacokinetic processes in the equilibrium apply to both labelled and unlabelled drug, and that labelled drug is absorbed and eliminated from the body in exactly the same manner as the unlabelled drug.

Methods

In the investigations patients of the Department of Medicine of the Medical Academy Erfurt were included. These patients underwent clinical treatment because of prethrombotic disorders, congestive heart failure and ischaemic heart disease. Phenprocoumon (Falithrom®), digitoxin and digoxin and the recently developed β_1-adrenoceptor blocking agent talinolol (Cordanum®) were used. The labelled form of the drugs were pure as determined (> 98 per cent) by thin-layer chromatography and by scanning. Digitoxin (specific activity $7.8 \cdot 10^7$ Bq per mg), digoxin ($7.4 \cdot 10^7$ Bq per mg) and phenprocoumon ($7.3 \cdot 10^5$ Bq per mg) were ^{3}H-labelled and talinolol (specific activity $8.9 \cdot 10^3$ Bq per mg) was ^{14}C-labelled. The synthesis of labelled drugs by Dr. Murawski (Berlin-Buch), Dr. Mittag (Dresden-Rossendorf), and Dr. Zerjatke (Dresden-Radebeul) is gratfully acknowledged (Bq= Becquerel; 1 Ci = $3.7 \cdot 10^{10}$Bq).

Results

Phenprocoumon

After loading doses, patients with latent thrombo-embolic disorders took maintenance doses of 1.5—3.0 mg phenprocoumon per day. The doses were chosen such that they inhibited the Quick values to more than 30 per cent of normal. The Quick value was measured daily [18, 19]. The investigations were started by administration of $3.7 \cdot 10^6$ Bq per 6 mg ^{3}H-phenprocoumon instead of the daily administered maintenance dose. Radioactivity and total phenprocoumon plasma levels were estimated daily. Total phenprocoumon (PPC) was determined fluorimetrically [21,22] and the urine metabolites were measured by TLC before and after β-glucuronidase incubation of the urine.
Under continous PPC intake the plasma concentration and Quick values remained unchanged (Figure 1). In contrast to total PPC concentration, plasma radioactivity declined monoexponentially. From this linear decline $^*T_{\frac{1}{2}}\beta$-values between 104 and 289 h with a mean of 181 ± 55 h were calculated (Table 1). Elimination of radioactivity in urine amounts to 8 per cent of total on the first day and to 3 per cent of total on the following days. The main metabolite was the glucuronide derivative with small amounts of unchanged PPC. The residue contains 5 to 10 per cent of total radioactivity excreted in urine. No correlation exists between the individual composition of urine metabolites and the corresponding elimination half-life.
No significant differences exist between the mean values of the half-life times measured in 10 patients after ^{3}H-PPC administration under steady-state conditions and those of 10 or 6 volunteers after PPC or ^{3}H-PPC intake as a single dose (Table 2).
In spite of continous PPC treatment, elimination of radioactivity was unchanged. Correlations were found between $^*T_{\frac{1}{2}}\beta$ and the mean maintenance doses and between the latter and "area under curve" (Figure 2). From the $^*AUC_0^\infty$-values the mean PPC plasma concentration can be calculated by Equation 1 [cf. 28]

$$\overline{C}_\infty = \frac{^*AUC_0^\infty \cdot F}{\tau} \qquad (1)$$

Group	N	Dose (mg)	^{3}H-Form	$T_{1/2}\beta$(h)	Conditions
Volunteers	10	12	No	153 ± 44	Single dose
Volunteers	6	12	Yes	140 ± 14	Single dose
Patients	10	6	Yes	181 ± 54	Steady-state
Patients	19	2—6	Yes	169 ± 34	Steady-state

Table 2: Comparison of half-life times following oral administration of phenprocoumon to volunteers and patients [*c.f.* 5, 6]

Patient	Maintenance dose ($\mu g \cdot kg^{-1} \cdot d^{-1}$)	^3H-phenprocoumon dose ($\mu g \cdot kg^{-1}$)	* $T_{1/2\beta}$ (h)	* AUC_0^∞ ($\mu g \cdot h \cdot ml^{-1}$)	Mean plasma level ($\mu g \cdot ml^{-1}$)	
					Measured	Calculated**
1 B.	21.4	85.7	160	141.6	0.85	1.33
2 K.	7.5	60.9	247	228.0	0.85	1.07
3 M.	36.9	101.3	185	115.2	0.80	1.57
4 M.	35.2	72.1	130	94.5	1.53	1.73
5 P.	20.1	97.3	289	178.8	1.80	1.39
6 S.	42.9	86.7	173	115.2	1.60	2.13
7 S.	53.6	107.5	104	86.4	1.48	1.79
8 S.	33.2	86.3	212	98.4	0.87	1.42
9 W.	35.3	94.2	165	132.0	2.12	1.85
10 W.	28.2	71.1	145	127.9	1.29	1.89

Table 1: Pharmacokinetic properties of phenprocoumon and prediction of plasma level

* Values calculated of the ^3H-phenprocoumon.
** Taking into consideration the maintenance dose.

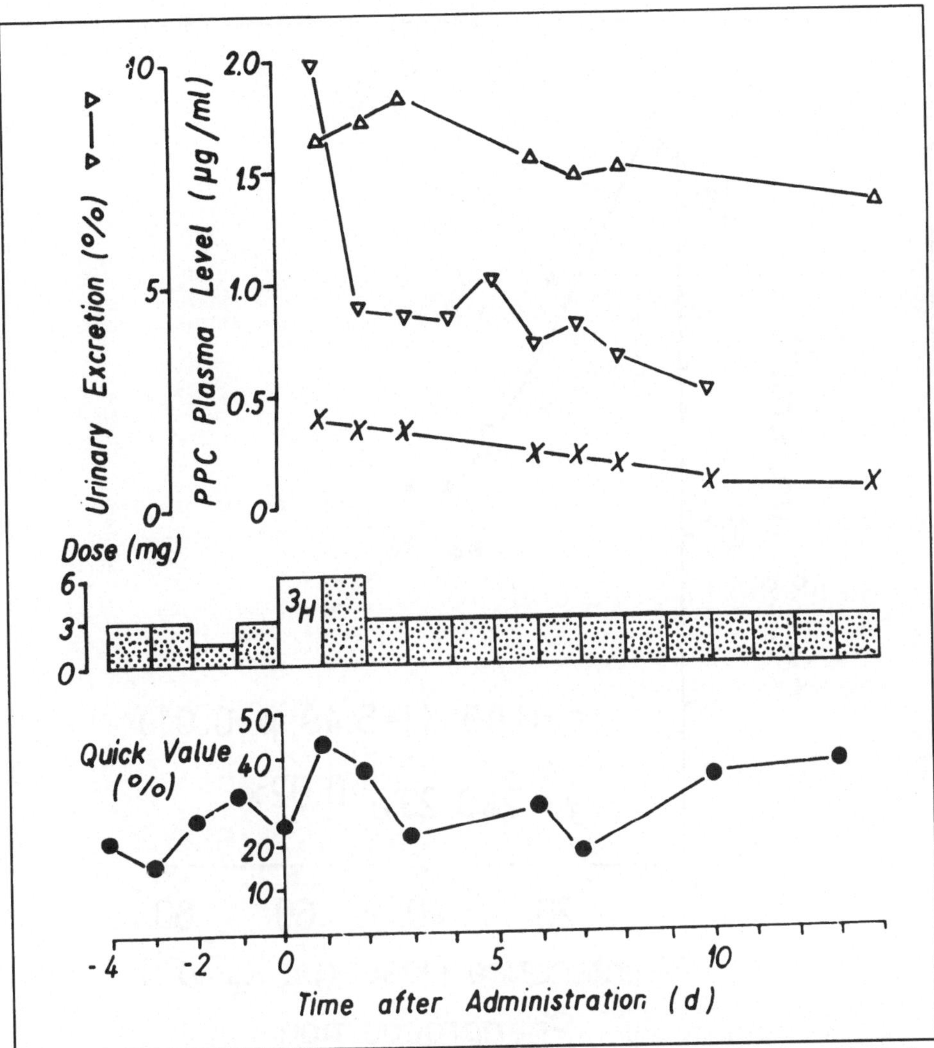

Figure 1: Time course of total PPC plasma concentration (Δ) and of prothrombin-complex activity during PPC treatment (dotted columns) in one patient. On the first day, ^{3}H-PPC (open column) was administered and on the following days, radioactivity of plasma (x) and activity excreted in urine (in % of administered dose, ⊲) were measured.

Too high PPC plasma levels were calculated because the administered radioactivity contained 2—4 times more PPC than the corresponding maintenance dose. When a correction is made for the amount of administered radioactivity in this calculation, the plasma levels in several patients are nearly equal to the measured ones (Table 1).

Digitoxin

Ten in-patients with different stages of congestive heart failure took maintenance doses of 0.1—0.15

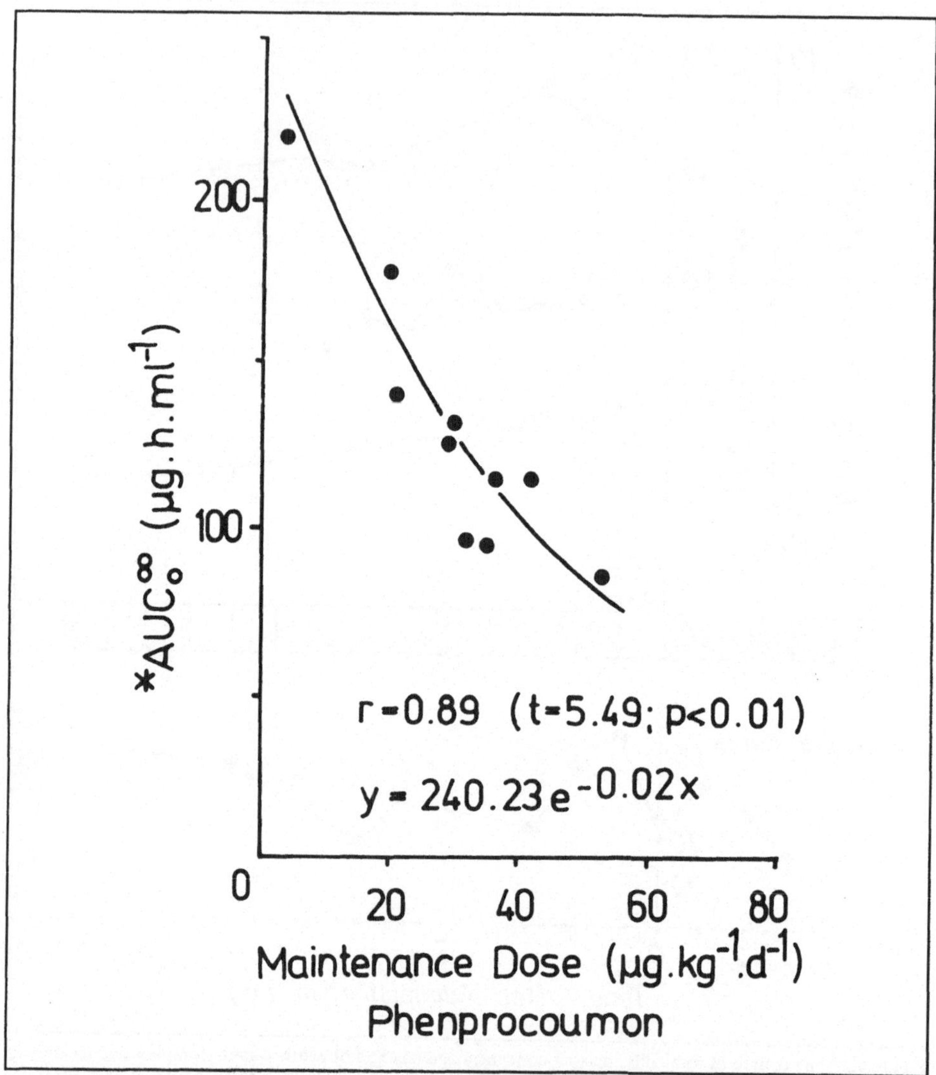

Figure 2: Relationship between maintenance dose of PPC and $^*AUC_0^\infty$ in 10 anticoagulated patients.

mg of digitoxin. The investigation was started by exchange of the maintenance dose for 3.7—4.6 · 10^6 Bq ^{3}H-digitoxin in 0.1 or 0.15 mg of the drug as an aqueous-ethanolic solution. During a period of 7 days the total glycoside plasma level was determined by the ^{86}Rb-technique [4, 13] and the decline of plasma radioactivity was measured. As seen from the experiment, radioactivity declined monoexponentially and independent of the total digitoxin plasma concentration (Figure 3). From the linear decline, elimination half-life times between 77 and 234 h with a mean of 138 h were calculated. The administered doses of ^{3}H-digitoxin amounted to 1.28 and 2.42 µg · kg^{-1}, and the initial concentration lay between 1.12 and 2.13 ng · ml^{-1} (Table 3).
Correlations existed between $^*T_{\frac{1}{2}}\beta$ and the amount of radioactivity excreted in urine as well as between $^*T_{\frac{1}{2}}\beta$ and total digitoxin plasma level (Figure 4). Using Equation 1 mean plasma concentrations were calculated and compared with the measured mean values (Table 3). With the exception of a single value, calculated and estimated levels were in good agreement.

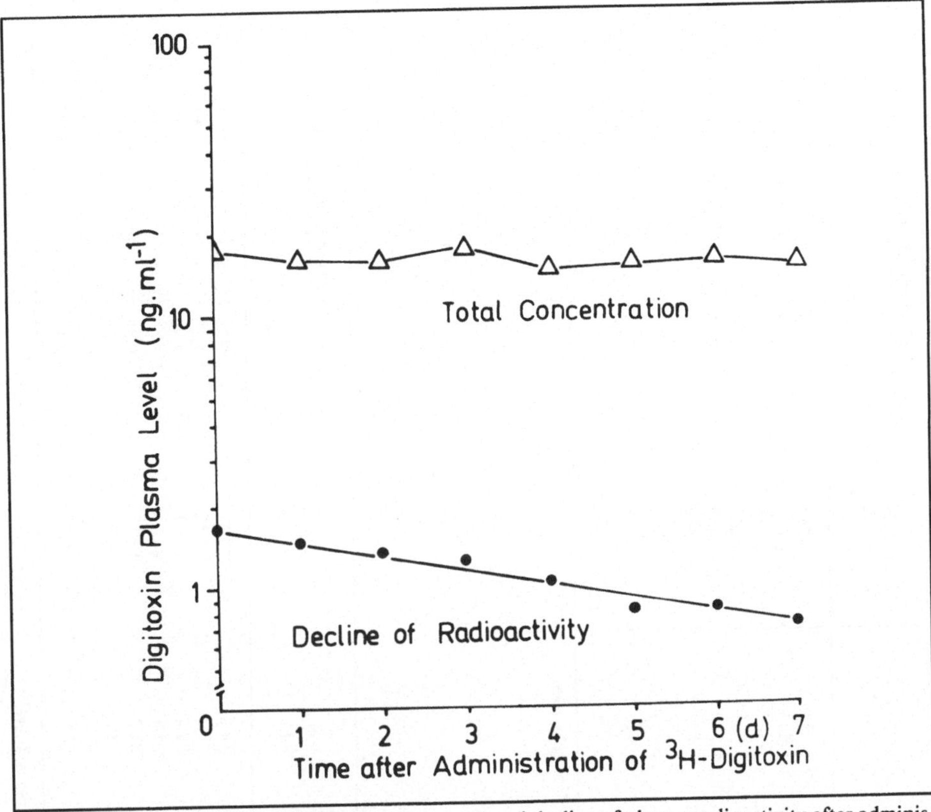

Figure 3: Time course of total digitoxin plasma level and decline of plasma radioactivity after administration of a single ^3H-digitoxin dose.

Digoxin

Ten patients were treated with digoxin instead of digitoxin. They took doses of 0.25 mg digoxin twice daily. The investigation was started by intake of $3.7 \cdot 10^6$ Bq per 0.25 mg drug as an aqueous-ethanolic solution. The previous digoxin dose as tablet was taken again 8—10 h later.
The mean elimination curve of ^3H-digoxin was elevated above the characteristic slope 12 to 24 h after administration (Figure 5). This enhanced mean value was caused by the second digoxin intake 8—10 h after starting the investigation due to redistribution of digoxin instead of ^3H-digoxin. In some patients a distinct increase in plasma radioactivity was observed. In 2 out of 10 patients the decline of radioactivity could not be measured over 72 h because the values of elimination phase decreased nearly to the range of background. At serum creatinine concentrations of 8 to 13 mg $\cdot$ L^{-1} the $^*T_{\frac{1}{2}}\beta$-values amounted to 9.2 and 38.6 h (Table 4). Correlations between $^*T_{\frac{1}{2}}\beta$ and the cumulative excretion of radioactivity were found when 8 of the 10 patients were included in the calculation. No correlations were found between the measured mean digoxin plasma level and the $^*AUC_0^\infty$-values nor between calculated and measured digoxin plasma levels (Table 4). This lack of correlation was caused possibly by limitations in evaluation of $^*T_{\frac{1}{2}}\beta$ and by the high degree of distribution of radioactivity.

Patient	Maintenance dose ($\mu g \cdot kg^{-1} \cdot d^{-1}$)	^3H-digitoxin dose ($\mu g \cdot kg^{-1}$)	$^*T_{1/2}\beta$ (h)	$^*AUC_0^\infty$ ($\mu g \cdot h \cdot ml^{-1}$)	Mean plasma level ($ng \cdot ml^{-1}$)	
					Estimated	Calculated
1 E.	1.34	1.34	119	0.341	18.4	15.1
2 F.	1.45	1.45	234	0.628	35.2	23.5
3 M.	1.79	1.79	170	0.355	9.2	13.3
4 P.	1.28	1.28	91	0.227	14.9	10.9
5 S.	1.46	1.46	172	0.628	24.0	23.5
6 D.	1.99	1.99	134	0.530	22.1	20.0
7 F.	2.42	2.42	77	0.227	12.7	9.5
8 F.	1.95	1.95	137	0.538	15.5	20.2
9 J.	1.84	1.84	139	0.560	18.5	21.0
10 K.	1.64	1.64	108	0.421	21.8	15.8

Table 3: Pharmacokinetic properties of digitoxin and prediction of plasma level

Patient	Maintenance dose ($\mu g \cdot kg^{-1} \cdot d^{-1}$)	^3H-digoxin dose ($\mu g \cdot kg^{-1}$)	$^*T_{1/2}\beta$ (h)	$^*AUC_0^\infty$ ($ng \cdot h \cdot ml^{-1}$)	Mean plasma level ($ng \cdot ml^{-1}$)	
					Estimated	Calculated
1 B.	9.8	4.9	14.6	13.27	0.85	0.77
2 C.	8.7	4.3	9.2	7.70	1.10	0.39
3 F.	6.7	3.3	28.2	14.64	1.89	1.22
4 F.	9.1	4.5	32.8	24.61	1.65	1.23
5 P.	6.7	3.4	21.7	19.10	0.86	0.96
6 S.	7.9	3.9	38.6	29.05	1.05	1.45
7 V.	9.1	4.5	30.5	19.80	0.81	0.99
8 W.	6.6	3.3	12.5	4.33	0.82	0.36

Table 4: Pharmacokinetic properties of digoxin and prediction of plasma level

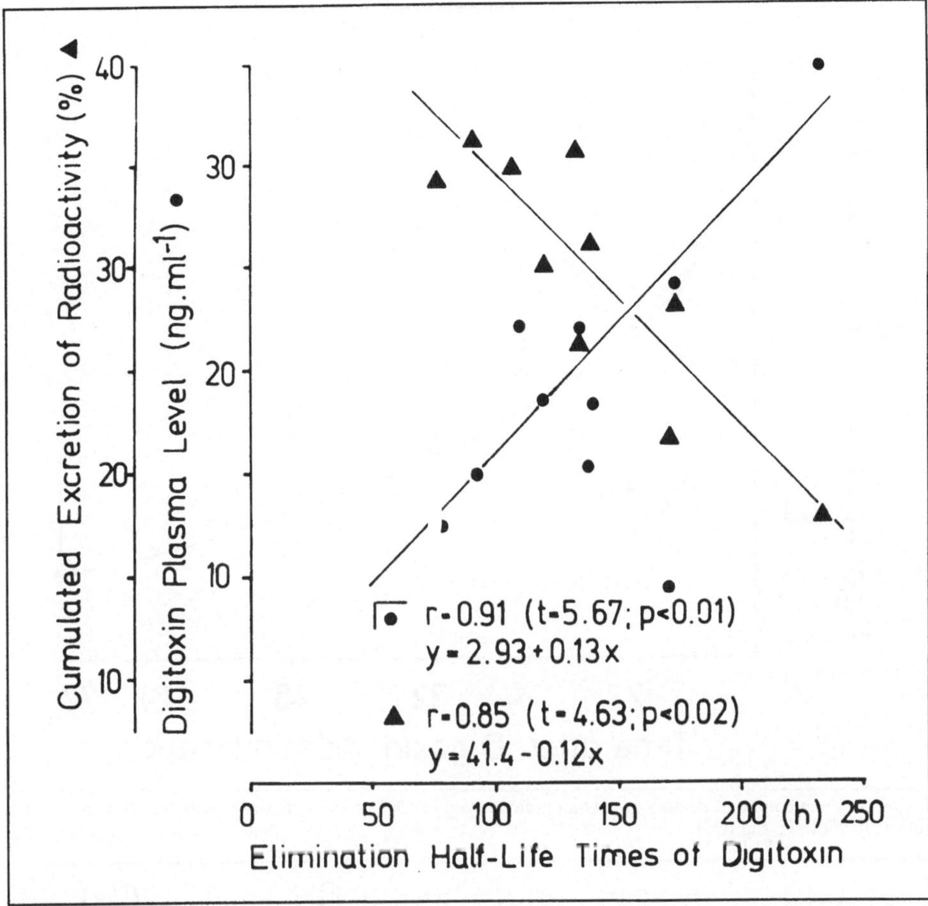

Figure 4: Relationships between $^*T_{1/2}\beta$ of ^3H-digitoxin and total digitoxin plasma level or cumulated excretion of radioactivity in urine in 10 digitalized patients.

Talinolol

In 1976, talinolol as a specific β_1-adrenoceptor blocking agent (*c.f.* Formula) was introduced into treatment of ischaemic heart disease and of various disturbances of heart rhythm. Pharmacokinetic data estimated by the use of a ^{14}C-labelled product resulted in a distribution half-life of 7 min, an apparent volume of distribution of 5.1 L · kg^{-1}, an initial concentration of 31.4 µg · L^{-1} and an elimination half-life of 1.8 h. Within 8 h 27.9 per cent and within 2 days 48.5 per cent of administered radioactivity was excreted in urine [7]. Two hours after i. v. injection radioactivity declines nearly to the background and thus, the values can be included into the calculations only with some reservation.

According to the dosage regimen 5 inpatients took orally 1.1 · 10^6 Bq ^{14}C-talinolol per 100 or 200 mg drug in aqueous solution. After initial high concentrations during the elimination phase, the measured plasma concentrations declined to low values which did not allow calculation of $^*T_{1/2}\beta$. The patients excreted 28.5 per cent of the administered radioactivity in urine within 2 days. The extent of excretion was in accordance with that of healthy volunteers after a single talinolol dose, thus, absorption of β_1-blocker in these patients was evident. The low plasma levels of ^{14}C-talinolol can be explained by its rapid absorption and distribution as well as by its rapid elimination.

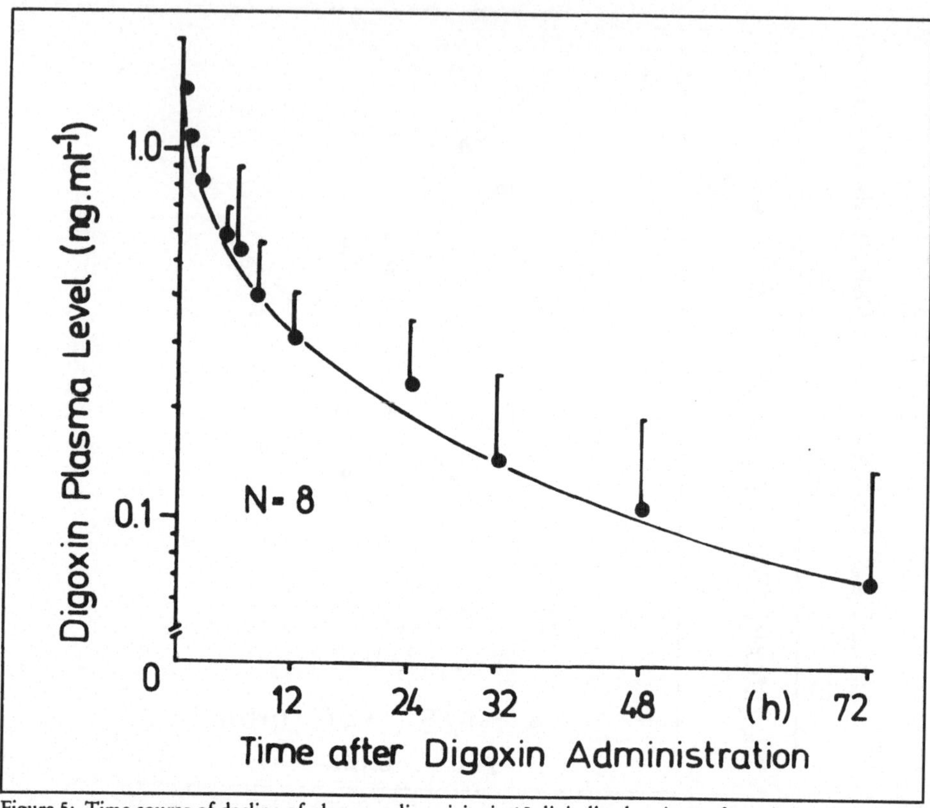

Figure 5: Time course of decline of plasma radioactivity in 10 digitalized patients after administration of a single dose of ^{3}H-digitoxin.

1-(4-cyclohexylureidophenoxy)-2-hydroxy- -3 tert.-butylaminopropane

Talinolol, Cordanum®

Formula: Talinolol

Discussion

The results show that pharmacokinetic data can be evaluated also in the patient who takes a drug under "steady-state" conditions. Furthermore, the investigations resulted in correlations between $^{*}AUC_0^{\infty}$ and the maintenance dose of phenprocoumon, and in the case of digitoxin and digoxin, between elimination half-life times and cumulated excretion of radioactivity. General prerequisites for the use of the proposed technique are: 1. The drug must be available in its unlabelled and labelled form (^3H or ^{14}C). 2. The specific activity must reach values which allow the administration in doses of $< 3.7 \cdot 10^6$ Bq in case of ^3H and $< 1.1 \cdot 10^6$ Bq in case of ^{14}C. 3. Radioactive labelling of the drug must be performed by synthesis and not by the Wilzbach technique.
With the technique proposed some kinetic parameters such as k_{el}, $\bar{C}_{\infty}$ *etc. can be calculated only by the use of the measured* $^{*}T_{\frac{1}{2}\beta}$-values. Estimation of c_0 becomes possible only after intravenous injection of the drug. Nevertheless, $^{*}c_0$-values of phenprocoumon, digitoxin and digoxin were evaluated after oral administration of the ^3H-drugs because they are absorbed from aqueous-ethanolic solutions rapidly and nearly completely (phenprocoumon and digitoxin > digoxin). The $^{*}T_{\frac{1}{2}\beta}$-values of the 3 drugs estimated under "steady-state" conditions agree with those described in the literature and calculated after single administration (Table 5). Only in the case of digoxin are the values lower than those found by other authors.

Drug	$T_{\frac{1}{2},\beta}$(h)	Patients (N)	References
Phenprocoumon	181 ± 54	10	Haustein *et al.* [6]
	153 ± 44	10	Haustein *et al.* [5]
	120	5	Meinertz *et al.* [15]
	157	4	Heni and Glogner [8]
	109 ± 25	53	Husted *et al.* [10]
Digitoxin	138 ± 46	10	*
	165	20	Gjerdrum [3]
	163	6	Vöhringer and Rietbrock [26]
	115	7	Lukas [14]
Digoxin	23.5 ± 10.7	8	*
	34.7	5	Nyberg *et al.* [16]
	48.4	6	Rabkin and Grupp [20]

Table 5: Elimination half-lives of phenprocoumon, digitoxin and digoxin

* Results of this investigation

This technique can be applied with particular advantage for phenprocoumon and digitoxin because of their nearly complete absorption (> 90 per cent; [1, 22]) and their high binding to plasma proteins (> 90 per cent; [9, 24]).
The labelled drug is exchanged for the unlabelled one quickly due to the high affinity for and the extent of binding to the plasma proteins. The forementioned kinetic processes seem to apply for both labelled and unlabelled forms of the drugs. The good agreement of the $^{*}T_{\frac{1}{2},\beta}$-values for digitoxin and phenprocoumon with the data of the literature is considered as confirmation of the working hypothesis that kinetic data can be measured also under continuous medication. For calculation of $^{*}AUC_0^{\infty}$ and of $^{*}V_{Cl}$ measurement of $^{*}c_0$ is required. This value must be considered with some reservation, if calculated after oral administration. These doubts are more applicable in case of digoxin than in those of phenprocoumon and digitoxin. The reason for the unsatisfactory (digoxin) or negative (talinolol) results is the high distribution volume of both drugs [7, 12] in the body. The limitations in evaluation of parameters of both drugs during their β-phase could be facilitated by administration of more radioactivity. However, this is not possible because of exposure of the patient to high radioactivity.
During the last few years many investigations have been performed in order to individualize pharmacotherapy. They all led to an accumulation of knowledge in the pharmacokinetic behaviour of drugs with concomitant procedures in calculating the plasma concentrations [*c.f.* 27, 28]. Our method recommended can be used for calculation of dosage schedules for long-term treatment. According to Equation 1, the maintenance dose can be calculated if this term is exchanged for the mean plasma concentration. In this case

$$D_M = \frac{{}^*V_{Cl} \cdot \overline{C}_\infty \cdot \tau}{F} \tag{2}$$

whereby the total body clearance can be calculated from

$$V_{Cl} = D_M / {}^*\mathrm{AUC}_0^\infty \; . \tag{3}$$

In case of drugs with low but reliable absorption percentages, a single intravenous injection of the labelled drug in a dose equivalent to the amount actually absorbed is proposed because only this procedure excluded factors of varying bioavailability. In addition, correct estimation of ${}^*c_0$ is given. The method is justified in case of drugs which possess narrow therapeutic range and/or in the case of drugs whose doses must be changed over short time intervals because of day to day fluctuations in parameters such as Quick value and blood pressure.

It has not yet been clarified whether or not the intraindividual elimination constant remains unchanged over a long period of time. Corresponding investigations in identical and fraternal twins show a certain amount of genetic control of this parameter [25]. In each case, however, changes of ${}^*T_{\frac{1}{2}}\beta$ are to be expected due to interactions with concomitantly administered drugs. Further investigations have to be done to clarify these details, and determination of $T_{\frac{1}{2}}\beta$ under the conditions of interactions might be also possible leading to useful dosage regimens under changed conditions.

Conclusions

1. Determination of pharmacokinetic parameters of a drug in patients on long-term treatment is possible when the drug in its radioactively labelled form is administered as a single dose. 2. The technique can be used mainly in case of drugs with high plasma protein binding. 3. Due to correlations between ${}^*\mathrm{AUC}_0^\infty$, ${}^*T_{\frac{1}{2}}\beta$ and total drug plasma concentration, mean plasma level can be calculated. 4. Because correlations exist between measured and calculated plasma concentrations of phenprocoumon and digitoxin, prediction of the maintenance dose on the basis of proposed mean plasma concentration becomes possible. 5. The technique recommended facilitates dosage calculations in patients on long-term treatment due to the individual elimination constant of a drug in each patient.

Abbreviations:

AUC_0^∞: area under curve, τ: interval between administration of 2 doses, F: fraction of the dose which is absorbed, D_L: loading dose, D_M: maintenance dose, V_{Cl}: plasma or serum ("body") clearance, $\overline{C}_\infty$: average steady-state plasma concentration; * means pharmacokinetic properties of the radioactively labelled form of the drug.

References

[1] Beerman, B., Hellstrom, K., and Rosen, A.: Fate of orally administered ^3H-digitoxin in man with special reference to the absorption; Circulation *43* (1971), 802—861

[2] Duhne, D. W., Greenblatt, D. J., Koch-Weser, J.: Reduction of digoxin toxicity associated with measurement of serum levels; Ann. intern. Med. *80* (1974), 516—519

[3] Gjerdrum, K.: Digitoxin studies—serum concentration during digitalization, maintenance therapy, and withdrawal. Estimation of proper maintenance dose; Acta Med. Scand. *191* (1972), 25—34

[4] Haustein, K.-O.: Methoden zur Bestimmung von Herzglykosiden: Möglichkeiten und Erfahrungen; Zschr. med. Labor.-Diagn. *20* (1979), 99—110

[5] Haustein, K.-O., Richter, M., und Vogel, G.: Zur Optimierung einer Langzeitbehandlung mit Phenprocoumon; Dt. Gesundh.-Wesen *30* (1975), 1514—1518

[6] Haustein, K.-O., Richter, M., Vogel, G., und Mittag, E.: Individualization of drug dosage during long-term treatment with phenprocoumon (Falithrom®); Int. J. clin. Pharmacol. *16* (1978), 372—276

[7] Haustein, K.-O., Fiehring, H., Oltmanns, G., Femmer, K.: On the clinical pharmacology of talinolol, a new β_1-adrenoceptor blocking agent; Int. J. clin. Pharmacol. *17* (1979), 465—470

[8] Heni, N., Glogner, P.: Pharmacokinetics of phenprocoumon in man investigated using a gas chromatographic method of drug analysis; Naunyn-Schmiedeberg's Arch. Pharmacol. *293* (1976), 183—186

[9] Hüthwohl, B., Jähnichen, E.: Displacement of phenprocoumon (Marcumar®) from albumin by sulfonylurea compounds, suramin and ioglycamic acid; Naunyn-Schmiedeberg's Arch. Pharmacol. *273* (1972), 204—212

[10] Husted, S., Andreasen, F., Foged, L.: Increased sensivity to phenprocoumon during methyltestosterone therapy; Europ. J. clin. Pharmacol. *10* (1976), 209—216

[11] Koch-Weser, J.: The serum level approach to individualization of drug dosage; Europ. J. clin. Pharmacol. *9* (1975), 1—8

[12] Koup, J. R., Greenblatt, D. J., Jusko, W. J., Smith, T. W., Koch-Weser, J.: Pharmacokinetics of digoxin in normal subjects after intravenous bolus and infusion doses; J. Pharmacokin. Biopharm. *3* (1975), 181—192

[13] Lowenstein, J. M., Corrill, E. M.: An improved method for measuring plasma and tissue concentrations of digitalis glycosides; J. Lab. clin. Med. *67* (1966), 1048—1053

[14] Lukas, D. S.: Some aspects of the distribution and disposition of digitoxin in man; Ann. N. Y. Acad. Sci. *179* (1971), 338—361

[15] Meinertz, T., Gilfrich, H.-J., Groth, U., Johnen, H.-G., Jähnichen, E.: Interruption of the enterohepatic circulation of phenprocoumon by cholestyramine; Clin. Pharmacol. Ther. *21* (1977), 731—735

[16] Nyberg, L., Andersson, K.-E., Bertler, A: Bioavailability of digoxin from tablets. II. Radioimmunoassay and disposition pharmacokinetics of digoxin after intravenous administration. Acta Pharmacol. Suecica *11* (1974), 459—470

[17] Oliver jr., G. C., Parker, B. M., Brasfield, D. L., Parker, C. W.: The measurement of digitoxin in human serum by radioimmunoassay; J. clin. Invest. *47* (1968), 1035—1072

[18] Owren, P. A.: Critical study of tests for control of anticoagulant therapy; Thrombos. Diathes. haemorrh. (Stuttg.) *9* (1963), 74—80

[19] Quick, A. J.: The development and use of prothrombin test; Circulation *19* (1959), 92—98

[20] Rabkin, S. W., Grupp, G.: A two compartment open model for digitoxin pharmacokinetics in patients receiving a wide range of digoxin doses; Acta Cardiol. *30* (1975), 343—351

[21] Richter, M.: Zur fluorimetrischen Bestimmung von Phenprokoumon im Blutplasma; Zbl. Pharm. *115* (1976), 611—614

[22] Seiler, K., Duckert, F.: Properties of 3-(1-phenyl-propyl)-4-oxycoumarin (Marcoumar®) in the plasma when tested in normal cases and under influence of drugs; Thrombos. Diathes. haemorrh. (Stuttg.) *19* (1968), 389

[23] Smith, Th. W., Haber, E.: Clinical value of the radioimmunoassay of the digitalis glycosides; Pharmacol. Rev. *25* (1973), 219—228

[24] Solomon, H. M., Reich, S., Spirit, N., Abrams, W. B.: Interactions between digitoxin and other drugs *in vitro* and *in vivo*; Ann. N. Y. Acad. Sci. *179* (1971), 362—369

[25] Vesell, E. S.: Factors causing interindividual variations of drug concentrations in blood; Clin. Pharmacol. Ther. *16* (1974), 135—148

[26] Vöhringer, H. F., Rietbrock, N.: Metabolism and excretion of digitoxin in man; Clin. Pharmacol. Ther. *16* (1974), 796—806

[27] Wagner, J. G.: Fundamentals of clinical pharmacokinetics. 1st Ed., 461 pp., Drug Intelligence Publications, Inc. Hamilton/Ill. 1975

[28] Wagner, J. G., Northan, J. I., Ahway, C. D., Carpenter, O. S.: Blood levels of drug at the equilibrium state after multiple dosing; Nature *207* (1965), 1391—1402

Aminoglycoside antibiotics: problems and methods

F. Follath, P. Spring, S. Vozeh, and M. Wenk

Clinical Pharmacology Division, Department of Medicine,
Kantonsspital, Basel, Switzerland

Aminoglycoside antibiotics play an important role in the treatment of infections with gram-negative bacteria. Gentamicin and tobramycin have been extensively used for several years, and more recently amikacin, sisomicin, and netilmicin were introduced to widen our therapeutic possibilities. These drugs are highly effective in septicemia and urinary tract infections, but their application is limited by a potential nephro- and ototoxicity. Much effort was therefore devoted to clarify the pharmacokinetic behaviour of aminoglycosides and to devise appropriate dosage regimens in different clinical situations. Measurement of serum levels was often recommended as a means to improve the safety of aminoglycoside treatment [1]. However, recent data on aminoglycosides [9, 13, 20] indicate that most of the previous studies did not completely describe the fate of these antibiotics in the human organism. The better understanding of aminoglycoside distribution and elimination is a direct consequence of an improved methodology for determination of drug levels and of a more refined data analysis. Therefore, it conforms to the subject of this symposium to review some of the problems connected with the use of these antibiotics and to discuss the practical importance of the currently proposed pharmacokinetic models.

Assay procedures

The introduction of radioenzymatic [10, 23] and radioimmunologic [2, 16] assays instead of the earlier microbiological methods not only improved the specificity and accuracy of aminoglycoside determination in serium and urine, but also enhanced the sensitivity of such measurements: whereas 0.2—0.5 mcg/ml is usually the lower concentration limit with agar diffusion assays, levels down to 10 ng/ml can be reliably measured by modern techniques. Today, specific RIA-kits are commercially available for gentamicin, tobramycin and amikacin, but for the other aminoglycosides separate methods have to be developed requiring much experience and skilful technique. An advantage of the radioenzymatic assay is that once introduced in a laboratory, almost all aminoglycosides can be determined in a very similar way since the necessary enzymes can be produced at the same place. Furthermore, as there is a strict linearity between drug concentration and the formed radiolabelled product, radioenzymatic assays are suitable for measure ment of a wide range of antibiotic concentrations. An excellent correlation between the radioimmunological and radioenzymatic assays could be demonstrated for gentamicin [17], sisomicin [25] and netilmicin [3]. High performance liquid chromatography, gaschromatography, and enzyme-immunoassay are the latest developments in this field, but their relative merits regarding clinical and experimental application are not yet established.

Pharmacokinetic models for aminoglycoside antibiotics

One of the main contributions of the improved laboratory techniques was the detection of a prolonged terminal elimination phase following single and multiple dosing of different aminoglycosides. SCHENTAG *et al* [20] demonstrated that gentamicin is present in serum and urine for several days after the final dose of prolonged treatment. They found terminal half lives over 100 hours even in patients without renal impairment. The same authors [21], and KAHLMETER *et al* [12] presented similar data on tobramycin. In a recent study of amikacin elimination after repetitive dosing, we could show that this drug is also retained in the body for prolonged periods, and only slowly excreted with terminal half lives of 46—81 hours [24]. It is apparent from these new data that a delayed elimination phase is a feature common to most aminoglycosides and therefore a multicompartment model is necessary to characterize their pharmacokinetic behaviour. Until recently, however, usually an open one or two compartment model was used to describe the elimination of gentamicin and tobramycin [19], amikacin [14], sisomicin [15] and netilmicin [11, 18]. Dominant half lives of about 2 hours, distribution volumes of 17—30% of the body weight and plasma clearances of 60—110 ml/min were given for all these antibiotics.
Looking at the discrepancies between earlier and newer aminoglycoside studies, the question arises whether the omission of the delayed elimination phase could be a practically relevant source of error? Our previously reported data on netilmicin in healthy volunteers [9] are suitable to illustrate the underlying methodological problem. After an *i. v.* dose of 3 mg/kg of netilmicin a slow elimination phase can be identified from serum concentrations and from urinary excretion rates in all subjects (Figure 1). By fitting the data to a *three compartment open model* we obtained the following pharmacokinetic parameters: $t_{1/2}\ \alpha$ 0.474 ± 0.12 h, $t_{1/2}\ \beta$ 1.99 ± 0.19 h, $t_{1/2}\ \gamma$ 36.89 ± 5 h, V_1 0.16 ± 0.02 l/kg, Vd_{ss} 0.679 ± 0.11 l/kg, and Cl_p 90.9 ± 13.9 ml/min. The early post-distribution phase (β) corresponds to the dominant elimination phase as described by others [11, 18], but this is followed by a prolonged terminal section of the elimination curve with a fractional area (AUC γ) reaching 12% of the total AUC. The second prominent finding is a 2—3 times higher steady-state distribution volume (Vd_{ss}) than in the cases studied by PECHERE [18] and JAHRE [11]. To prove that these differences are mainly due to the duration of serum and urinary sampling and to the type of pharmacokinetic analysis, we calculated the pharmacokinetic parameters in the same individual by an *open two compartment* model, using only drug levels obtained up to the 8th hour. The results were as follows: $t_{1/2}\ \beta$ 2.11 ± 0,25 h, V_1 0.16 ± 0.03 l/kg, Vd_{ss} 0.25 ± 0.013 l/kg, and Cl_p 97.91 ± 15.39 ml/min. By this approach our values are similar to those in the studies cited above. Thus, our findings with netilmicin further underline the fact that drug uptake into a tissue compartment is a basic feature of aminoglycoside pharmacokinetics which can be demonstrated even after single intravenous doses, when sensitive analytical techniques are employed and sampling periods are sufficiently extended. The magnitude of aminoglycoside retention in the organism is indicated by the high values of distribution volumes.

Toxicity and tissue levels of aminoglycosides

Experimental and clinical findings suggest that aminoglycoside toxicity is a dose related phenomenon. However, there is considerable uncertainty about the relative importance of serum levels, total dose and duration of treatment [1].
Excessive serum levels are generally regarded as a major cause of renal or auditory damage, but it is still debated whether the peak or trough levels are more relevant. It is equally possible that the area under the serum concentration time curve during a dosing interval is the main risk factor. While these questions remain open, it can be shown that the deep tissue compartment will usually not influence aminoglycoside serum concentrations to a clinically relevant degree. Since the area under the serum concentration curve during the terminal phase only amounts to a small fraction of the total AUC, plasma clearance (Cl) and the mean serum concentrations ($\overline{C}_{ss}$) will remain in a similar range whether the two or three compartment model is used for data analysis:

$$Cl = \text{dose/AUC}$$
$$\overline{C}_{ss} = \text{AUC/T}$$

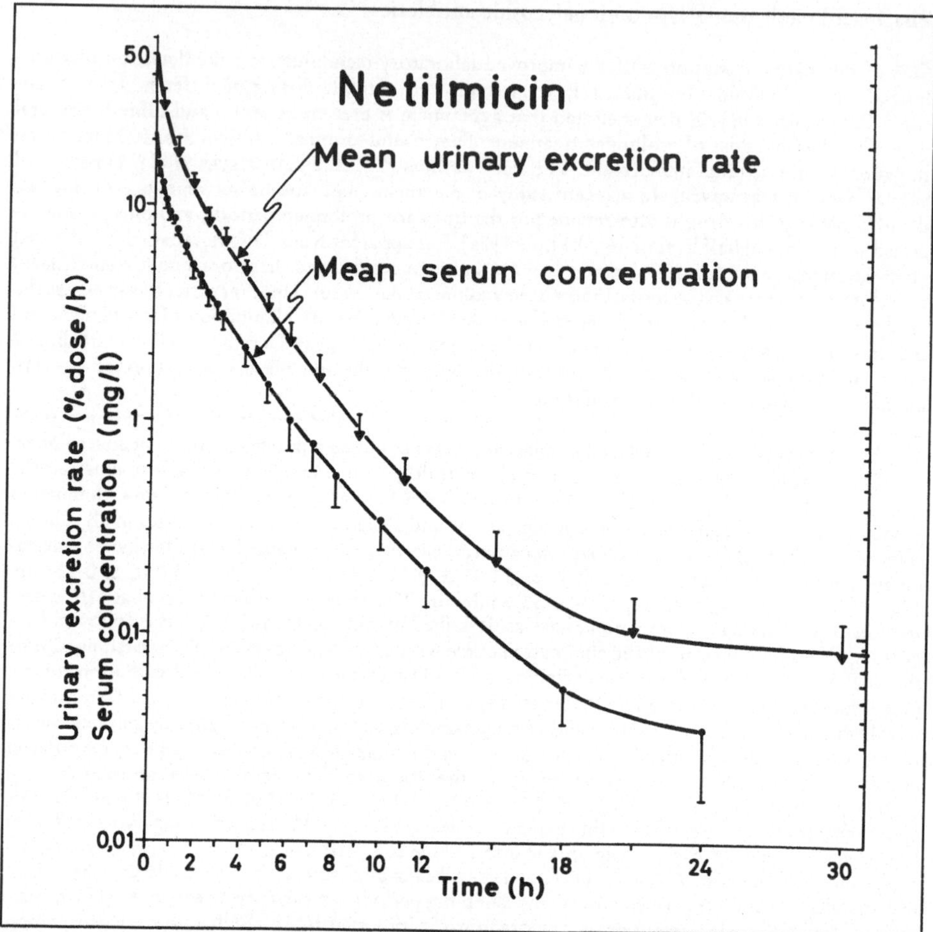

Figure 1: Mean serum concentration and urinary excretion rate of netilmicin in 6 healthy volunteers.

where T is the dosing interval. The consequence of a larger steady-state distribution volume might, on the other hand, be quite different. Following a prolonged treatment Vd_{ss} is proportional to the average amount of drug in the body:

$$A_b = \overline{C}_{ss} \cdot Vd_{ss},$$

therefore, aminoglycoside tissue levels would be considerably underestimated if the terminal phase of the elimination curve were not taken into account. Recent findings indicate that the amount of drug in the body might be more relevant to toxicity than serum concentration values. SCHENTAG *et al* have reported that calculated gentamicin and tobramycin tissue contents, as predicted by a multi-compartment model, correlate well with measured levels obtained at autopsy [20, 21]. Amikacin was also shown to accumulate in the body [7]. Furthermore, animal experiments indicate that the inner ear pharmacokinetically behaves as a part of the deep compartment [8]. Concentrations of gentamicin and tobramycin in the perilymphe rise slower but persist longer than corresponding serum concentrations. Thus, for this group of antibiotics the correct pharmacokinetic model provides some explanation for the well known toxic side-effects.

Is there an optimal dosage regimen for aminoglycosides?

The final point for discussion is, how the new insight into the pharmacokinetic behaviour of aminoglycosides should influence their clinical use. To find an answer to this question we simulated serum concentrations and drug amounts in the tissue compartment for prolonged gentamicin treatment, using the recently published pharmacokinetic data of SCHENTAG [20]. In a case with a normal creatinine clearance, gentamicin doses of 80 mg given 8-hourly will generally result in optimal therapeutic serum levels, but drug retention in the deep tissue compartment will occur and progressively increase up to 10 days (Figure 2). In a patient with a creatinine clearance of 50 ml/min similar serum concentration and accumulation curves are obtained when the maintenance dose is reduced to 40 mg and the dosing interval is prolonged to 16 hours, which corresponds to the expected elimination half life at this clearance value [6]. In contrast, in a case with severe renal failure (Cl_{cr} = 5 ml/min) drug uptake into the deep compartment continues at a high rate even after ten days and serum concentrations also progressively increase despite prolongation of the dosing interval to 34 hours and reduction of the maintenance dose to 40 mg. This simulation experiment illustrates the current therapeutic dilemma: A dosage regimen required to maintain serum concentrations in an effective range inevitably leads to a continuous drug accumulation in the body, especially in the renal tissue, where toxic damage can occur. Thus, and in addition to avoid excessive serum concentrations, it would seem logical to limit the duration of aminoglycoside treatment to the shortest possible period. However, even a strictly limited course of aminoglycoside treatment does not guarantee freedom from toxicity. Investigations of CHAUVIN*et al* [4] have shown that gentamicin concentrations in the rat kidney rise within hours to high levels and reach a plateau within one week. A similar early aminoglycoside fixation to the human kidney could also occur, and much faster than expected from the pharmacokinetic model. In fact, SCHENTAG*et al* recently presented some evidence suggesting that a higher rate of drug transfer into the peripheral tissue compartment could identify patients with a special predisposition to renal toxicity [5, 22].
The example of aminoglycoside antibiotics illustrates that a careful consideration of methodological aspects is necessary when pharmacokinetic data are analysed. Wide variations may result from differences in the duration of serum and urine sampling and from technical differences in drug level determinations. The choice of the adequate pharmacokinetic model for a given drug should also depend on the related clinical problems.

References

[1] Barza, M., and Lauerman, M.: Why monitor serum levels of gentamicin? Clin. Pharmacokinetics: 3: 202—215 (1978)

[2] Broughton, A., Strong, J. E., Pickering, L. K., and Bodey, G. P.: Radioimmunoassay of iodimated tobramycin. Antimicrob. Agents Chemother.: 10: 652—656 (1976)

[3] Broughton, A., Strong, J. E., Pickering, L. K., Knight, J., and Bodey, G. P.: Radioimmunoassay and radioenzymatic assay of a new aminoglycoside antibiotic, netilmicin. Clin. Chem.: 24: 717—719 (1978)

[4] Chauvin, J. M., Rudhardt, M., Blanchard, P., Gaillard, R., and Fabre, J.: Le comportement de la gentamicine dans le parenchyme rénale. Schweiz. Med. Wschr.: 108: 1020—1025 (1978)

[5] Colburn, W. A., Schentag, J. J., Jusko, W. J., and Gibaldi M.: A model for prospective identification of the prenephrotoxic state during gentamicin therapy. J. Pharmacokin. Biopharm.: 6: 179—186 (1978)

[6] Dettli, L.: Drug dosage in patients with renal disease. Clin. Pharmacol. Ther.: 16: 274—280 (1974)

[7] Edwards, C. Q., Smith, C. R., Baughman, K. L., Rogers, J. F., and Lietman P.: Concentrations of gentamicin and amikacin in human kidneys. Antimicrob. Agents Chemother.: 9: 925—927 (1976)

[8] Federspiel, P.: Zur Ototoxizität des Tobramycins. Infection, Suppl. 1: 50—57 (1975)

[9] Follath, F., Spring, P., Wenk, M., Benelt, L. Z., and Dettli, L.: Comparative pharmacokinetics of sisomicin and netilmicin in healthy volunteers. In: Current Chemotherapy, Vol. II: pp. 997—980, Amer. Soc. Microbiology, Washington D.C., 1978

[10] Holmes, R. K., and Sanford, J. P.: Enzymatic assays for gentamicin and related aminoglycoside antibiotics. J. Infect. Dis.: 129: 519—527 (1974)

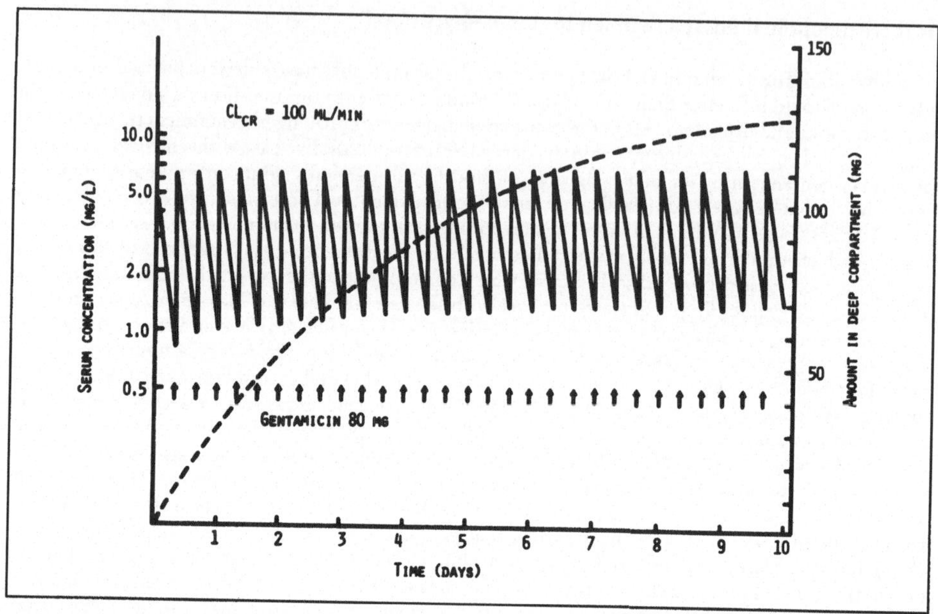

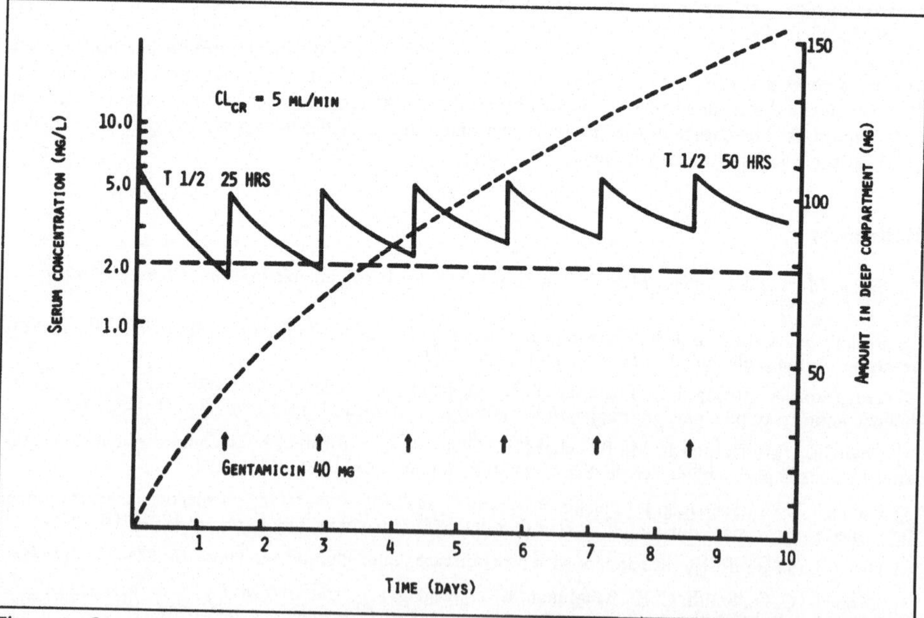

Figure 2: Computer simulation of gentamicin serum concentrations and drug amounts in the deep compartment in a patient with normal renal function (above), and in a patient with renal failure (below).

[11] Jahre, J. A., Fu, K. P., and Neu, H. C.: Kinetics of netilmicin and gentamicin. Clin. Pharmacol. Ther.: 23: 591—597 (1978)

[12] Kahlmeter, G., Jonsson, S., and Kamme, C.: Multiple compartment pharmacokinetics of tobramycin. In: Current Chemotherapy, Vol. II, pp. 912—915, Amer. Soc. for Microbiology, Washington D. C. (1978)

[13] Kahlmeter, G., Jonsson, S., and Kamme, C.: Longstanding posttherapeutic gentamicin serum and urine concentration in patients with unimpaired renal function. J. Antimicrob. Chemother.: 4: 132—152 (1978)

[14] Kirby, W. M. M., Clarke, J. T., Libke, R. D., and Regamey, C.: Clinical pharmacology of amikacin and kanamycin. J. Infect. Dis.: 134: Suppl., 312—315 (1976)

[15] Lode, H., Kemmerich, B., Koeppe, P., and Langmaack, H.: Vergleichende Pharmakokinetik und klinische Erfahrungen mit einem neuen Aminoglykosid-Derivat: Sisomicin. Dtsch. Med. Wschr.: 100: 2144—2150 (1975)

[16] Mahon, W. A., Ezer, J., and Wilson, T. W.: Radioimmunoassay for measurement of gentamicin in blood. Antimicrob. Agents Chemother.: 3: 585—589 (1973)

[17] Minishew, B. H., Holmes, R. K., and Baxter, C. R.: Comparison of a radioimmunoassay with and enzymatic assay for gentamicin. Antimicrob. Agents Chemother.: 7: 107—109 (1975)

[18] Pechere, J. C., Dugal, R., and Pechere, M. M.: Kinetics of netilmicin in man. Clin. Pharmacol. Ther.: 23: 677—684 (1978)

[19] Regamey, C., Gordon R., and Kirby, W. M.: Comparative pharmacokinetics of tobramycin and gentamicin. Clin. Pharmacol. Ther.: 14: 396—403 (1973)

[20] Schentag, J. J., Jusko, W. J., Vance, J. W., Cumbo, T. J., Abrutyn, E., de Lattre, M., and Gerbracht, L.: Gentamicin disposition and tissue accumulation on multiple dosing. J. Pharmacokin. Biopharm.: 5: 559—577 (1977)

[21] Schentag, J. J., Lasezkay, G., Cumbo, T., Plaut, M. E., and Jusko, W. J.: Accumulation pharmacokinetics of tobramycin. Antimicrob. Agents Chemother.: 13: 649—656 (1978)

[22] Schentag, J. J., Plaut, M. E., Cerra, F. B., Wels, P. B., Walczak, P., and Buckley, R.: Aminoglycoside toxicity in critically ill surgical patients. J. Surg. Res.: 26: 270—279 (1979)

[23] Smith, A. L., Waitz, J. A., Smith, D. H., Oden, E. M., and Emerson, B. B.: Comparison of enzymatic and microbiological gentamicin assays. Antimicrob. Agents Chemother: 6: 316—319 (1974)

[24] Vozeh, S., Wenk, M., Spring, P., and Follath, F.: Verzögerte Ausscheidung der Aminoglykosid-Antibiotika: Bedeutung für die klinische Anwendung. Schweiz. Med. Wschr.: to be published (1979)

[25] Watson, R. A. A., and Wenk, M.: New ^{125}I tracers in netilmicin and sisomicin radioimmunoassay. In: Current Chemotherapy, Vol. II, pp. 906—907, Amer. Soc. Microbiology, Washington D. C. (1978)

Preliminary observations of the pharmacokinetics of oral prednisolone

W. A. C. McAllister, J. V. Collins, J. Morley

Department of Clinical Pharmacology, Cardiothoracic Institute,
Brompton Hospital, Fulham Road, London, SW3.

Prednisolone has been in clinical use since 1955 in a number of conditions, and it is estimated that 5 million people in the United States are currently taking this drug. Through the years prescribing practice has been based on the assumption that the pharmacokinetics of prednisolone were dose independent. Little work has been done to elucidate to what extent kinetics might underly differences in patient reactivity to these drugs. With the advent of methods for measuring plasma prednisolone it becomes possible to evaluate these problems in normal volunteer subjects and patients without recourse to intravenous injection of radioactive substances.
Accordingly we have undertaken a study of prednisolone kinetics over a wide dosage range using a radio-immunoassay having cross-reactivity with cortisol in our laboratory of only 1.9%.

Methods

Five healthy male volunteers (age 23—25 years; weight 68—84 kg) were selected after giving informed consent to take part in the study. None of the subjects were on any form of drug therapy but four of the five were smokers. All abstained from alcohol for 24 hours before and after initiation of each study and from tea and coffee for twelve hours following tablet ingestion. Subjects fasted overnight and were given doses of 5, 10, 20, 40 and 80 mg of prednisolone in random order with intervals of at least a week between each dose. They remained fasted for four hours after ingestion and thereafter standardised meals were taken at 4 and 8 hours. Blood samples were taken via an indwelling catheter in the forearm at 0.5, 1, 2, 3, 4, 6, 8, 10 and 24 hours. Plasma samples were separated and frozen immediately for future assay. No untoward effects were noticed by any of the subjects.

Assay procedure

The radio-immunoassay used was described by Chakraborty *et al* (1976) [1] and has been modified by them, in that plasma is extracted using ethyl acetate which is evaporated to dryness and the residue dissolved in buffer. We used antiserum kindly donated for this study by these workers. In preparation of the antigen they conjugated prednisolone—21—hemisuccinate to bovine serum albumin by the mixed anhydride method. Antiserum was raised to this in female Suffolk cross sheep. All assays were performed by one operator and the consistency of the assay was checked by measuring pooled samples of plasma to which prednisolone had been added. A standard curve was constructed with concentration from 0.1 to 1000 ng. Log dose was plotted against counts per minute and prednisolone levels were interpolated on the straight portion of the curve. Plasma was appropriately diluted when values for undiluted plasma were expected outside this range.

Results and conclusion

1) The area under the plasma concentration time curve (Figure 1) was calculated using the linear trapezoidal rule and confirmed by Spline-Akima method using a digital high speed computer. Those areas were a linear function of the dose administered (Figure 2) however the regression line does not pass through the origin.
2) The volume of distribution and clearance increased with increasing dose.
3) The half lives by log-linear regression increased with increasing dose.
4) Peak concentrations were a linear function of dose administered (Figure 3) but again the regression line does not pass through the origin.

Discussion

Pickup *et al.* [2] found, like us, that with increasing dose of prednisolone there is a prolongation of the plasma half life and an increase in the volume of distribution and plasma clearance of prednisolone. We took this as evidence of dose dependent pharmacokinetics of prednisolone and have therefore confirmed in our oral study the findings of Pickup *et al.* in their intravenous study. It has been shown by Tanner *et al.* [3] that intravenous and oral prednisolone have approximately equivalent bioavailability therefore allowing calculation of apparent volume of distribution and systemic clearance in this oral study.

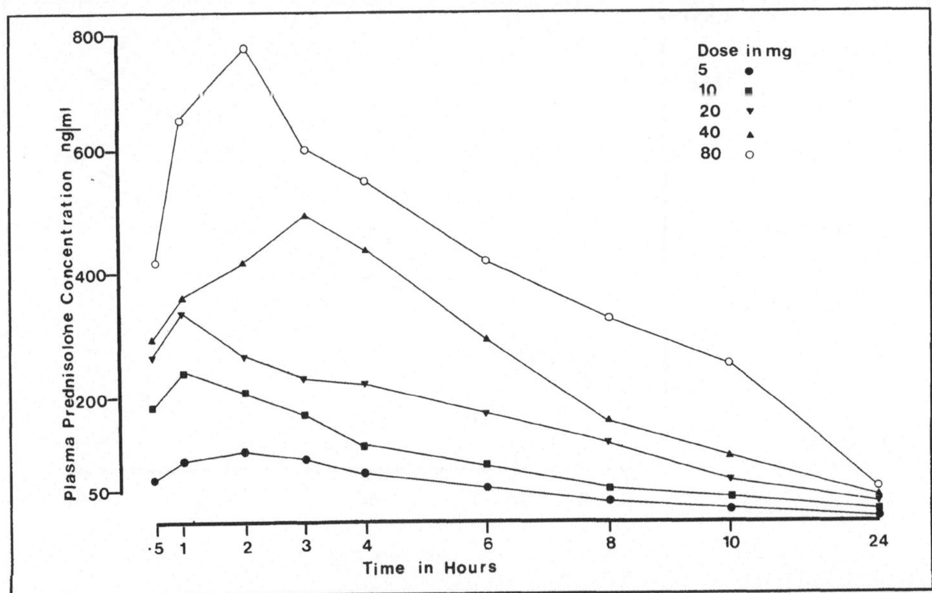

Figure 1: Demonstrating plasma prednisolone concentrations (ng/ml) over a twenty four hour period following ingestion of 5, 10, 20, 40 and 80 mg prednisolone in one individual.

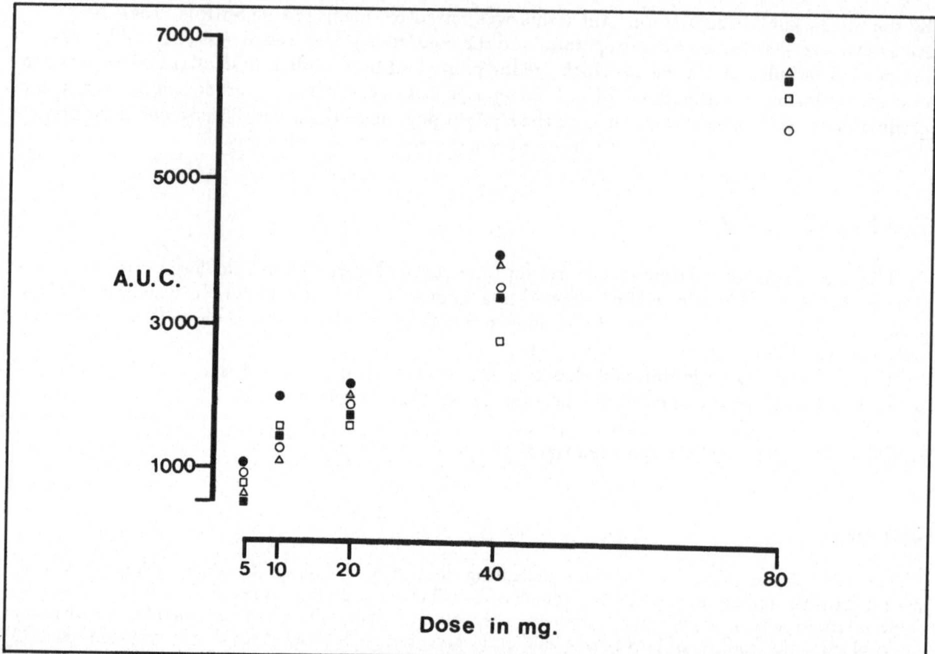

Figure 2: Demonstrating area under the plasma concentration time curve (AUC) (ng/ml/hour) in all five subjects at 5, 10, 20, 40 and 80 mg doses.

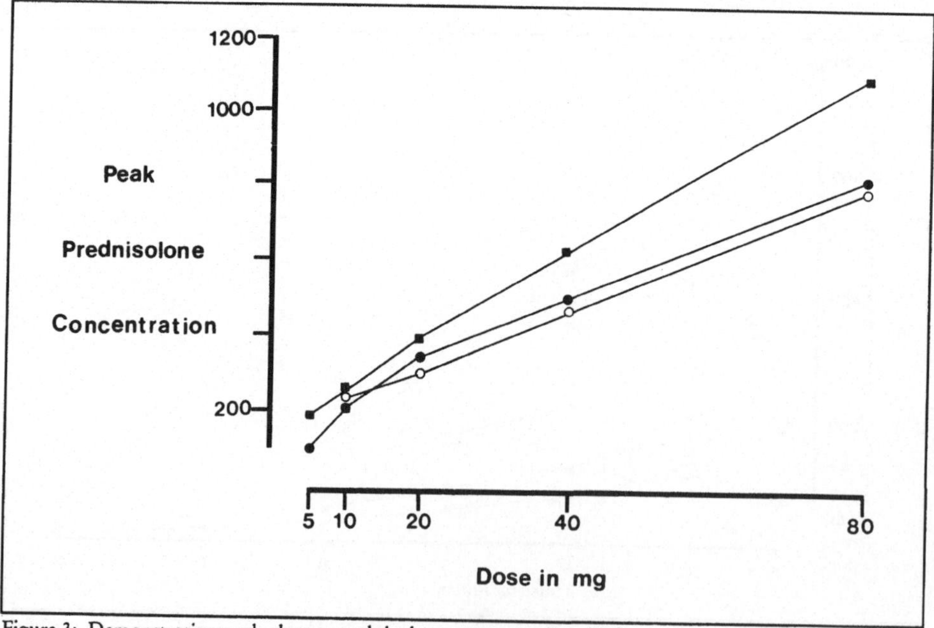

Figure 3: Demonstrating peak plasma prednisolone concentrations in three subjects at 5, 10, 20, 40 and 80 mg doses.

References

[1] Chakraborty, J. English, J., and Marks, V. A radio-immunoassay method for prednisolone, Brit. J. Clin. Pharmacol. *3*, 903—906 (1976).

[2] Pickup, M. E., Lowe, J. R., Leatham, Patricia A., Rhind, Valerie M., Wright, V., and Downie, W. W. Dose dependent pharmacokinetics of prednisolone. Europ. J. Clin. Pharmacol. *12*, 213—219 (1977).

[3] Tanner, A., Bochner, F., Coffin, J., Halliday J., and Powell, L. Dose dependent prednisolone kinetics. Clin. Pharm. Ther. *25*, 571—578 (1979).

Chapter 5

Drug monitoring and dosage prediction

The statistical basis for forecasting individual pharmacokinetics*

Lewis B. Sheiner, Stuart Beal, Barr Rosenberg, Vinay Marathe
From the Division of Clinical Pharmacology, Department of Medicine, and the Department of Laboratory Medicine of the School of Medicine, University of California, San Francisco, California, and the School of Business Administration, University of California, Berkeley, California

To accurately forecast, or predict the pharmacokinetics of a drug in an individual patient implies that one can accurately forecast the plasma drug concentration (PDC) time course that one will see in response to an arbitrary dosage regimen. Why might one wish to do this? The reasons concern clinical management of patients as well as research.

For clinical purposes, the dosage of certain drugs, such as phenytoin, are regulated, at least in part, so as to achieve PDC's within a certain range. Such a drug is one of those we have previously called drugs for which a "Target concentration strategy" is appropriate [1]. For such drugs, it is obvious that if one is able to forecast the drug-dose-to-PDC relationship accurately, one may more accurately choose the dosage that will result in the desired target. Another clinical use of accurate PDC forecasts is monitoring. If predictions deviate from observations by amounts larger than expected, one may wish to ask whether the patient's physiology (kinetics) have changed, and if so, why? The forecasts, or rather their errors, here serve an alerting or diagnostic function. A similar use can be made of the aggregate of forecasts from many patients: if, for example, in a certain period of time, forecasts begin to be systematically lower than observed, across many patients, one may be tempted to ask whether the drug preparation's bioavailability has changed, or if the drug concentration measuring laboratory is functioning adequately. This, too, is a clinical use.

There are also research uses. As before, discrepancies between forecasts and observations may highlight groups of patients whose kinetics differ from others, and, indeed, one may propose possible reasons and "test" them using the forecasting system.

Thus, there are a number of reasons for wanting to be able to forecast individual pharmacokinetics, and much effort has been expended by many researchers in pursuit of this goal (for review, see [1]). It is important to note, that for all the uses discussed, accurate and precise forecasts (that is, unbiased forecasts with small typical error magnitudes, as measured by the error standard deviation) are crucial. A poor forecasting scheme will lack the necessary sensitivity to be of any of the above uses. The following question, then, must be addressed: how does one produce accurate and precise forecasts? In order to answer this question, we must consider a general scheme for forecasting: one first

*Work supported in part by USDHEW grant GM 16496

formulates a model for the general case. In pharmacokinetics, this would mean to adopt a certain pharmacokinetic model, for example, the two-compartment mammillary model, for a given drug. Next one must *initialize the model* for the individual in question, by somehow estimating that patient's values for the parameters (constants) of the model. In pharmacokinetics, this would mean estimating an individual's clearance (*Cl*), volume of distribution (Vd), and so forth, for a given drug. The next part of the task is not quite so obvious, but, as we shall see, is of major importance: After the control action has been administered, one may measure outcome, and use this to *revise* the individual parameter estimates, thereby improving the model through *feedback*. In pharmacokinetics, one would administer a dosage, measure a PDC, and use this measured value to improve future forecasts. Thus, forecasting involves three crucial steps: model formulation, initializiation, and revision.
In pharmacokinetics, the first task, model formulation, is essentially a research one, involving study of a drug's pharmacokinetics in various populations to arrive at an adequate model through intuition, experience, trial-and-error, and testing of the various possibilities. We will not discuss this further, but will assume from now on that the type of model has already been chosen. We are left with two tasks: model initialization and revision. We have previously pointed out [2] that these tasks involve knowledge of a number of population pharmacokinetic parameters. We must first, therefore, define these. They are of three types.
First, there are "regression" parameters. These are constants that describe the average relationship between physiology and pharmacokinetics. So, if we state that

$$Cl_j = \Theta_l \, Cl_j^{Cr} + \Theta_2$$

where Cl_j is drug clearance in the jth patient and Cl_j^{Cr} is his creatinine clearance, then Θ_l *and* Θ_2 are population parameters, the first expressing the average proportionality between creatine clearance and renal clearance of drug, and the second expressing average non-renal clearance.
Next, we recognize that equations such as that above are not exact; the true parameters of the jth patient will differ, to some degree, from the average value given by any equation even though the equation attempts to correct for certain causes of inter-individual variability (renal function). The typical magnitude of the discrepancies between the actual parameter values for individuals and the predicted value, as measured by their standard deviations (the "inter-individual differences standard deviation") is another type of population parameter. It measures essentially, how well we can know a patient's parameter using only *a priori* information (such a sex, age, weight, or creatinine clearance).
Finally, even if we knew an individual's *average* parameter values perfectly, there would still be a discrepancy between a measured PDC and the value predicted from the model using these correct individual parameters. This residual random error arises from a number of sources: for example, PDC laboratory measurement error, day-to-day intra-individual parameter variation, and lack of ability of the chosen model to exactly describe pharmacokinetics. The typical magnitude of this error, as measured by its standard deviation (the "residual error standard deviation"), is also a population parameter.
Before considering how these population parameters can be used for model initialization and revision, we note that it is not at all obvious how to get values for the population parameters. Clearly, they must come from study of patient groups, but classical pharmacokinetic study of many, perhaps quite ill patients, is possibly unethical, probably difficult, and certainly costly.
We have proposed a methodology for deriving these parameter values from routine clinical pharmacokinetic data (i. e., PDC's measured in the course of patient care) plus some easily obtained additional data, and have used this methodology in a few cases [2, 3]. It appears to be effective, and promises to ease somewhat the problems of obtaining good estimates of population parameters.
Now, assuming we have estimates of the above types of population parameters, as well as a formulated model, we can proceed to discuss how model initialization and revision proceeds.
It is almost intuitive that for model initialization, one simply substitutes the patient's own values for the observable variables (such as creatinine clearance) into the average relationships (e. g., the equation above) quantified by the regression parameters. These are the *initial* individual parameter estimates, and they are used in the chosen pharmacokinetic model to forecast the PDC that will result from any given dosage. Such a forecasting approach, however, corresponds to asserting that the PDC will assume its modal value, rather than its mean value, the usually desired forecast. However

[1] forecasting the mean would be difficult, involving an integration step, and [2] if the interindividual differences are fairly symmetrically distributed and certain other conditions are approximately met, the mode will not be too different from the mean. Simplicity, tradition, and good performance dictate the continued choice of this approach: it is the basis of all nomograms for adjusting initial dosage of aminoglycoside antibiotics (e. g., [4]) and digoxin (e. g., [5]) to name only a few. Unlike initialization, feedback model revision, when there are only 1 or 2 measured PDC's available has attracted little attention, and there is no accepted, "classical" method. A frequently used, ad hoc, method is to keep all parameters but one (usually clearance) at their initial estimates and to use a single measured drug level to "solve" the pharmacokinetic model for the one parameter to be estimated. When one must solve for two parameters simultaneously, as one must for phenytoin, certain graphical procedures have been proposed [6]. All of these methods share certain disturbing characteristics. First, the PDC information is ignored for those parameter estimates fixed to initial values, while for the parameter(s) re-estimated using the PDC(s), the initial estimates are ignored: this seems rather contradictory. Second, it is not clear how one chooses which parameters to fix, and which to re-estimate, yet therapeutic implications may differ. Third, the statistical properties of such ad hoc procedures are not known, but it is certain that they do not correspond to optimal strategies unless one is willing to make certain patently incorrect assumptions (e. g., that the residual error standard deviation and the fixed parameters' interindividual difference standard deviations are all zero). This lack of statistical optimality does not, of course, mean that the revised parameter estimates so obtained will fail to produce acceptable PDC predictions in an absolute sense; only that one *must* be able to improve on those predictions using some other method.

Under certain reasonably realistic assumptions, there is a relatively easily obtained parameter estimate revision approach that is near optimal. It is called an Empirical Bayes approach, and we have previously presented it in the literature [2].

Rather than fix some parameters and alter others, the method alters all parameter estimates simultaneously: it adjusts parameter estimates in light of (any number of) measured PDC's in inverse proportion to their initial certainty (i. e., the larger the interindividual difference standard deviations, the more a parameter estimate may be altered), but also, of course, in proportion to the degree to which a unit shift in the parameter estimate serves to produce a better prediction of the observed PDC's. One additional feature is that the method also takes into account the residual error standard deviation: parameter estimates are adjusted to bring forecasts *close* to observations, but not to reproduce them exactly, because the method recognizes that the measured value is not an exact reflection of the true mean individual parameters. All other things being equal, the larger the residual error standard deviation, the less the system adjusts parameter estimates. This is because a large residual standard deviation implies "noisy" measurements that lack a great deal of information. Conversely, a small residual error standard deviation forces parameter estimates to be extensively revised so that the forecast matches the observation relatively well.

We have tried this forecasting approach only in a limited number of instances; the most extensive being a study involving digoxin. The results are reported in [7]. In brief, the results were gratifying, and sometimes surprising.

With regard to the ability to estimate plausible individual parameter values (it must be remembered that this is not the point of the approach; it is rather to produce accurate and precise PDC forecasts: the revised parameter estimates are merely a means to that end), the system performed well: parameters were adjusted appropriately. For example, using steady-state PDC's for feedback caused no change in the individual estimates of volume of distribution (Vd), but only in clearance. This is appropriate behavior since steady-state PDC's will not change due to changes in Vd alone. It is gratifying, but predictable, that the system does not alter parameter estimates arbitrarily.

With regard to PDC forecasts, we found that use of one measured PDC for forecast revision allowed more accurate future forecasts than use of all observable data: sex, age, height, weight and serum creatinine. When 2 PDC's were used for feedback revision, forecasts became almost as accurate and precise as theoretically possible (i. e., error magnitude was only slightly larger than residual error magnitude: this error, of course, can never be eliminated through feedback).

In summary, a unified scheme for forecasting individual PDC's includes three essential steps: *formulating* the appropriate pharmacokinetic model, *initializing* it for an individual by estimating his parameters from observable features such as weight and serum creatinine, and *revising* this estimate after observing the PDC resulting from the dosage administered. After model formulation, the next two steps involve knowledge of population pharmacokinetic parameters describing the relationships between physiology and kinetics, and also describing the typical magnitude of persistent interindividual kinetic variability, as well as the typical magnitude of intraindividual residual "error" in the PDC-dosage relationship. If these be known, near optimal methods can be devised for the initialization and revision steps.

References

[1] Sheiner LB, Tozer TN: Clinical Pharmacokinetics—the use of plasma concentrations of drugs. *In* Melmon KL & Morrelli HF (eds.) Clinical Pharmacology, Macmillan, 2nd Edition, 1978.

[2] Sheiner LB, Rosenberg B & Melmon KL: Modelling of individual pharmacokinetics for computer-aided drug dosage. Comp. & Biomed. Res. *5*: 441, 1972.

[3] Sheiner LB, Rosenberg B & Marathe V: Estimation of population characteristics of pharmacokinetic parameters from routine clinical data. J. Pharmacokin. & Biopharmaceut. *5*: 445, 1977.

[4] Cutler RE, Gyselynck A, Fleet WP & Flory AW: Correlation of serum creatinine concentration and gentamycin half-life. J.A.M.A. *219*: 1037, 1972.

[5] Jelliffe RW, Buell J & Kalaba R: Reduction of digitalis toxicity by computer-assisted glycoside dosage regimens. Ann. Int. Med. *77*: 891, 1972.

[6] Ludden TM, Allen JP, Valotsky WA et al.: Individualization of phenytoin dosage regimens. Clin. Pharm. Therap. *21*: 287, 1977.

[7] Sheiner LB, Beal SL, Rosenberg B & Marathe VV: Forecasting individual pharmacokinetics. Clin. Pharm. Therap., in press 1979.

Prospective *versus* retrospective studies on the variance of digoxin plasma levels

Norbert Heinz and Carmen I. Flasch
Medizinische Forschung, Beiersdorf AG, Unnastr. 48, D-2000 Hamburg 20

Introduction

Two years ago we began studies on the statistical computations of plasma digoxin concentrations (PDC). According to the general literature, and the work of WAGNER and coworkers [6], multiple linear regression with PDC as the dependent variable seems to be the most suitable method for mathematical analysis. Initially, multiple linear regression was performed using our own program on the IBM 370/148 [4]. In the meantime several clinical studies of various designs have been conducted and lately we have used the excellent Biomedical Computer Programs (BMDP) of the University of California, Los Angeles [5] with a marked improvement in data analysis (in comparison to that obtained using the initial program).

Method

The population studied included hospitalized patients requiring digitalis for treatment of all types of severe heart failure associated with both sinus rhythm or chronic arrhythmia.
The studies A and B had retrospective design, and study D prospective design with patients taking β-acetyldigoxin, whereas the patients of the prospective study C received digoxin. The equivalence of the bioavailability data on the β-acetyldigoxin* and the digoxin** tablets used in these studies was the premise for computing all plasma digoxin concentrations (PDC) in the same manner [2, 3]. There was no selection of the patients according to their renal function. Patients taking quinidine, cholestyramine or antacids were excluded from the prospective studies. The clinical data are listed in Table 1. The plasma PDC were determined by radioimmunoassay.
In this table the arithmetic means and the ranges of all variables are listed. In the case of the creatinine and digoxin plasma levels a prior logarithmic transformation for all following calculations has been used (see below). In order to allow more perspicuity in this table the retransformed antilogs are given, *i. e.* the corresponding means are now of the geometric type.
The data analysis was performed with the aid of the Biomedical Computer Programs of UCLA [5].
In this study we were concerned with two main topics:

* NOVODIGAL®
** DIGACIN® } Beiersdorf AG, Hamburg

Study	type	n	age	height (m)	weight (kg)	antilog creatinine (mg/100 ml)	dose (mg/die)	antilog c_{ss} (ng/ml)
A	retrosp. mono-center	213	35—93 69	1.44—1.90 1.64	36—125 62	0.4—11.6 1.2	0.2 —0.6 0.3	0.50—5.30 1.50
B	retrosp. multi-center	1136	13—92 69	1.41—1.95 1.67	34—150 63	0.4—15.3 1.3	0.05—0.6 0.3	0.10—4.80 1.32
C	prosp. multi-center	494	18—95 69	1.30—1.87 1.64	30—111 63	0.4— 3.1 1.0	0.1 —0.4 0.3	0.13—4.80 1.20
D	prosp. mono-center	102	32—86 70	1.39—1.84 1.64	36—100 62	0.7— 2.8 1.1	0.1 —0.4 0.25	0.10—2.47 0.84

Table 1 (Explanation see text)

1. multiple linear regression
2. residual analysis

1: A multiple linear regression relates a dependent variable to the linear combination of several independent variables:

$$y = b_0 + b_1x_1 + b_2x_2 + \ldots + b_px_p + \varepsilon$$

"y" represents the value of the dependent, the predictand, variable—in this case the plasma digoxin concentration (PDC). $x_1, x_2 \ldots x_p$ stand for the independent variables (the predictor variables); dose of digoxin, serum creatinine and serum potassium concentrations, reciprocal of body weight and height and for age and sex. As an index of the relationship between y and x_p the multiple correlation coefficient is used. The coefficient of determination (100 r^2) gives the percentage of the total variance of the plasma digoxin concentrations which is accounted for by the linear combination of the variables mentioned above.

2: When the independent variables $x_1, x_2 \ldots x_p$ are given, the dependent variable (PDC) can be calculated by the regression equation. The difference between the value actually measured (y) and this value predicted by formula ($\hat{y}$) is defined as "residual." The residuals for each case are computed as

$$(y - \hat{y}) = (y - \bar{y} - b_1(x_1 - \bar{x}_1) - \ldots - b_p(x_p - \bar{x}_p)$$

The standardized residuals used in this study are obtained by dividing each residual by its standard error.

In the ideal or theoretical situation, there will be no difference between observed and predicted values of the target variable. However, it is to be expected that the residuals will be normally distributed with mean $\bar{x} = 0$.
Logarithmic transformation of the PDC provided a more normally distributed group of data, and similar findings are to be seen in the literature. Beyond that we have always used logarithms because of an additional reason: It is to be expected that the study population and that of the retrospective studies in particular include a certain percentage of non-compliant patients, that is patients who have taken less than the prescribed digoxin dose. Accordingly, the measured PDC would be much smaller than those predicted by the regression equation based on the nominal maintenance doses. These "false" low PDC can be identified more easily after transformation (Figure 1). In such cases the standardized residuals have abnormally large negative values which can be used as the basis for eliminating these patients. At a very early stage of examination of the data this procedure allows the detection of outliers with regard to the PDC. In no case however was this procedure used to exclude possible outliers under the predictor variables offered by the BMDP.

Results and discussion

For each study the residual analysis and consecutive outlier elimination were carried out until all cases with the standardized residual less or equal to — 2.8 were deleted. The effect of this procedure on the original PDC distribution is shown in Table 2.

study/type	steps of residual analysis	n	antilog c_{ss} (ng/ml)	skewness	kurtosis	$100\ r^2$ (%)
$A_{(R)}$	0	213	1.5	0.03	− 0.75	18
$B_{(R)}$	0	1136	1.3	− 1.12	1.91	11
	I	1115	1.4	− 0.67	0.35	13
	II	1103	1.4	− 0.57	0.16	14
$C_{(P)}$	0	494	1.2	− 0.58	1.74	33
	I	489	1.2	− 0.29	0.85	38
	II	487	1.2	− 0.18	0.59	38
$D_{(P)}$	0	102	0.8	− 1.13	3.27	20
	I	100	0.9	− 0.29	0.43	21

Table 2

Especially in regard to the multicenter studies (B and C) with large numbers of cases, the deletion of several outliers gave an approximation to a nearly normal distribution of the PDC indicated by the values of skewness and kurtosis approaching closer to zero. Simultaneously the coefficients of determination were increased.
The distribution of the standardized residuals of the retrospective study B is represented in Figure 1. Part A includes the residuals of all cases before outlier elimination. It is apparent that there exists

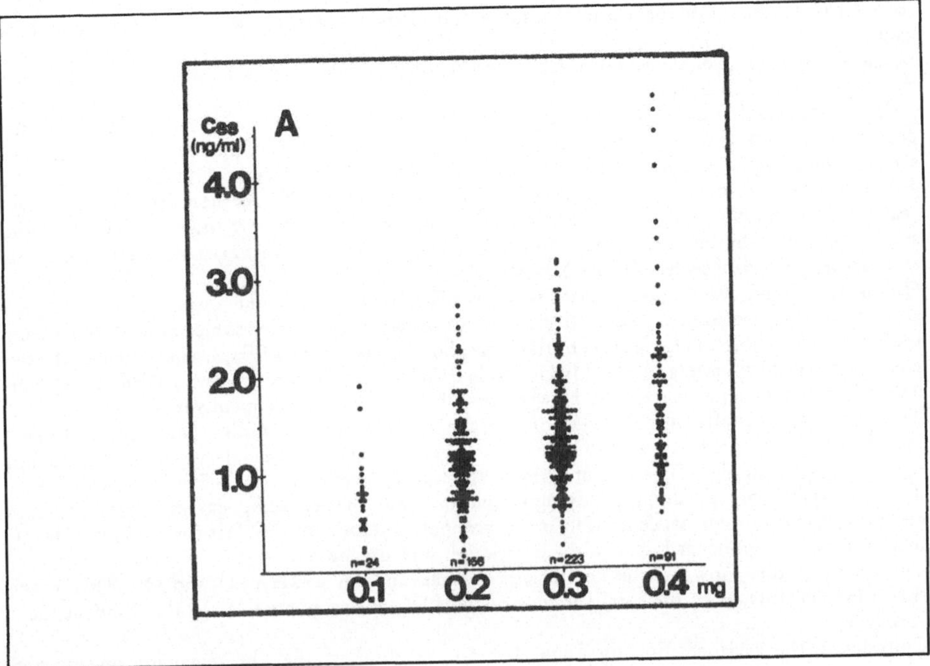

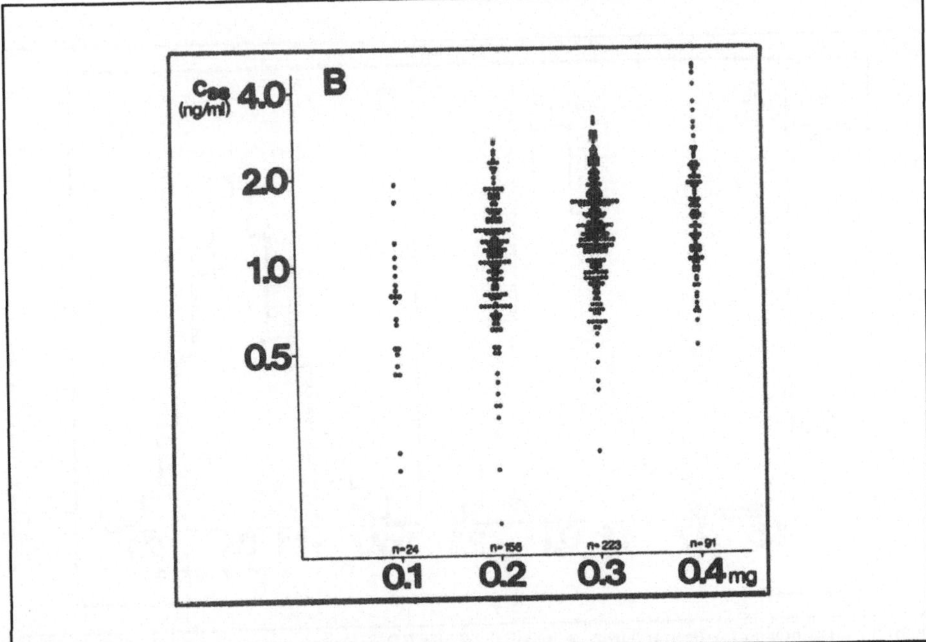

Figure 1: Arithmetic (A) and geometric (B) means of the PDC in steady state related to the digoxin maintenance dose.

some PDC values whose logarithms are more than three standard deviations from the predicted values.
Because of the low probabilities of these large negative residuals it is to be assumed that these patients have not taken the prescribed dose.
Indeed it appears that the 1136 patients of the retrospective study represent a rather heterogeneous population composed of two groups. One group is assumed to consist of patients who take the prescribed tablets regularly. This will be the essential group for our mathematical calculation. The other group includes non-compliant patients having abnormally low PDC. As these latter cases are revealed by the residual analysis, this computation may be used to improve the homogeneity of the study population. In the retrospective studies where a high degree of heterogeneity may exist, this method proves very effective (Table 2/Figure 2).
On the other hand, several outliers with very low PDC and explicable only by non-compliance, can also be found in prospective studies. In study C for instance, the elimination of only seven patients leads to a nearly normal distribution of the logarithms of the original PDC, as indicated by the decreasing values of skewness and kurtosis in Table 2. Moreover, the increased coefficient of determination shows a stronger correlation between the PDC and the independent variables.
There are still some differences between prospective and retrospective studies. The results in Table 3 indicate that in the prospective studies the coeffiecents of determination always are higher than in the retrospective studies. The two studies however show agreement in the predictive value of the individual variables of the multiple linear regression equation. All four studies gave the dose of digoxin and the serum creatinine concentration as the strongest determinant variables for the PDC. The effect of age as a significant factor in the correlation was also noted.
The present studies show multiple coefficients of determination between 14% and 38%. That means that these percentages of the total variance of the PDC are accounted for by the 7 independent variables.
Considering the variances S^2_{log} in Table 4 it can be observed that the remaining unexplained variances in the retrospective studies are twice as high as those of the prospective studies.

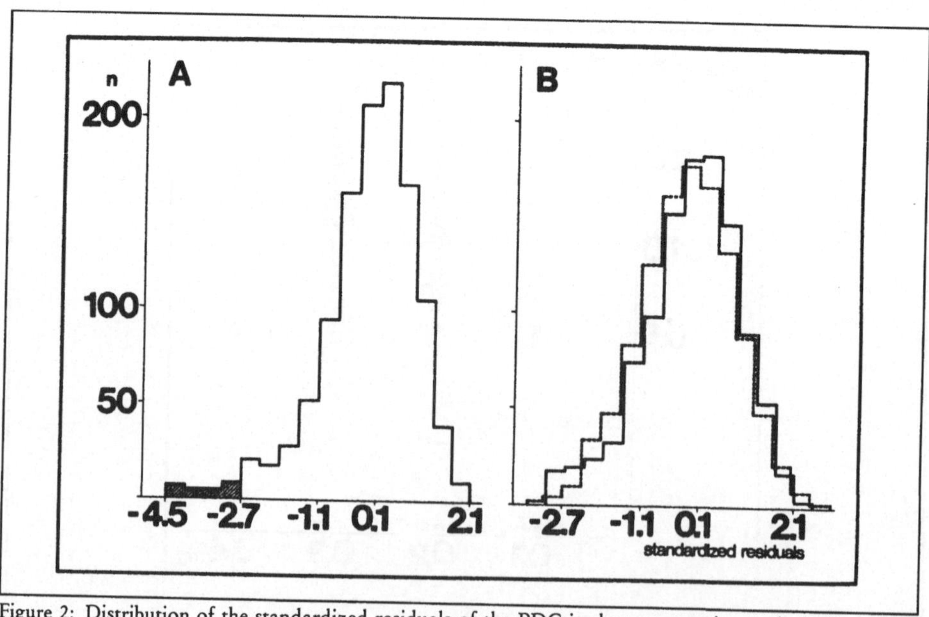

Figure 2: Distribution of the standardized residuals of the PDC in the retrospective study B; Part A: all cases (n = 1136). Part B: after two steps of deleting cases with standardized residuals less or equal to −2.8 (n = 1103); ——— normal distribution.

100 r^2 (%)								
study	multiple	sex	age	height	weight	dose	log creat.	potas.
$A_{(R)}$	18	0.7	1.4	0.3	1.4	6.7**	6.9**	1.3
$B_{(R)}$	14	1.2**	3.2**	0.1	0.5*	4.9**	4.4**	2.5**
$C_{(P)}$	38	0.8*	3.2**	0.0	2.8**	17.4**	11.4**	0.0
$D_{(P)}$	21	3.7*	4.8*	0.0	0.0	3.5*	6.6**	1.8

Table 3

study	S^2_{log} I	S^2_{log} II	$S^2_{log} \times r^2$	$S^2_{log}(1 - r^2)$
$A_{(R)}$	0.051	0.051	0.009	0.042
$B_{(R)}$	0.080	0.058	0.008	0.050
$C_{(P)}$	0.043	0.037	0.014	0.023
$D_{(P)}$	0.044	0.032	0.007	0.025

Table 4: Variances of PDC before (I) and after (II) residual analysis and outlier elimination

Finally, the relationship between PDC, digoxin and creatinine clearances is defined in a very similar manner for both types of study (Figure 3). Whilst the importance of renal function as a factor in determining the correct digoxin dosage is well known, the data show that less variability in PDC could be achieved if more attention was given to estimates of creatinine clearance.

Acknowledgements

The authors are indebted to Mrs. Jarmila Simova for advice and the carrying out of the statistical analysis as well as to Mrs. Renate Gassen and to Miss Ursula Baer for technical assistance.

Literature

[1] Cockcroft, D. W., Gault, M. H.; Nephron *16*, 31 (1976).

[2] Flasch, H.; Klin. Wschr. *53*, 873 (1975).

[3] Flasch, H., Asmussen, B. und Heinz, N.; Arzneimittelforsch. *28*, 326 (1978).

[4] Heinz, N. und Rietbrock, N.; Europ. J. clin. Pharmacol. *15*, 109 (1979).

* $p < 0.05$
** $p < 0.001$

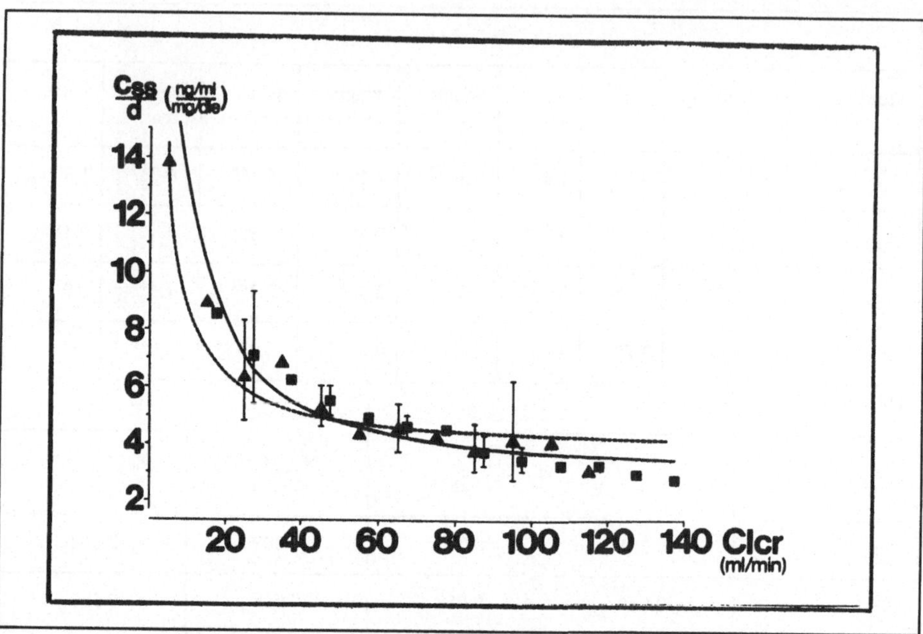

Figure 3: The relationship between the calculated creatinine clearances* and the quotient of the geometric mean of the steady-state PDC (c_{ss}) and the individual daily dose of digitalis.

$$\text{* creatinine clearance} = \frac{(140 - \text{age}) \times \text{body weight (kg)}}{72 \times \text{serum creatinine (mg/100 ml)}}$$

(COCKCROFT and GAULT [1])

..... ▲ retrospective study A

——— □ prospective study C

[5] University of California, Los Angeles. BMDP—77, Biomedical Computer Programs* P. Series, University of California, Mass., Berkeley, Los Angeles, London 1977.

[6] Wagner, J. G., Yates, J. D., Willis III, P. W., Sakmar, E. und Stoll, R. G.; Clin. Pharmacol. Ther. *15*, 291 (1974).

* Programs were developed at the Health Sciences Computing Facility, UCLA, sponsored by NIH Special Research Resources Grant RR-3; revision of the programs: Sept. 1977.

Techniques for evaluating the steady-state serum concentration—Dose relationship in phenytoin Therapy

Peter W. Mullen
Department of Pharmacology, Materia Medica and Therapeutics,
Stopford Building, University of Manchester, Oxford Road, Manchester M13 9PT, U.K.

Introduction

Although introduced in 1938 [16], phenytoin (5,5-diphenylhydantoin) still remains a drug of choice in the treatment of *grand mal* epilepsy. In addition to continuing investigations aimed at elucidating its mode of action [21], numerous studies over the years have contributed to a much greater appreciation of the dispositional characteristics peculiar to this drug. Recently acquired knowledge obtained from serum phenytoin concentration monitoring [1, 2, 9, 11, 13, 15, 22, 23] has provided pharmacokinetic explanations for the prescribing problems occasionally encountered when a patient's dosage is altered in an attempt to achieve optimal anti-epileptic therapy. In this paper I shall review some recent pharmacokinetic findings and techniques pertaining to the steady-state serum concentration—dose relationship in phenytoin therapy.

In the compliant patient, any difficulties experienced in attaining an optimal dosage schedule could be associated with two related aspects of phenytoin's disposition in the body:

i) the drug undergoes extensive biotransformation by the liver mixed-function oxidase enzyme system [3, 5] at different rates in different individuals [15] and,

ii) in the case of phenytoin, this enzyme system appears to be readily saturable at doses employed clinically resulting, *in vivo*, in nonlinear or "dose-dependent" pharmacokinetics [1, 9, 10, 15, 23]. Thus, following a large single dose the observed nonlinear serum phenytoin concentration—time curve is best described by the classical Michaelis-Menten Equation 1 [17] in its integrated form (2) [1, 9, 10, 15, 24]:

$$v = \frac{dC_t}{dt} = -\frac{V_{max} \cdot C_t}{K_m + C_t} \tag{1}$$

$$C_0 - C_t + K_m ln(C_0/C_t) = V_{max} \cdot t \tag{2}$$

where, V_{max} is the theoretical maximal rate of elimination (in units such as mg/L/h, and K_m, the Michaelis-Menten constant, is the serum concentration at ½ V_{max}.

C_t represents the serum concentration at any time, t.

When $t = 0$, $C_t = C_0$.

Simulated serum concentration—time curves for a drug eliminated by Michaelis-Menten kinetics are shown in Figure 1, where $V_{max} = 6.0$ mg/L/day, $K_m = 6$ mg/L and $C_0 = 5$, 10 or 15 mg/L. Of greater relevance to long-term anti-epileptic therapy is the finding that as a consequence of its saturation kinetics there is a nonlinear relationship between steady-state serum phenytoin concentration (C_{ss}) and dose [2, 15, 23] of the form illustrated in Figure 2. It is this relationship between C_{ss} and dose which accounts for any difficulties in achieving serum phenytoin concentrations within the "therapeutic range" of 10—20 mg/L, [4, 11] widely regarded as being consistent with optimal phenytoin therapy. It is obvious from Figure 2 that once C_{ss} approaches the lower end of the therapeutic range (*i. e.* 8—10 mg/L) an additional increase in dose results in a disproportionately large increase in the steady-state serum concentration. Moreover, as demonstrated by BOCHNER *et al.* [2] and RICHENS and DUNLOP [23], the 'steepness' of the concentration—dose curve can vary considerably from patient to patient due to individual differences in the MICHAELIS-MENTEN parameters K_m and D_{max} (see below). For phenytoin and other drugs eliminated by MICHAELIS-MENTEN kinetics, the serum concentration—dose relationship in the steady-state can be represented by Equation 3 [12—14, 19, 20, 25]:

$$C_{ss} = \frac{D \cdot K_m}{D_{max} - D} \tag{3}$$

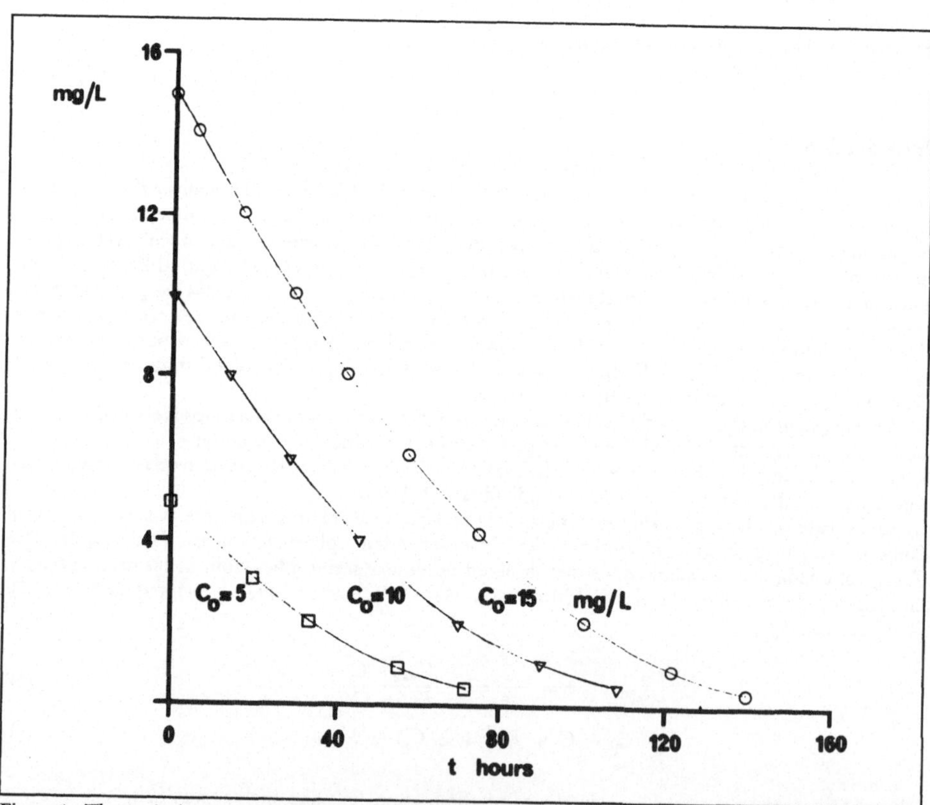

Figure 1: Theoretical serum concentration—time curves for a drug such as phenytoin displaying nonlinear elimination kinetics. Each of the three curves shown (starting concentrations of 5, 10 and 15 mg/L) were obtained using the integrated form of the MICHAELIS-MENTEN Equation 2 in which V_{max} and K_m values of 6.0 mg/L/day and 6.0 mg/L, respectively were substituted. Note that at higher concentrations an apparent zero-order decay phase is observed.

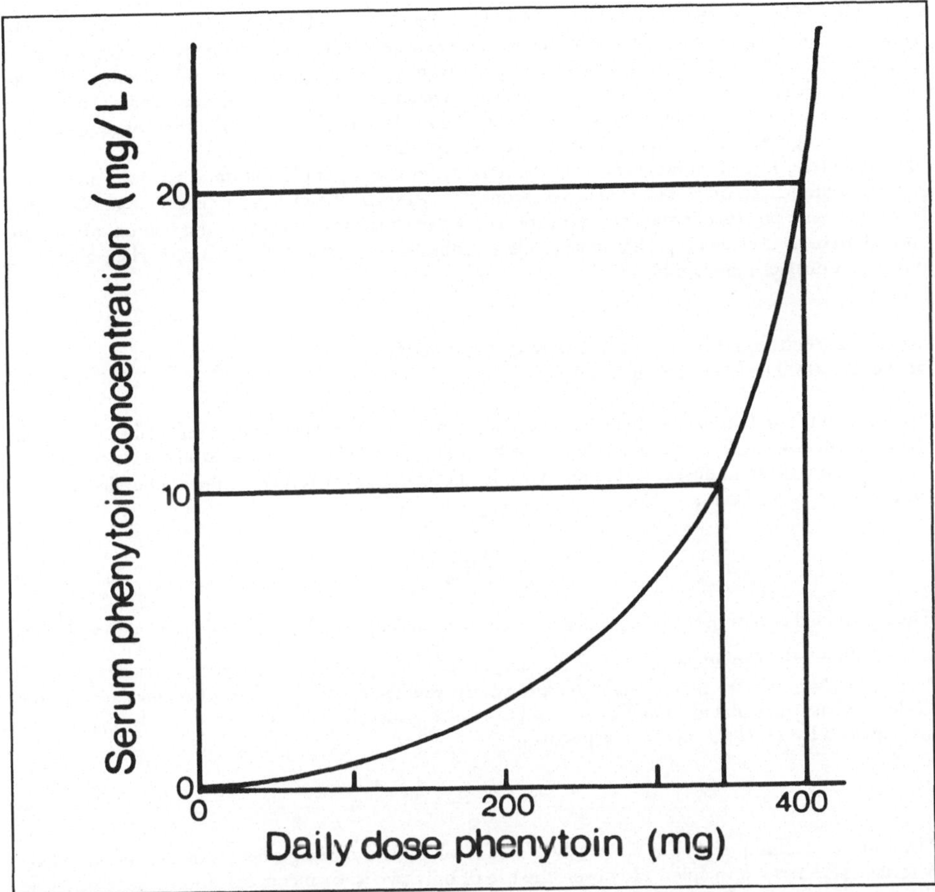

Figure 2: The theoretical relationship between steady-state concentration and daily dose of phenytoin as reported by MAWER, MULLEN, RODGERS, ROBINS and LUCAS, *Br. J. Clin. Pharmacol. 1,* 163—168 (1974) [15] (Reproduced with permission). Similar nonlinear curves relating steady-state serum concentration and dose have been observed in patients. [2, 23]

which is merely a rearranged form of Equation (1) with D (dose in mg/day), D_{max} (the theoretical maximal daily dose under steady-state conditions) and C_{ss} replacing v, V_{max} and C_t, respectively. Mean K_m and D_{max} values of 5.9 mg/L and 355 mg/day, respectively were obtained in a recent study of 127 children and adults suffering from epilepsy; D_{max} (but not K_m) was positively correlated with both patient age and body surface area [22].

Pharmacokinetic techniques used to predict desired steady-state serum concentrations in phenytoin therapy

The RICHENS and DUNLOP nomogram [23]:

By combining the K_m values pertaining to the steady-state concentration—dose relationship in four patients with a mean ($n = 15$) K_m value obtained in this laboratory from concentration—time data

following a 600 mg dose of sodium phenytoin [15], RICHENS and DUNLOP [23] constructed a nomogram for predicting the daily dose required to achieve a steady-state serum phenytoin concentration of either 15 or 20 mg/L. This technique has the advantage that it enables the physician to estimate the desired dose from a single known steady-state serum concentration. A recent improved version of the nomogram devised by RAMBECK *et al* [22] allows the clinician to predict the dose required to achieve a range of desired steady-state phenytoin concentrations.
Unfortunately, since a nomogram is constructed from mean population data it would not be expected to predict accurate *individualized* serum phenytoin concentrations in every case. Nevertheless, when only one steady-state concentration on a particular dose is known, the revised nomogram should serve as a valuable preliminary guide to complement clinical observations when altering a phenytoin dosage schedule [22, 23].

Graphical techniques based on linear rearrangements of the MICHAELIS-MENTEN equation:

In an attempt to individualize phenytoin therapy, LUDDEN *et al* [13] proposed a method to determine the values of K_m and D_{max} characteristic of each patient provided at least two steady-state concentrations (C_{ss}) on different doses (D) are known. The method uses the following linear equation (a rearranged form of Equation 3 [13]):

$$D = -K_m \frac{D}{C_{ss}} + D_{max} \tag{4}$$

Thus, provided two or more D, C_{ss} values are available, a simple plot of D (ordinate) against $\frac{D}{C_{ss}}$ (abscissa) will readily provide estimates of K_m (slope) and D_{max} (ordinate intercept). Once the patient's MICHAELIS-MENTEN parameter values are known, the predicted dose required to achieve any desired C_{ss} level is easily calculated using Equation 5 [13] which is merely Equation 1 in which v, V_{max} and C_t are replaced by D, D_{max} and C_{ss}, respectively:

$$D = \frac{D_{max} \cdot C_{ss}}{K_m + C_{ss}} \tag{5}$$

The LUDDEN technique [13] is obviously a means of individualizing phenytoin dosage based on MICHAELIS-MENTEN principles. However, the use of only two known concentration—dose values in Equation 4 will give D_{max} and K_m values of questionable reliability particularly if these two data points are close together. Moreover, as discussed below, Equation 4 may not in fact provide the best estimates of D_{max} and K_m if one assumes that most experimental (analytical) error is inherent in C_{ss} rather than D.
In their work LUDDEN *et al* [13] used Equation 4 because this Equation had previously been shown to give the most reliable estimates of the MICHAELIS-MENTEN parameters, K_m and V_{max} pertaining to enzyme kinetics [7]. Although several linear algebraic rearrangements of Equation 1 can be written, the values of K_m and V_{max} obtained from each will differ unless the data conforms to a "true" (*i. e.* no error) MICHAELIS-MENTEN relationship. Of course, in actual enzyme kinetic studies, experimental error is inherent in the rate (v) of reaction values. Therefore, as pointed out by DOWD and RIGGS in 1976 [7], commonly used equations (especially the $\frac{1}{v}$ versus $\frac{1}{C_t}$ plot) which utilize the reciprocal of v tend to 'magnify' the error inherent in this variable, leading occasionally to spurious values of K_m and V_{max}.
In the relationship between dose and steady-state serum phenytoin concentration the latter becomes the dependent (and error containing) variable. Hence intuitive reasoning indicates that the following Equation:

$$C_{ss} = D_{max} \cdot \frac{C_{ss}}{D} - K_m \tag{6}$$

should produce estimates of D_{max} and K_m better than those obtained by Equation 4 [20]. Indeed, assuming that any error in D is negligible (*i. e.* complete patient compliance and a constant fraction of drug absorbed) compared to that found in C_{ss}, experiments using computer generated data have demonstrated that Equation 6 is in fact superior not only to Equation 4, but to other linear rearrangements [14] of Equation 3 as well [20]. Whether or not such equation differences are meaningful in practive however, remains to be established. In any case, regardless of the linear equation employed, the K_m and D_{max} values obtained from two or more concentration—dose data must then be substituted in Equation 3 along with the desired steady-state concentration so that the required dose can be calculated.

The direct linear plot (DLP) technique [18—20]:

The direct linear plot was originally described in 1974 by Eisenthal and Cornish-Bowden [6, 8] as an easy, reliable means of determining the K_m and V_{max} values of enzyme reactions. Its first pharmacokinetic application was in phenytoin dosage prediction [18, 19]. The DLP technique is extremely simple to use since it requires no calculations but merely a pencil, a sheet of ordinary graph paper and a ruler; nevertheless, good estimates of K_m and D_{max} are obtained [6, 8, 18—20].
Utilization of the DLP in phenytoin therapy requires, like the graphical procedures described in the previous section, a minimum of two known steady-state serum phenytoin concentrations on two different doses [18—20]. To use the DLP technique, the first two quadrants are delineated on a sheet of graph paper with the abscissa and ordinate axes labelled 'Concentration' and 'Dose', respectively. (Strictly speaking, the axes should be labelled K_m and D_{max} since the DLP is based on solving simultaneous equations of the form $D_{max} = \frac{D}{C_{ss}} \cdot K_m + D$ obtained by rearranging Equations 3 or 5 [6, 8, 18—20].
Each value of C_{ss}, arbitrarily given a negative sign, is marked on the 'Concentration' axis and then joined to its corresponding 'Dose' point on the ordinate by a line which is extended into the first quadrant. The intersection point (s) of such lines in the first quadrant determines the values of K_m and D_{max} on the 'Concentration' and 'Dose' axes, respectively (see Figure 3). From a strictly functional viewpoint however, the actual values of D_{max} and K_m do not need to be ascertained since normally only the (median) intersection point in the first quadrant is used in dosage prediction. Thus, a line drawn from the intersection point in the first quadrant to any desired C_{ss} value on the negative abscissa will cut the 'Dose' axis at the dose required, thereby obviating the need to substitute the values of K_m and D_{max} into Equation 5 [18, 19]. Although theoretically all concentration—dose data obeying Equation 3 should intersect at a common point in the first quadrant, in practice, due to experimental error, a number of intersection points may be observed when several concentration—dose lines are drawn [20]. Therefore, as more steady-state concentration—dose data are obtained, the best intersection point to use will be that representing the *median* of ½ n (n — 1) intersections, where n is the number of lines (see references 6, 8 and 20).
Studies using computer generated data to compare various techniques for relating steady-state serum phenytoin concentration and dose have shown that the DLP technique is superior to most of those based on linear rearrangements of Equation 3 [20]. (Of all graphical procedures investigated only Equation 6 was found to give estimates of K_m and D_{max} better than those obtained with the DLP [20]). Moreover, since the DLP technique is based on non-parametric estimates of K_m and D_{max} a single outlying value, due to analytical error in the determination of one steady-state concentration, will not alter the overall ('true') value of K_m and D_{max} when several concentration—dose data are used. In other words, when several concentration—dose data have been collected over the long-term, the DLP technique will readily indicate a single C_{ss} value which is inconsistent with a particular Michaelis-Menten relationship [20].
Speaking of the long-term, one advantage of the DLP in addition to its simplicity is that new concentration—dose data can be added as they become available, thus providing a permanent graphical record on which to base more and more precise individualized dosage predictions [18, 19]. By keeping such a simple graphical record, any appreciable changes in the values of K_m and D_{max} which might occur due to patient noncompliance or the introduction of concomitant therapy (induction or inhibition of phenytoin's metabolism causing changes in D_{max}) would become apparent [19, 20].

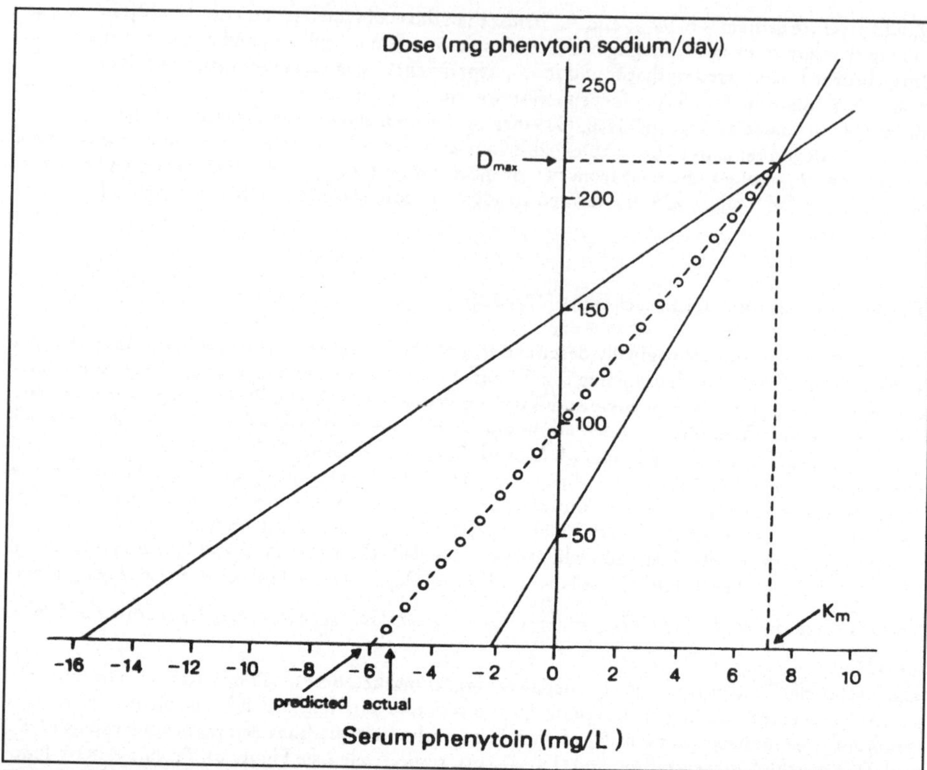

Figure 3: The direct linear plot (see text for details) as applied to the steady-state serum phenytoin concentration—dose data obtained for one patient. [23] From the intersection point of the highest and lowest concentration—dose values, a steady-state serum concentration of 6.0 mg/L is predicted on a dose of 100 mg/day in this case. (Reproduced with permission from *Br. J. Clin. Pharmacol. 4,* 733P—734P [1977])

Concluding Comments

With the availability of 25 mg capsules of sodium phenytoin it should now be possible to attain serum phenytoin concentrations consistent with optimal therapy in any patient, bearing in mind that the time to reach the steady-state will tend to increase with an increase in daily dose. Although not a substitute for clinical acumen, dosage individualization techniques such as the DLP [17, 18] should serve, nevertheless, as valuable tools in realizing the maximal therapeutic potential of this drug. The requirement of steady-state concentrations on two different doses however, should not limit their application since, after all, phenytoin is taken for long (often life-long) periods and frequent serum concentration monitoring is already generally accepted as being an essential part of successful antiepileptic drug therapy.

References

[1] Atkinson, A. J., Shaw, J. M: Pharmacokinetic study of a patient with diphenylhydantoin toxicity. *Clin. Pharmacol. Ther. 14,* 521—528 (1973).

[2] Bochner, F., Hooper, W. D., Tyrer, J. N., Eadie, M. J.: Effect of dosage increments on blood phenytoin concentrations. *J. Neurol, Neurosurg. Psychiatry 35,* 873—876 (1972).

[3] Borga, O., Garle, M., Gutová, M.: Identification of 5-(3,4-diphydroxyphenyl-5-)phenlyhydantoin as a metabolite of 5,5-diphenylhydantoin (phenytoin) in rats and man. *Pharmacology 7,* 129—137 (1972).

[4] Buchthal, F., Svensmark, O., Schiller, P. J.: Clinical and electroencephalographic correlations with serum levels of diphenylhydantoin. *Arch. Neurol. 2,* 624—630 (1960).

[5] Butler, T. C.: The metabolic conversion of 5,5-diphenylhydantoin to 5-(p-hydroxyphenyl)5-phenylhydantoin. *J. Pharmacol. Exp. Ther. 119,* 1—11 (1957).

[6] Cornish-Bowden, A., Eisenthal, R.: Statistical considerations in the estimation of enzyme kinetic parameters by the direct linear plot and other methods. *Biochem. J. 139,* 721—730 (1974).

[7] Dowd, J. E., Riggs, D. S.: A comparison of estimates of Michaelis-Menten kinetic constants from various linear transformation. *J. Biol. Chem. 240,* 863—869 (1965).

[8] Eisenthal, R., Cornish-Bowden, A.: The direct linear plot. A new graphical procedure for estimating enzyme kinetic parameters. *Biochem. J. 139,* 715—720 (1974).

[9] Garrettson, L. K., Jusko, W. J.: Diphenylhydantoin elimination kinetics in overdosed children. *Clin. Pharmacol. Ther. 17,* 481—491 (1975).

[10] Gerber, N., Wagner, J. G.: Explanation of dose-dependent decline of diphenylhydantoin plasma levels by fitting to the integrated form of the Michaelis-Menden equation. *Res. Commun. Chem. Pathol. Pharmacol. 3,* 455—466 (1972).

[11] Kutt, H., McDowell, F.: Management of epilepsy with diphenylhydantoin sodium. *J. Am. Med. Assoc. 203,* 969—972 (1968).

[12] Ludden, T. M., Allen, J. P., Schneider, L. W., Stavchansky, S. A.: Rate of phenytoin accumulation in man: A simulation study. *J. Pharmacokinet. Biopharm. 6,* 399—415 (1978).

[13] Ludden, T. M., Allen, J. P., Valutsky, W. A., Vicuna, A. V., Nappi, J. M., Hoffman, S. F., Wallace, J. E., Lalka, D., McNay, J. L.: Individualization of phenytoin dosage regimens. *Clin. Pharmacol. Ther. 21,* 287—293 (1977).

[14] Martin, E., Tozer, T. N., Sheiner, L. B., Riegelman, S.: The clinical pharmacokinetics of phenytoin. *J. Pharmacokinet. Biopharm. 5,* 579—596 (1977).

[15] Mawer, G. E., Mullen, P. W., Rodgers, M., Robins, A. J., Lucas, S. B.: Phenytoin dose adjustment in epileptic patients. *Br. J. Clin. Pharmacol. 1,* 163—168 (1974).

[16] Merritt, H. H., Putnam, T. J.: Sodium diphenyl hydantoinate in the treatment of convulsive disorders. *J. Am. Med. Assoc. 111,* 1068—1073 (1938).

[17] Michaelis, L., Menten, M. L.: Die Kinetik der Invertinwirkung. *Biochem. Z. 49,* 333—369 (1913).

[18] Mullen, P. W.: A novel graphical procedure for individualizing phenytoin therapy. *Br. J. Clin. Pharmacol. 4,* 733P—734P (1977).

[19] Mullen, P. W.: Optimal phenytoin therapy: A new technique for individualizing dosage. *Clin. Parmacol. Ther. 23,* 228—232 (1978).

[20] Mullen, P. W., Foster, R. W.: Comparative evaluation of six techniques for determining the Michaelis-Menden parameters relating phenytoin dose and steady-state serum concentrations. *J. Pharm. Pharmacol. 31,* 100—104 (1979).

[21] Perry, J. G., McKinney, L., De Weer, P.: The cellular mode of action of the anti-epileptic drug 5,5-diphenylhydantoin. *Nature 272,* 271—273 (1978).

[22] Rambeck, B., Boenigk, H. E., Dunlop, A., Mullen, P. W., Wadsworth, J., Richens, A.: Predicting phenytoin dose—a revised nomogram. *Therap. Drug Monitor. 1,* 325—333 (1979).

[23] Richens, A., Dunlop, A.: Serum phenytoin levels in management of epilepsy. *Lancet 2,* 247—248 (1975).

[24] Wagner, J. G.: Properties of the Michaelis-Menten equation and its integrated form which are useful in pharmacokinetics. *J. Pharmacokinet. Biopharm. 1,* 103—121 (1973).

[25] Wagner, J. G.: Time to reach steady-state and predicition of steady-state concentrations for drugs obeying Michaelis-Menten elimination kinetics. *J. Pharmacokinet. Biopharm. 6,* 209—225 (1978).

Drug monitoring in a clinical pharmacy laboratory: methods and case discussions

Tom B. Vree and Eppo van der Kleijn
Department of Clinical Pharmacy
Roelof van Dalen and Jules S. F. Gimbrère
Intensive Care Unit
Theo A. Thien and Frans T. M. Huysmans
Department of Internal Medicine, Division of Nephrology
Jan C. M. Hafkenscheid
Laboratory for Clinical Chemistry, Department of Internal Medicine
Theo H. M. Arts
Central Animal Laboratory
Sint Radboud hospital, University of Nijmegen, Nijmegen
The Netherlands.

Drug monitoring in small volumes (100 µl) of body fluids

The laboratory of Clinical Pharmacy in the Sint Radboud hospital at Nijmegen is charged with analyses on body fluids of drugs used in the hospital. The discrimination between routine and research analyses becomes vary vague when blood and urine concentration values are requested from patients with for instance liver- and kidney diseases or from severe hypertensive patients. In all these cases much research has to be carried out before the pharmacokinetics in all these situations are understood.
Several years ago we changed from gas chromatography to High Performance Liquid Chromatography for the analysis of the majority of drugs. It became possible to carry out the analysis in as little as 100 µl of plasma and in 5—10 µl of urine. With these small volumes and by simple precipitation of the proteins with perchloric acid we can reach the sensitivity limit of 300 ng/ml. When, as will be shown with the benzodiazepines, lower concentrations are expected, enrichment, by one simple extraction and evaporation step, can lower the limit to 30 ng/ml. The HPLC equipment of the laboratory consists of 4 Spectra Physics 3500B machines and 3 "home made" machines. The columns used are all Lichrosorb RP8, particle size 5 u and by merely varying the solvent, we are able to analyse all the compounds mentioned.
The routing in the development of an analysis proceeds as follows: first HPLC analysis, then construction of the calibration curves followed by an animal experiment in order to check the kinetics of the drug and to check whether the method is reliable or not. Volunteers then take the drug for analysis of the kinetics of distribution, metabolism and renal excretion in healthy persons before samples from patients reach the laboratory.
The small sample volume of plasma makes it possible to collect blood with a simple finger-tip punc-

ture, which can be done by a collegue or by oneself. The advantage is that about 15—20 samples can be taken at time intervals according to the pharmacokinetics of the drug, even at night time at home. Some of the results obtained with this procedure are included below.

Methods

Apparatus:

A Spectra Physics 3500B high-performance liquid chromatograph was used, equipped with a spectrophotometer with variable wavelength detection (model 770). The detector was connected to a lmV recorder (BD 7; Kipp and Zonen, Emmen, The Netherlands). A stainless-steel column, 10 cm × 4.6 mm I.D., packed with Lichrosorb RP8, particle size 5 µm, was used. The injection loop was 100 µl size.
The solvents used for the analysis of the drugs and their metabolites are described elsewhere [4—10].

Subjects and patients:

The subjects who participated in these studies are employees of the Departments of Clinical Pharmacy and of Nephrology of the hospital. The patients in the study on Cephalosporins are recruited from the Intensive Care Unit.
Full details of each analysis are given elswhere [4—10].

Results and case discussions

Diazoxide

Figure 1 shows the kinetics of diazoxide in a healthy physician of the Department of Nephrology. Diazoxide appears to exhibit a relatively short halflife time of elimination of 17 hrs. However, in severe hypertensive patients this $T_{\frac{1}{2}}$ ranges from 40—50 hrs. In the first 15 hrs after intravenous administration a plateau in the plasma concentration curve is observed, an effect which is more pronounced in patients. The saliva concentration is lower and parallels the plasma concentration. In the urine only 16.5% is excreted unchanged. At first sight there is no direct correlation between renal excretion or clearance and urine flow. The relationship between renal excretion rate (µg/min) and plasma concentration (µg/ml) appears linear, showing an average renal clearance of about 5 ml/min. This renal clearance is controlled by tubular reabsorption phenomena as the renal clearance of Diazoxide is related to the urine flow ($r = 0.81$) and not to the urinary pH ($r = 0.25$). Tubular secretion does not occur because co-medication of probenecid has no influence on the renal clearance of diazoxide in man. [4]

Benzodiazepines

Quite different problems are encountered with benzodiazepines such as Diazepam which is metabolized into N-desmethyldiazepam, oxydiazepam and oxazepam. Two metabolic pathways are involved, N-oxidation and C-hydroxylation. For severeal years only Diazepam and N-desmethyldiazepam could be analysed, but just recently we succeeded in separating all 4 benzodiazepines in one simple run [5]. Diazepam in a dog is very quickly metabolized to N-desmethyldiazepam, which can be expected since N-oxidation is a very fast process. C-hydroxylation of N-desmethyldiazepam into oxazepam is some what less rapid, and as soon as oxazepam is formed, it is conjugated and oxazepamglucuronide becomes the second important metabolite [5]. The direct hydroxylation of diazepam is also a slow process and is followed instantaneously by N-oxidation to oxazepam and glucuronidation. This is the reason why only a small amounts of oxydiazepam-glucuronide can be detected. N-desmethyldiazepam is slowly hydroxylated at the C_3-position to oxazepam, which is rapidly glucuronidated (Figure 2). Which of the stereo isomers (+) or (−) oxazepamglucuronide is preferentially formed is not yet known [3]. The rapid conversion of oxydiazepam into its glucuronide and oxazepam is an intrinsic property of the compound itself (Figure 3). The rate of the N-oxidation is about

the same order as that for the glucuronidation. The rapid glucuronidation of oxazepam in the dog is also an intrinsic behaviour of the compound. Free oxazepam is hardly excreted in the urine (0.07%), oxazepamglucuronide is the main compound excreted (24.5% in 7 hrs).
In volunteers it was interesting to see whether oxazepam was glucuronidated and excreted faster than oxydiazepam. Both compounds were therefore administered orally together in small doses (6—14 mg) and the

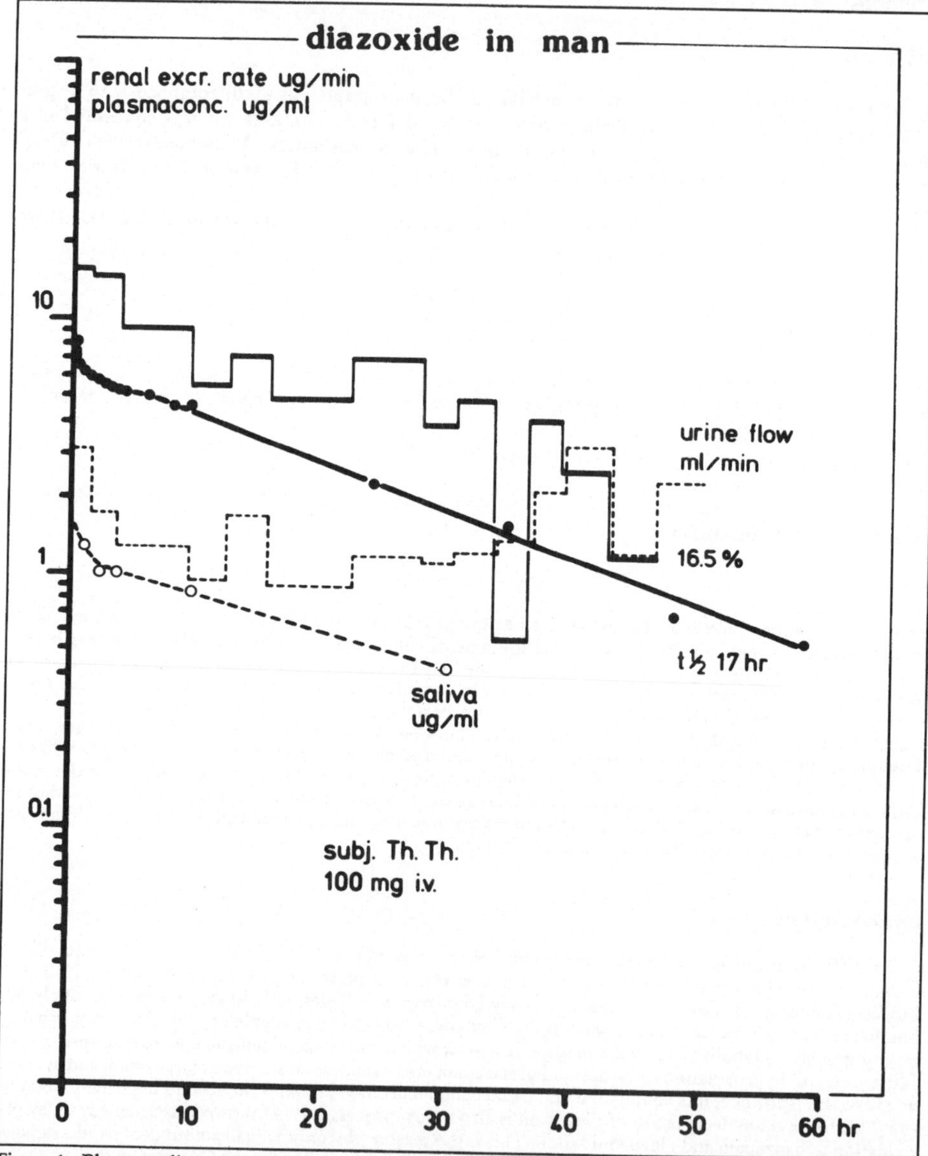

Figure 1: Plasma, saliva concentration and renal excretion rate—time profiles of diazoxide after an intravenous dose of 100 mg in a volunteer.
There appeared to be a constant ratio between the plasma and saliva concentration (ratio 4.8). The urinary pH in this experiment has been kept alkaline (pH 7.70 ± 0.49 SD)

renal excretion was followed for 60 hrs. Both compounds exhibit almost the same half life time of elimination (7 hrs). In addition, oxazepam occassionally exhibits diurnal behaviour (Figure 4). It can be observed that during night time the renal excretion rate of oxazepamglucuronide is much lower than during day time. When we put the day time curves together, the half life of elimination of the day time curve is 3 hrs, while that of the total curve is 6.5 hrs. It is not certain whether this is the result of decreased enzyme activity or decreased renal excretion. When the two drugs are ingested simultaneously side effects occur resembling alcohol intoxication followed by drowsiness and sleep. When the compounds are administered separately in these small doses, these effects are not noticed.

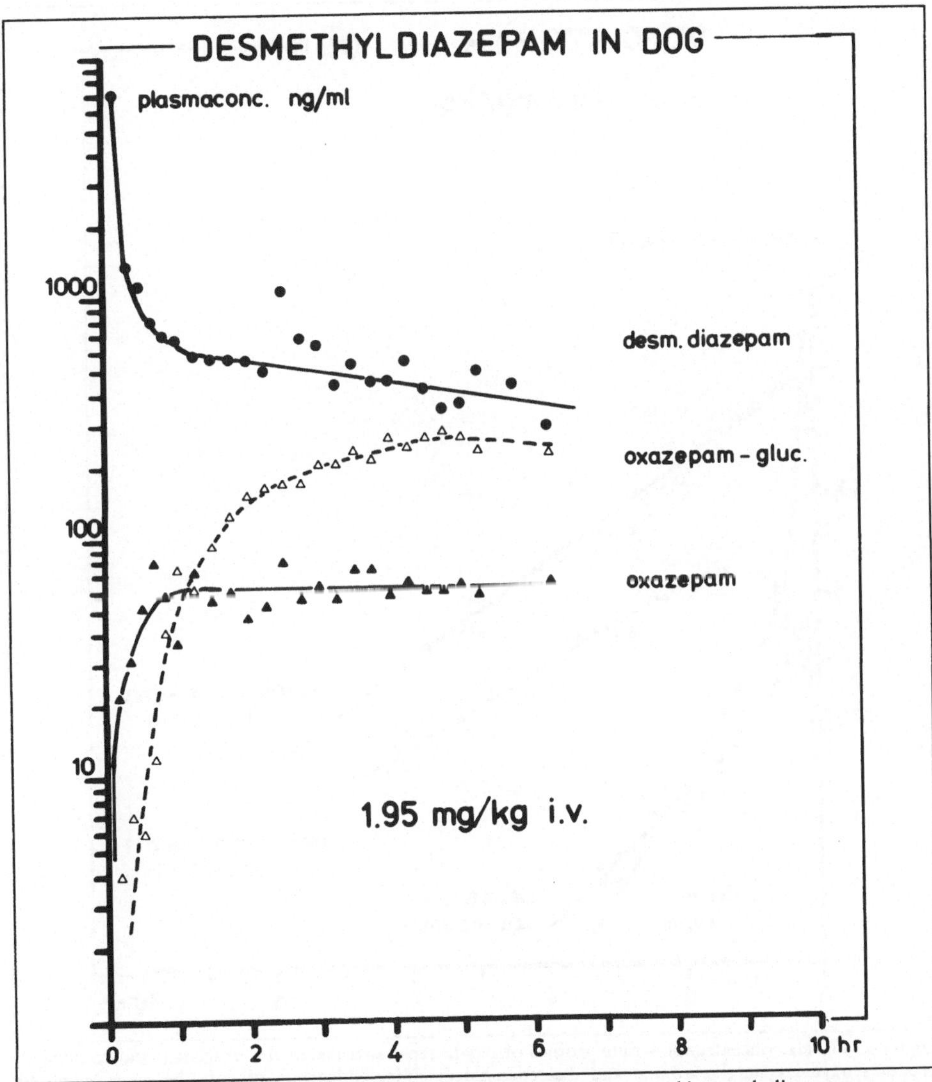

Figure 2: Plasma concentration—time profiles of N-desmethyldiazepam and its metabolites oxazepam and oxazepamglucuronide in a beagle dog after intravenous administration of N-desmethyldiazepam.

Sulphonamides

The HPLC technique offers the possibility of measuring the parent compound as well as the N_4-acetyl derivatives [6]. The study was started when the Intensive Care Unit addressed the laboratory with the question whether it was possible and meaningful to measure plasma concentrations of co-trimoxazole (Bactrimel®), sulphamethoxazole and trimethoprim. At this moment questions of acetylation and renal excretion processes are subjects of studies with other para-amino phenolic compounds. As is known, sulphadimidine shows the best differences between *'fast'* and *'slow'* acetylators (Figure 5). The $T_{½}$ of elimination of sulphadimidine, in a 'fast' acetylator is 1.5 hr, and in a 'slow' acetylator 5.5 hrs. The variation in the $T_{½}$ of the main metabolite N_4-acetylsulphadimidine in 'fast' and 'slow' acetylators range from 5—7 hrs. In clinical practice

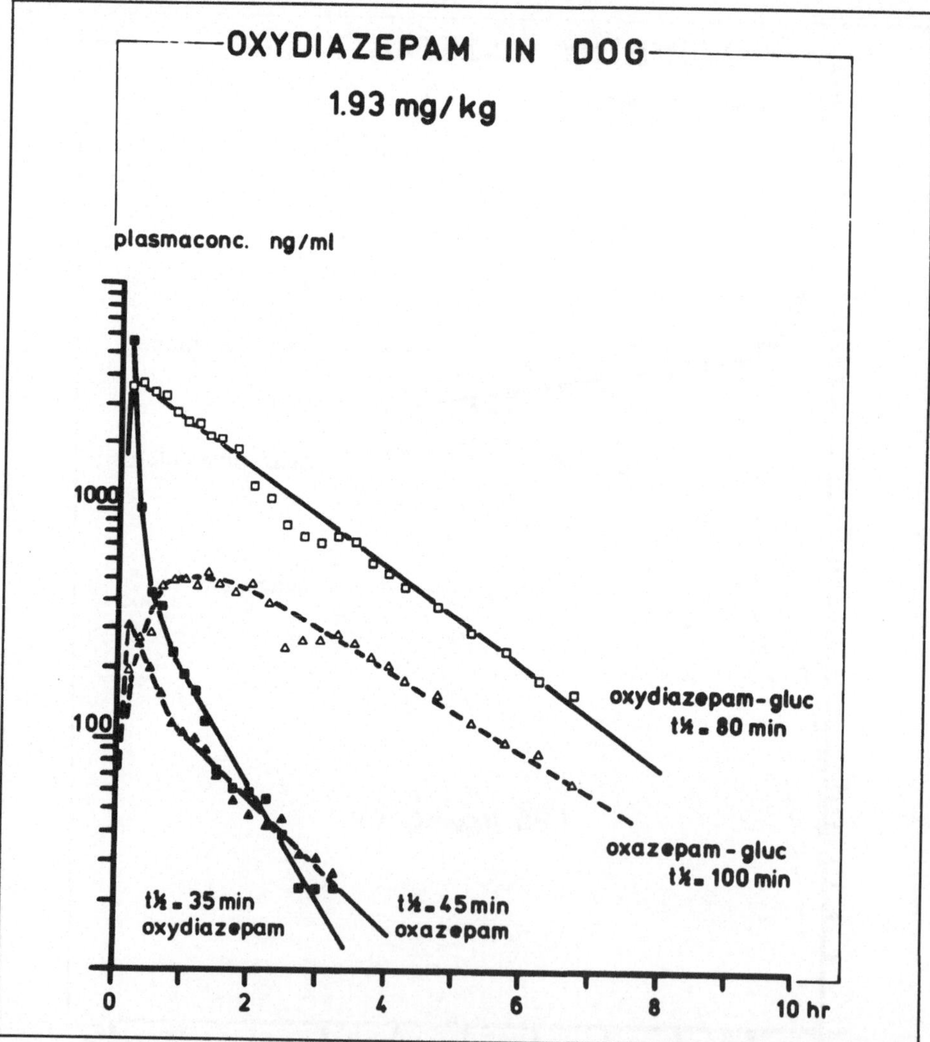

Figure 3: Plasma concentration—time profiles of oxydiazepam, its metabolite oxazepam and conjugated products oxydiazepamglucuronide and oxazepamglucuronide. Glucuronidation is the main metabolic pathway. Renal excretion of the glucuronides is the main pathway in excretion as little free drug is excreted.

there appears no standard method for *acetylator phenotyping*. At this moment 11 different methods or modifications, without any rationale, have been described. One of the oldest and widely used methods to express acetylation is to calculate the N_4-acetylsulphonamide derivative as a percentage of the total amount of sulphonamide in a single plasma or urine sample. The best way however to express the percentage of N_4-acetylsulphonamide derivative is to construct a percentage N_4-acetylderivative-time profile for a sufficiently long time period. The result is a more reliable separation between 'fast' and 'slow' acetylators (Figure 6). The picture looks like an infusion of N_4-acetylsulphadimidine and in fact may be regarded as a metabolite infusion. When the percentage N_4-acetylsulphonamide is plotted logarithmically, the residual curves give the rate of acetylation and again the $T\frac{1}{2}$ of 'fast' acetylation is 2 hrs, while that of the 'slow' acetylators is 5.5 hrs [7].

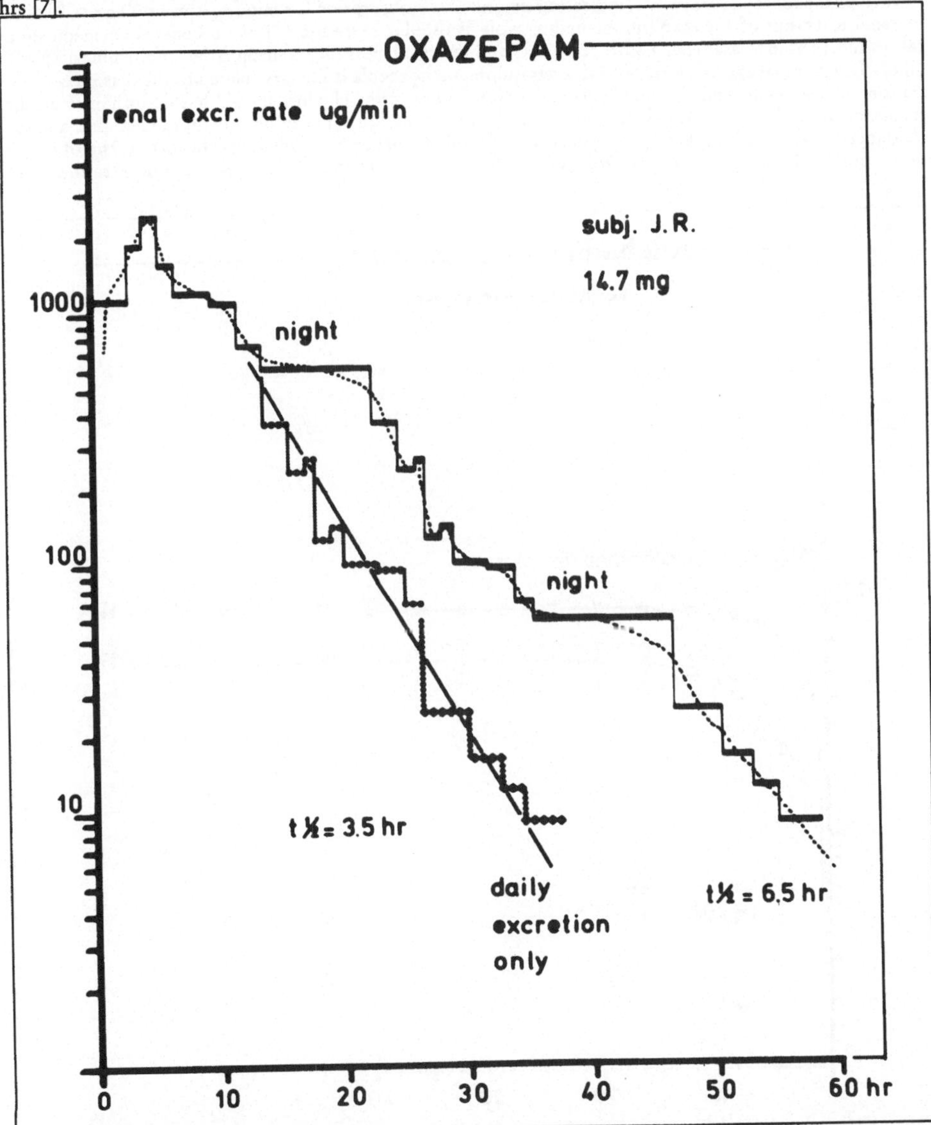

Figure 4: Renal excretion rate of oxazepamglucuronide in a human volunteer after an oral dose of 14.7 mg oxazepam. Note the difference in renal excretion rate during day and night time.

Sulphamethoxazole in contrast shows no difference between 'fast' and 'slow' acetylation. Thus there is no need for phenotyping to adjust the dosage [8].

In Figure 7 the differences in rate of acetylation between different sulphonamides (-dimidine, -pyridine, and -diazine) are shown. Sulphadimidine and sulphapyridine show the largest differences between 'fast' and 'slow' acetylators, although their mechanism of acetylation is different. Sulphadiazine cannot be used for phenotyping.

When N_4-acetylsulphamethoxazole is administered as a parent compound, it is eliminated by renal excretion only, with an elimination half-time of 3.5 hrs [9]. This half-time is much shorter than when N_4-acetylsulphamethoxazole is eliminated as the metabolite of sulphamethoxazole (9 hrs). The urine flow has no influence on the renal excretion rate, indicating that tubular reabsorption is a minor pathway. The mechanism of renal excretion of N_4-acetylsulphamethoxazole is tubular excretion [1] as probenecid co-medication causes the $T\frac{1}{2}$ to increase from 3.5 hrs to 7.0 hrs and the renal clearance to drop from 49 ml/min to 15 ml/min [10]. The renal excretion rate of N_4-acetylsulphamethoxazole is linearly related to the plasma concentration and the renal clearance and is normally about 49 ml/min. The urinary pH has no influence on the renal clearance of N_4-acetylsulphamethoxazole. As no correlation between the creatinine clearance and the clearance of N_4-acetyl sulphamethoxazole can be found, it must be concluded that the mechanism of excretion is purely tubular [1]. A linear relationship between renal excretion rate and plasma concentration is not

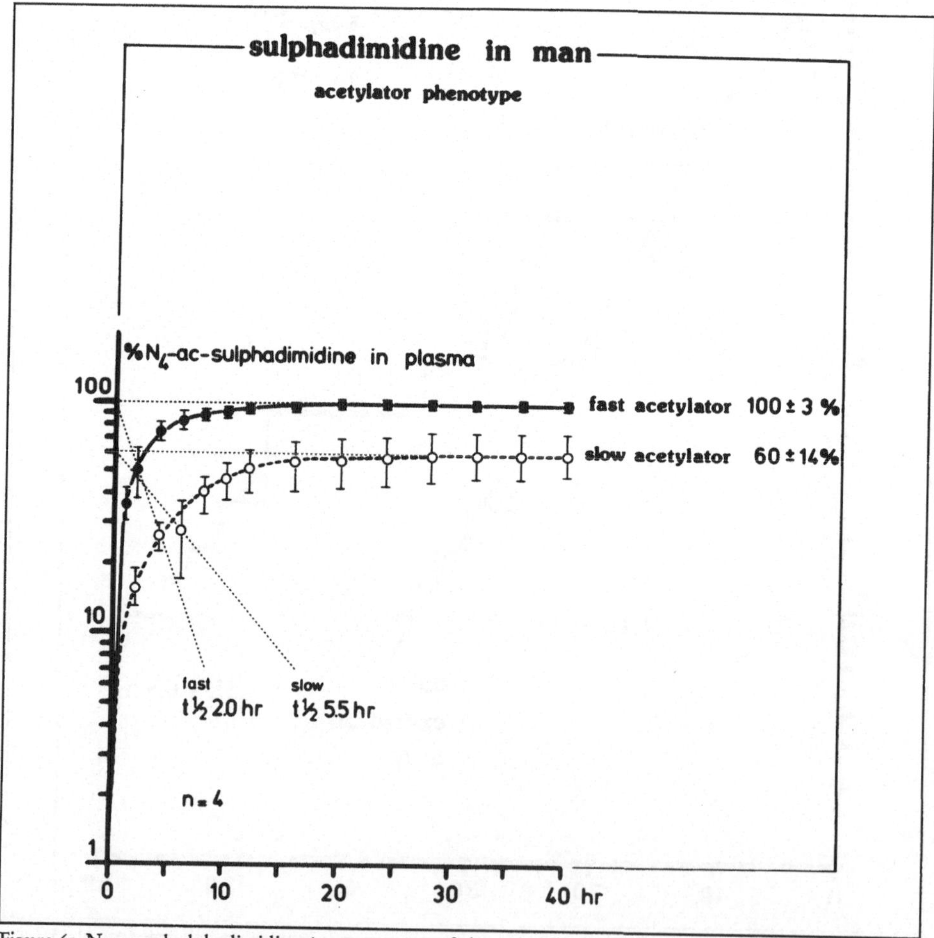

Figure 6: N_4-acetylsulphadimidine (as percentage of the sum of parent compound and metabolite)—time profiles in 'fast' and 'slow' acetylators.

always apparent. N4-acetylsulphamethoxazole as metabolite may show a totally different behaviour. In Figure 8 two different excretion processes may be distinguished. The solid line represents the situation when the plasma concentration of N4-acetylsulphamethoxazole is still rising as result of mainly metabolism. Then, at the maximum plasma concentration there is a change in renal clearance until the elimination phase is dominating. In the final elimination phase, the renal clearance is just half that of the initial process (20 over 51 ml/min). These 'loop' phenomena may be the result of a time constant in reaching equilibrium in the renal excretion. The fact that some kidneys do and others do not show these phenomena, and that sometimes the initial process is slower than the latter process, obscures the mechanisms of renal excretion. The curves of sulphapyridine show capacity limited phenomena of parent drug and its metabolite N4-ace-

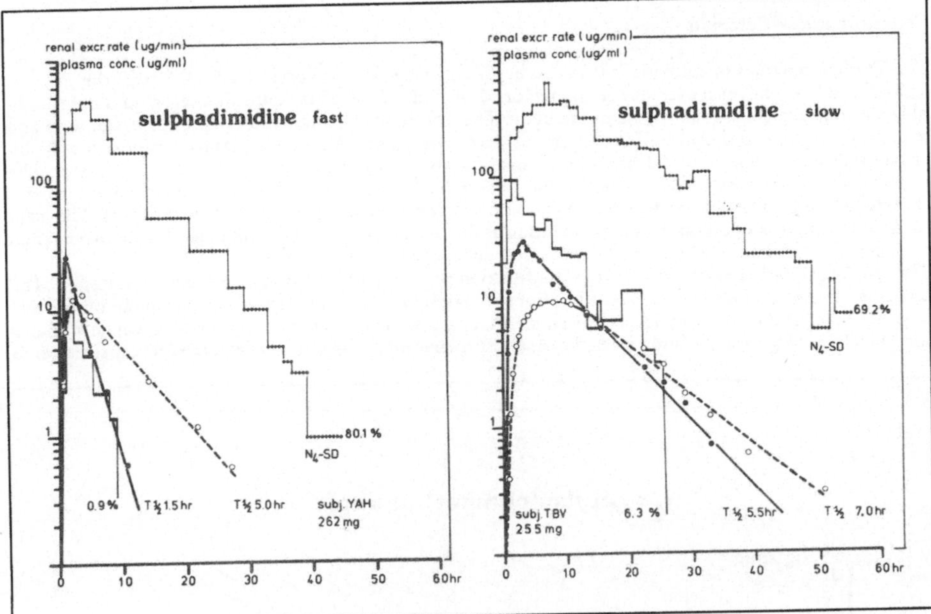

Figure 5: Plasma concentration and renal excretion rate—time profiles of sulphadimidine and N4-acetylsulphadimidine in a 'fast' acetylator (left) and 'slow' acetylator (right). Note the difference between the T½ of elimination of sulphadimidine in the 'fast' (T½ = 1.5 hrs) and 'slow' acetylator (T½ = 5.5 hrs).

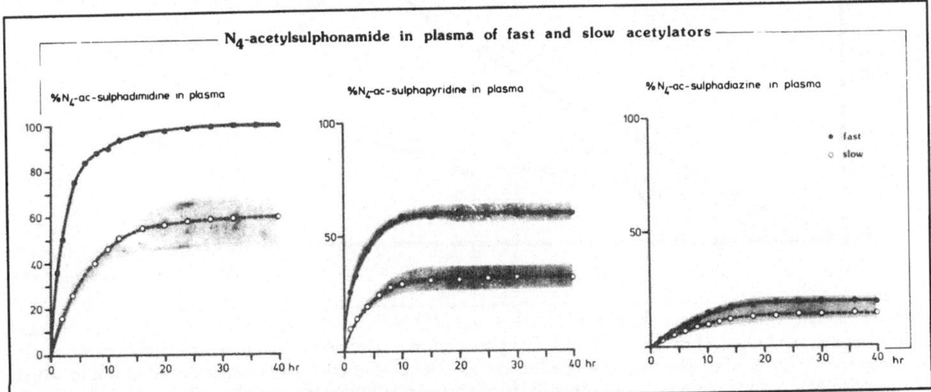

Figure 7: Percentage of N4-acetylsulphadimidine, N4-acetylsulphapyridine and N4-acetylsulphadiazine—time curves in 'fast' and 'slow' acetylators.

tylsulphapyridine. The curve of sulphapyridine shows capacity limited tubular secretion and reabsorption [2]. As stated before, each kidney has its own capacity limits and excretes the sulphonamides in its own specific way. All investigated N_4-acetylsulphonamide derivatives are excreted by tubular excretion. Their clearance cannot be related with the creatinine clearance, nor with urine flow or urine pH. The tubular excretion can be inhibited by probenecid. In fact, it appears that the renal clearance of N_4-acetylsulphamethoxazole can be reduced from 50 ml/min to 15 ml/min. Sulphamethoxazole itself shows the same renal clearance rate with or without probenecid accounting for about 5 ml/min. The influence of probenecid and the mechanism of tubular excretion can elegantly be demonstrated with the antibiotic cefoxitin, a new member of the cephalosporins.

Cephalosporins—Cefoxitin

The $T_{½}$ of elimination of cefoxitin is 0.5—1.0 hr. With probenecid in doses of 1.5—2.0 gram the $T_{½}$ is increased to 2 hrs. The renal excretion accounts for 100% of the dose. This means that cefoxitin is not metabolized during the short time-course in the body. The difference in elimination rate of cefoxitin with and without probenecid is shown in Figure 9. In this particular patient the normal plasma curve tends to be biphasic with a nominal $T_{½}$ of 1.3 hr. With co-medication of probenecid the $T_{½}$ increases to 2.0 hrs. The plasma concentration of probenecid is also shown and the $T_{½}$ of probenecid is 7 hrs. Inhibition of cefoxitin elimination only appears when the plasma concentration of probenecid is higher than 25 µg/ml. The main route of elimination of probenecid is metabolism, as the renal clearance of the compound is about 5 ml/min and only about 5% of the dose can be recovered unchanged from the urine.
The renal clearance constant of cefoxitin is a function of glomerular filtration and tubular secretion. The cefoxitin clearance at low plasma concentrations is mainly tubular secretion with a maximum of 447 ml/min. At higher plasma concentrations, the glomerular part of the clearance becomes visible, which accounts for 84 ml/min (Figure 10c). With co-medication of probenecid in the same patient, the tubular secretion is

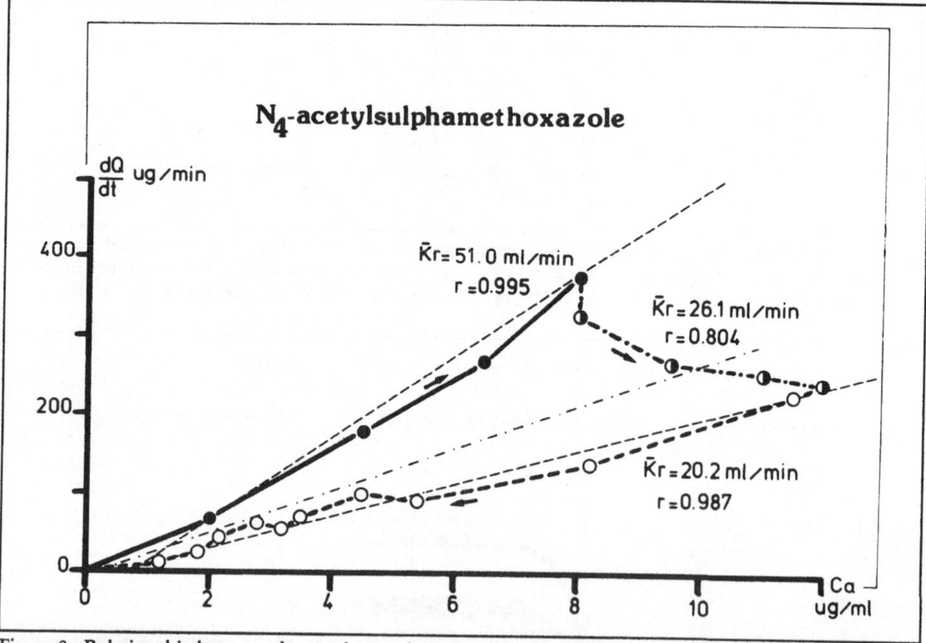

Figure 8: Relationship between the renal excretion rate (dQ/dt) and plasma concentration (C_A) of N_4-acetylsulphamethoxazole in a human volunteer. The proportionality constant, being the renal clearance, is different in the different time periods during elimination. The closed circles represent the situation in which N_4-acetylsulphamethoxazole is predominantly formed from sulphamethoxazole and in which its plasma concentration is still rising. The open circles represent the situation in which the metabolite is mainly excreted and the plasma concentration is decreasing.

blocked and the resulting clearance is only caused by glomerular filtration as shown by the dashed line. It turned out that in this case the glomerular filtration of the compound is 79 ml/min, which means that probenecid does not affect the glomerular filtration. It only blocks the anion transport mechanisms of the tubules and in this way inhibits the tubular transport of cefoxitin. The renal clearance of cefoxitin seems to depend on urine flow. The net tubular excretion is about 450 ml/min, but since the clearance is flow dependent, there must also be a considerable reabsorption by the tubules (Figure 10a). Creatinine is less flow dependent than cefoxitin. Creatinine is cleared 80% by glomerular filtration and 20% by tubular secretion. Also the correlation ($r = 0.596$) between the creatinine clearance and the urine flow is much lower than for cefoxitin ($r = 0.769$).

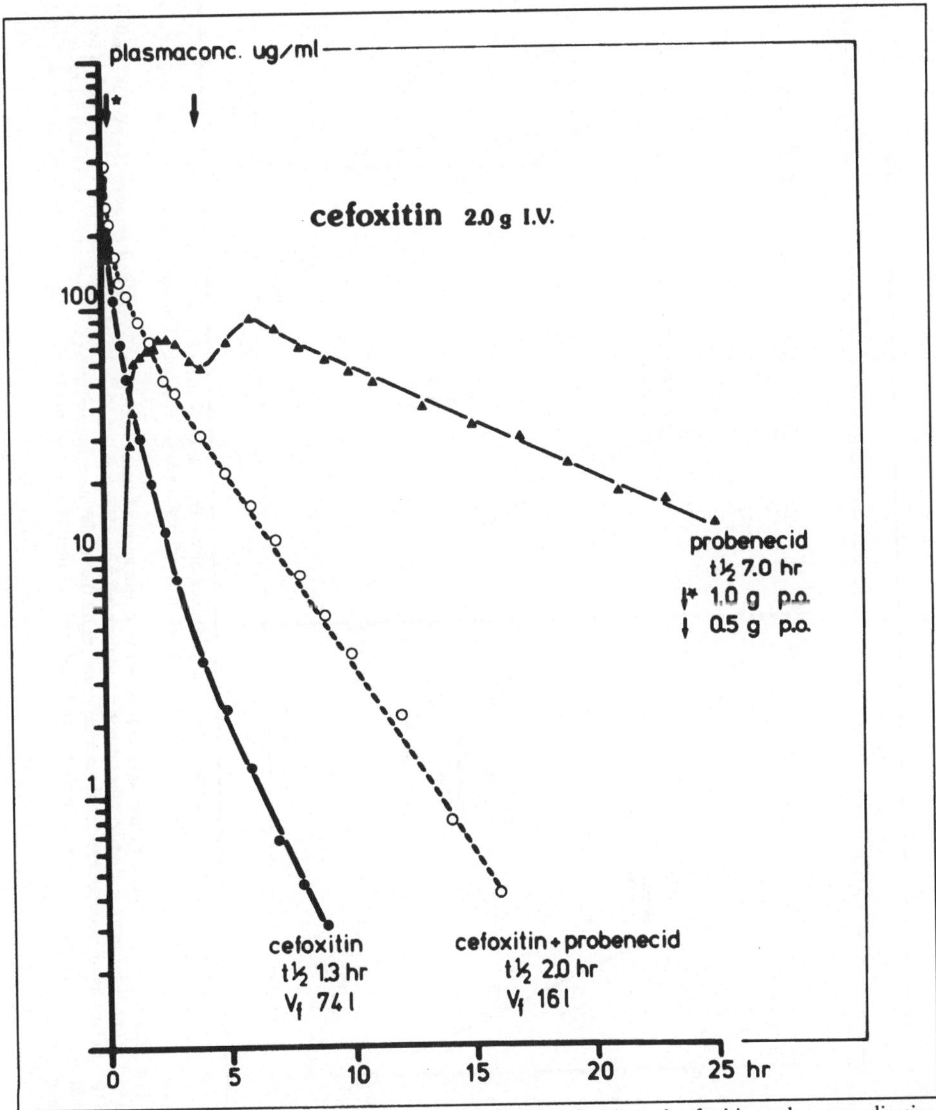

Figure 9: Plasma concentration—time curves of probenecid, cefoxitin and cefoxitin under co-medication of probenecid.

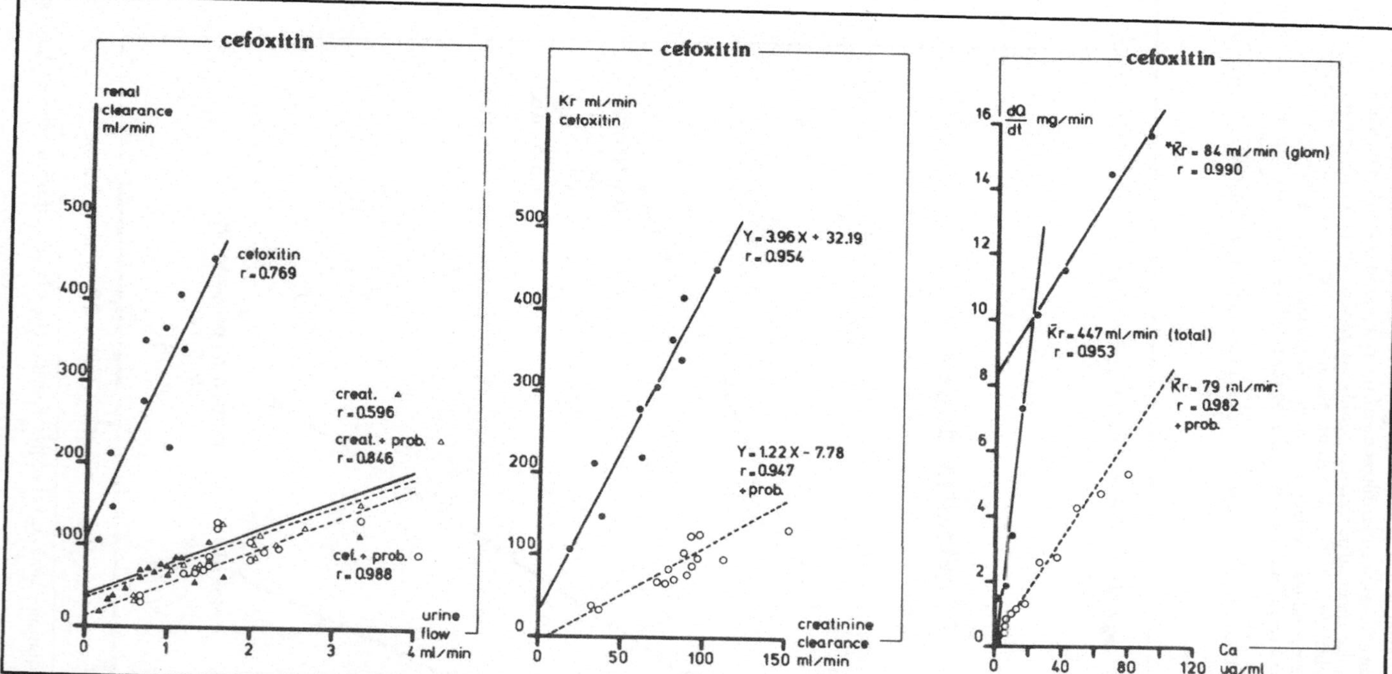

Figure 10a: Relationship ($r = 0.769$) between the renal clearance of cefoxitin and creatinine ($r = 0.596$) with the urine flow. These relationships also exists under co-medication of probenecid, though the actual values of the clearance and the slope of the regression line of cefoxitin (+ probenecid) is much lower ($r = 0.846$).
Figure 10b: Relationship between the renal clearances of cefoxitin and creatinine with ($r = 0.947$) and without ($r = 0.954$) probenecid co-medication. With probenecid co-medication the ratio between cefoxitin and the creatinine clearance is 1.22, indicating that the cefoxitin is cleared by glomerular filtration only.
Figure 10c: Relationship between the renal excretion rate (dQ/dt) and plasma concentration (C_A) of cefoxitin with and without probenecid as co-medication. Note that the glomerular part of the renal excretion of cefoxitin accounts for 84 ml/min ($r = 0.990$), which is 79 ml/min ($r = 0.982$) under the co-medication of probenecid.

The dashed lines represent the same situation under influence of probenecid. The steep regression line of the cefoxitin—urine flow relationship is reduced (open circles) and is now within the range of regression lines of creatinine. Also the regression line of creatinine with probenecid is somewhat lower. This is the second indication that the tubular secretory function is completely occupied by probenecid and that in this case cefoxitin and creatinine are excreted by the same glomerular filtration process. When the renal clearance of both cefoxitin and creatinine are dependent on the same parameter, 'urine flow,' then of course the renal clearance of cefoxitin is related to the creatinine clearance. From Figure 10b it can be seen that the cefoxitin clearance is about 4 times the creatinine clearance. With probenecid, the cefoxitin clearance is 1.2 times the creatinine clearance. Thus from these ratios it can be calculated that the tubular secretion rate of cefoxitin is 3.2 times the glomerular filtration rate.
The presence of probenecid in the body does not necessarily imply inhibition of the tubular secretion. As stated before the minimal plasma concentration of probenecid at which inhibition can be noticed is 25 µg/ml. In patient HR, shown in Figure 11, probenecid was administered in two separate doses of 1.0 gram followed by 0.5 gram 5 hrs later. 2 grams of cefoxitin was injected intravenously and the $T_{\frac{1}{2}}$ of elimination of cefoxitin appeared to be 1.5 hrs. The $T_{\frac{1}{2}}$ of probenecid is 6.25 hrs 26 hours after the first injection of cefoxitin at a probenecid concentration of about 4—5 µg/ml. A second dose of 2 grams of cefoxitin was injected

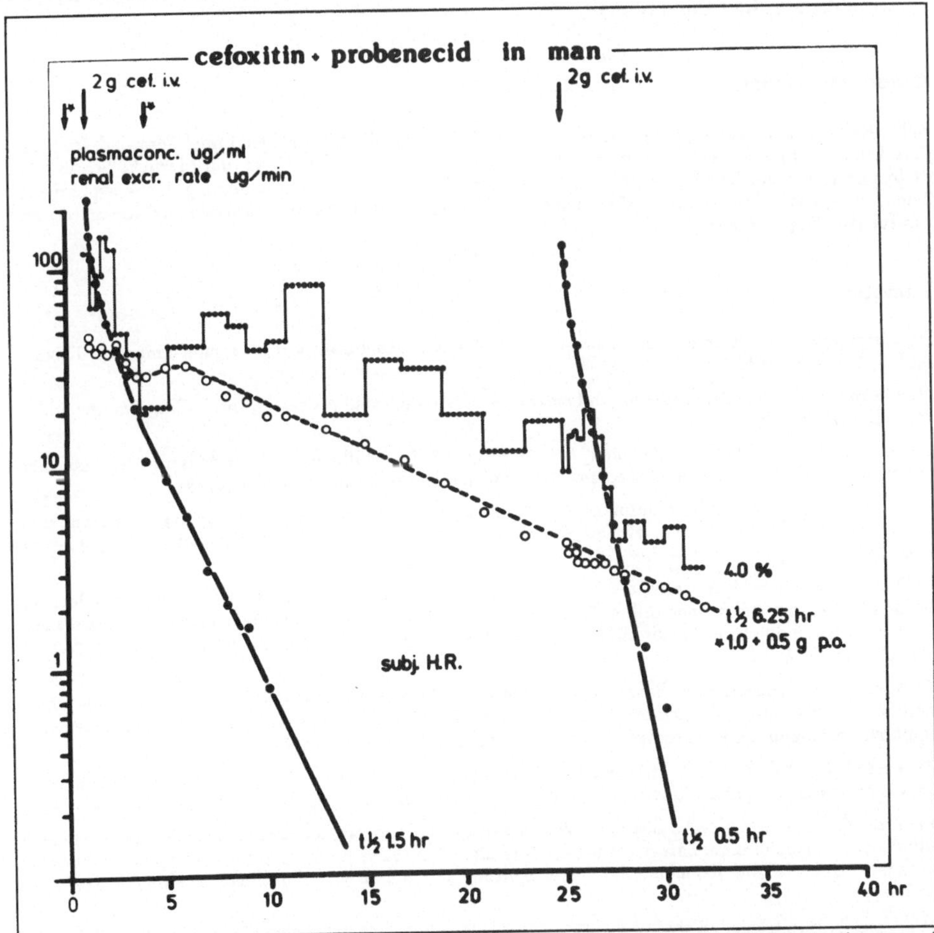

Figure 11: Plasma concentration-time curves of cefoxitin and probenecid and the renal excretion rate of probenecid. Note that cefoxitin is inhibited only in the first dose when the plasma concentration of probenecid is high (> 25 µg/ml).

intravenously, which resulted in a T½ of elimination of 0.5 hrs. Thus it might be concluded that only at high (> 25 μg/ml) plasma concentrations of probenecid is the tubular secretion of cefoxitin inhibited. Renal excretion of probenecid as shown in the figure proceeds as usual, 4% is excreted unchanged.

Conclusion

The small volume of biological fluid required for the analysis enables blood samples obtained with the simple fingertip puncture to be used. However, blood samples alone are not enough. Blood samples provide the overall elimination constant, but without urine samples one of the elimination parameters is completely missed. Therefore it is desirable to take as many blood and urine samples as possible, in order to measure renal clearance phenomena. The renal parameters of each drug should be completely understood before a drug is administered to a patient with impaired kidney function. The few examples shown in this article, obtained through cooperation with the clinical departments, are taken from larger studies and are meant to give an idea how the department of Clinical Pharmacy works in the Sint Radboud hospital.

Acknowledgements

Bill O'Reilly, Chiel Hekster, Pieter Guelen, Marijn Oosterbaan, Fred Schobben, Emiel Termond, Ita Baars, Joke Damsma, Joke Reekers, Francis Hurkmans, Tineke Lenselink, Rita Dirks and Marijcke Schoots van de Siepkamp are thanked for skilful assistance, helpful discussions and volunteering in the experiments. The nursing staff of the Intensive Care Unit and Clinical Departments are acknowledged for correct and careful sampling of the patients.

Literature:

[1] Despopoulus, A.; A defenition of substrate specificity in renal transport of organic anions. J. Theoret. Biol. *8*, 163—192 (1965)

[2] Garrett, E. R., Pharmacokinetics and clearances related to renal processes. Int. J. Clin. Pharmacol. *16*, 155—172 (1978)

[3] Ruelius, H. W., Tio, C. O., Knowles, J. A., McHugh, S. L., Schillings, R. T., and Sisenwine, S. F.; Diastereoisomeric glucuronides of oxazepam. Drug Metabolism & Disp. *7*, 40—43 (1979)

[4] Vree, T. B., Lenselink, B., Huysmans, F.T.M., Fleuren, H.L.J., and Thien, Th. A.; Rapid determination of Diazoxide in plasma and urine of man by means of high performance liquid chromatography. J. Chromatog. Biomed. Appl. *164*, 220—234 (1979)

[5] Vree, T. B., Baars, A. M., Hekster, Y. A., van der Kleijn, E., and O'Reilly, W. J.; Simultaneous determination of diazepam and its metabolites N-desmethyldiazepam, oxydiazepam and oxazepam in plasma and urine of man and dog by means of high performance liquid chromatography. J. Chromatog. Biomed. Appl. *162*, 605—614 (1979)

[6] Vree, T. B., Hekster, Y. A, Baars, A. M., Damsma, J. E., and van der Kleijn, E.; Determination of trimethoprim and sulphamethoxazole (Co-trimoxazole) in body fluids of man by means of high performance liquid chromatography. J. Chromatog. Biomed Appl. *146*, 103—112 (1978)

[7] Vree, T. B., O'Reilly, W. J., Hekster, Y. A., Damsma, J. E., and van der Kleijn, E.; Determination of the acetylator type and pharmacokinetics of some sulphonamides in man. Clin. Pharmacokin. (1980) In press.

[8] Vree, T. B., Hekster, Y. A., Baars, A. M., Damsma, J. E., and van der Kleijn, E.; Pharmacokinetics of sulphamethoxazole in man. Effects of urinary pH and Urine flow on metabolism and renal excretion of sulphamethoxazole and its metabolite N_4-acetylsulphamethoxazole. Clin. Pharmacokin. *3*, 319—329 (1978)

[10] Vree, T. B., Hekster, Y. A., and van der Kleijn, E.; Clinical pharmacokinetics of sulphonamides. In: The serum concentration of drugs. Ed. F. Merkus. Exerpta Medica, Elsevier, 1979.

Drug utilisation and single and multiple dose pharmacokinetic and pharmacodynamic studies in assessing the influence of old age on drug action

I. H. Stevenson
Department of Pharmacology and Therapeutics
Nivewells Hopsital and Medical School

Although the elderly have often been thought to be more sensitive than younger patients to the action of many drugs, there is a marked lack firstly, of actual data which supports this and secondly, of evidence as to any mechanisms which may operate. In a programme to examine the influence of old age on drug action several different approaches have been used as follows:

(1) Drug Utilisation Studies

In a retrospective survey of the records of hospitalised patients receiving warfarin, warfarin dose was found to decrease significantly with age whereas the anticoagulant effect increased, despite the lower dose. A further prospective study in out-patients also produced evidence of an increased warfarin dose-effect relationship in the elderly.

(2) Drug Plasma Steady-State Levels

Studies carried out in out-patients attending a thyroid clinic demonstrated that the steady state plasma levels of propranolol increased significantly with age of patient and that age was the most important single determinant of plasma propranolol steady state level.

(3) Single Dose Pharmacokinetic Studies

Evidence has been obtained of a decreased elimination (plasma half-life or clearance) of antipyrine, phenylbutazone, aspirin and quinine in elderly subjects. With warfarin on the other hand, no alteration in either of these parameters occurred. In a study to assess possible age-related changes in the effects of inducing agents, the plasma elimination of antipyrine and quinine was determined in young and elderly subjects before and after 2 weeks treatment with hypnotic doses of the inducing agent dichloralphenazone. The plasma clearance of both drugs was significantly increased post-dose in the young but not in the elderly group.

(4) Single Dose Pharmacodynamic Studies

In young and elderly patients given a single dose of warfarin, the hypoprothrombinaemic response was found to be greater in the elderly group. Further investigation indicated that at the same plasma warfarin level the suppression of the clotting factor synthesis was greater in the elderly group.

(5) Multiple Dose Pharmacodynamic Studies

In hyperthyroid patients on propranolol therapy, the ratio percentage reduction in exercise heart rate/plasma propranolol steady state concentration was used as an index of sensitivity to propranolol and was found to correlate negatively with age, suggesting a reduced sensitivity to propranolol in the elderly.

Chapter 6

Liver function tests and hepatic drug metabolism

Liver function tests and elimination of drugs in man

Ulrich Klotz

Dr. Margarete Fischer-Bosch-Institut für Klinische Pharmakologie,
Auerbachstr. 112, 7000 Stuttgart 50

Introduction

The intensity and duration of a drug's action is dependent on its rate of elimination. For many compounds this process takes place in the liver. Therefore the characterisation of liver function is important for a safe and effective drug treatment. Alterations in liver function can intensify or diminish the therapeutic and toxic effects. From a prospective drug surveillance study of 1280 patients the frequency of adverse drug reactions was higher in 333 patients with clinical and/or histopathological evidence of liver cirrhosis than in 188 with other liver diseases ($p<0.01$) and than in 759 patients without liver disease ($p<0.0001$). Side effects were more common for drugs biotransformed by the liver [10]. The large, well known interpatient variability in the response to a standard dose might be, at least partially, due to differences in liver function. Consequently, in recent years many attempts were made to individualize drug therapy based upon pharmacokinetic considerations. As a result of these pharmacokinetic studies it became apparent that many factors influence the hepatic elimination of drugs, such as genetic constitution, environment (pollutants), nutrional status, age, sex, smoking habits or concomitantly given drugs. Various disease states, which alter the protein bindung or cardiac output, can also influence the disposition of drugs. Liver function varies widely within any diagnosed group of patients. Difficulties also occur in the selection of the correct and comparable control individuals. Many investigators have studied changes in the half-life ($T_{1/2}$) under the assumption that this parameter directly reflects drug metabolism or excretion by the liver. While this may indeed be a correct presumption for a few drugs with specific characteristics it is not generally valid. This is because $T_{1/2}$ is dependent on both the total body clearance ($\overline{Cl}$) of the drug and its apparent distribution volume (Vd_β):

$$T_{1/2(\beta)} = \frac{0.693 \times Vd_\beta}{\overline{Cl}}$$

Physiological variables, such as hepatic blood flow, drug metabolizing activity/capacity and plasma binding also determine the elimination of drugs. Certain diseases may affect more than one of these determinants, and thereby exaggerate or dampen any effect associated with altered hepatocyte function alone. The clearance concept is of particular value in this regard, since it is independent of distributional changes and is a direct measure of the efficiency of drug removal from a biological fluid. Pharmacokinetically, total body clearance ($\overline{Cl}$) can be calculated, independent of the compartment model used, by the equation:

$$\overline{\mathrm{Cl}} = \frac{i.\,v.\ \text{dose}}{\mathrm{AUC}_{0\to\infty}}$$

Physiologically, $\overline{\mathrm{Cl}}$ may be defined relative to the hepatic blood flow Q and the extraction ratio E, which is dependent on the arterial (c_a) and venous (c_v) drug concentration across the organ:

$$\overline{\mathrm{Cl}} = Q \times E \text{ with } E = \frac{c_a - c_v}{c_a}$$

If only the liver is involved in the elimination of the drug, $\overline{\mathrm{Cl}}$ represents the hepatic clearance ($\mathrm{Cl_H}$). In these considerations it is important that clearance is based upon blood concentrations. It is usually assumed that only the unbound drug can be cleared by the liver. If this is true, and since this fraction can be altered in some patients, it may be more appropriate to consider the clearance of free drug.

Results and discussion

Many attempts have been made to develop predictive tests for the characterization of the degree of alteration in hepatic function, especially for patients with liver disease. Initially, correlations were attempted between observed changes in $T_{1/2}$ or $\overline{\mathrm{Cl}}$ and biochemical laboratory tests. Only few successful correlations with drug elimination have been established, albumin, bilirubin and prothrombin time exhibiting the highest discriminating value. Different model drugs which are removed by the liver were utilized for a test predicting alterations in drug elimination.

Based on their clearance values hepatic elimination of drugs can be characterised either as blood flow dependent or blood flow independent. For so called high clearance drugs, such as propranolol, lidocaine or pethidine, hepatic blood flow will be an important determinant. For measuring the blood flow through this drug metabolizing organ various direct or indirect methods have been applied in man [12]. It was demonstrated by Wilkinson and Shand [16] that low clearance drugs in contrast to high-clearance drugs will be hardly effected by changes in hepatic blood flow. In addition hepatic blood flow can be changed by different physiological, pathological and pharmacological factors [11].

For some drugs, which are mainly eliminated by acetylation, two genetically determined phenotypes exist. For treatment with isoniazid, hydrallazine, dapsone, procainamide or certain sulfonamides, differentiation of the patients into slow and fast acetylators can help to define or to adjust the proper dose. We have determined with sulfapyridine the acetylation rate in patients with Morbus Crohn and colitis ulcerosa to reduce the incidence of side effects which are almost exclusively directed to slow acetylators [2].

For the characterisation of the metabolic capacity different approaches have been made, such as determination of galactose elimination capacity, cytochrome P-450 content and enzyme activities in biopsy samples, antipyrine clearance and radioactive breath tests. Alterations in the metabolic capacity will have distinct effects on the plasma concentrations of drugs, dependent on the clearance rate of the compound. Drugs with flow-independent elimination will be effected to a greater extent than drugs with a high clearance rate. The mentioned tests have been primarily applied to healthy subjects and patients with different types of hepatic dysfunction. Therefore the following data will be a reflection of this situation. The content of cytochrome P-450 and the activity of typical liver enzymes were measured in biopsy samples of different patients [15]. The impairment has to be rather severe before significant changes in these parameters of liver function could be demonstrated. On the other side disturbing effects of drugs given concomitantly cannot be ruled out completely. It is well-known that certain drugs can induce liver enzymes and thereby changing liver function. In biopsy material of healthy subjects [14] a difference in the content of cytochrome P-450 was observed if drug-free individuals were compared with those taking metabolism inducing drugs (Figure 1). For the assessment of enzyme induction γ-glutamyl-transpeptidase in plasma, d-glucaric acid, 6-β-hydroxycortisol and 17-hydroxycorticosteroid urinary excretion have frequently been employed. In a study by Ohnhaus and Park with antipyrine, phenobarbitone and rifampicin, a significant correlation ($p < 0.001$) was found only between the clearance of antipyrine and 6-β-hydroxycortisol [13]. Similarly Freundt [3] could not find a correlation between the 24 hour urinary excretion of d-glucaric acid and the metabolic formation of 4-aminoantipyrine. The determination of the galactose elimination capacity has been used by some investigators, but this method only gave a significant correlation to the clearance of antipyrine when different patients were combined in one group [1].

Well established methods are represented by the model drugs aminopyrine and antipyrine. Both compounds, used either for pharmacokinetic analysis or radioactive breath tests were used in numerous studies to characterize the liver function of the patients studied. In most studies the relationships between the elimination of these model drugs and other therapeutic agents were also evaluated. Since the $14CO_2$-breath tests necessitate the administration of labelled compounds (*e.g.* aminopyrine, galactose, glycodiazine, glycocholate, diazepam, phenacetin, ethanol), attempts have been made to overcome this limiting factor by using sta-

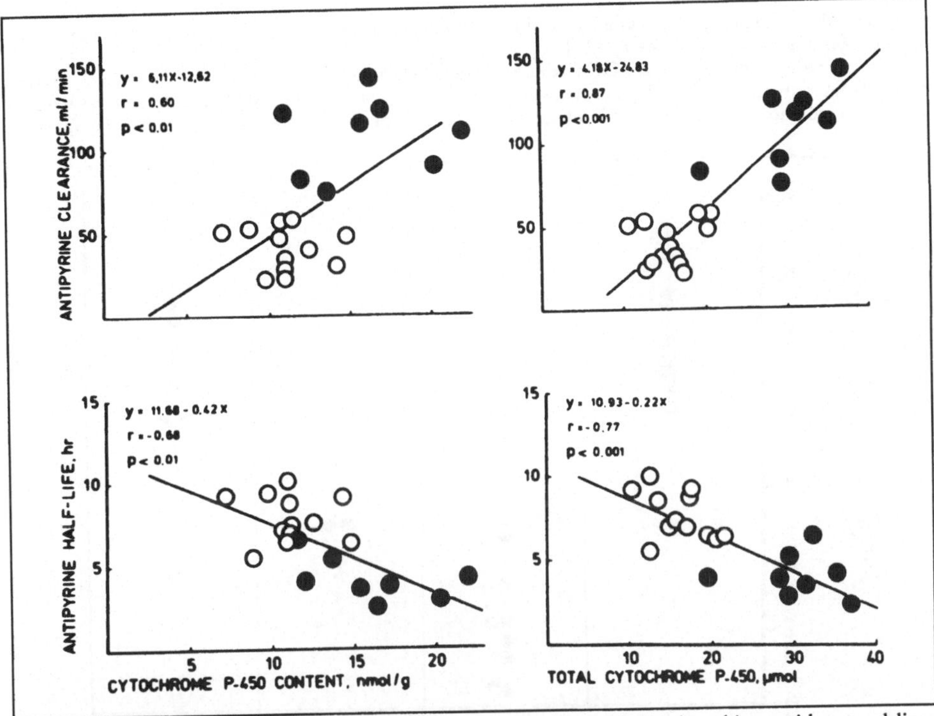

Figure 1: Correlation between antipyrine kinetics and cytochrome P-450 in subjects with normal liver parenchyma. Closed circles represent subjects with inductive drugs and open circles those without history of inducing drugs (from H. I. Pirttiaho et al; 14)

bile isotopes such as ^{13}C-labelled aminopyrine, galactose, trioctanoate and glycocholate. The validity of the radioactive breath analysis has been established from comparative pharmacokinetic analyses of different drugs. For instance it was shown for diazepam [6] or aminopyrine [5, 6] that the amount of radioactive CO_2 expired in the air was proportional and linearly correlated with the elimination rate of the corresponding drug.

In different groups of patients [4, 5, 6] it could be also demonstrated that the percentage of exhaled $^{14}CO_2$ was dependent on the liver function (Figure 2, 3).

Since the determination of the antipyrine clearance or half-life is easy to perform and much data is now available, it can be regarded as almost the standard liver function test. In numerous studies, relationships between this compound and different therapeutic agents (*e. g.* with propranolol; 19) could be documented. Surprisingly a linear correlation was even found between indocyanine green, the model compound characterizing hepatic blood flow, and the clearance of antipyrine (Figure 4). Moreover, our own studies in cirrhotic patients with antipyrine and the high-clearance antiarrhythmic drug lorcainide demonstrated a relationsship between the clearances of these two drugs [9]. However, if the percentage of the impairment was compared, it became obvious that the clearance of antipyrine was significantly (p = 0.0003) more strongly effected than the clearance of lorcainide (Figure 5).

In addition, in most studies, the previously mentioned correlations became only significant, if normals and diseased patients were regarded as one group. Therefore it seems that antipyrine clearance serves as a good qualitative test, but that the quantitative predictive value might be limited, especially if the drugs belong to groups having different types of hepatic elimination.

For routine clinical work the pharmacokinetic or radioactive analyses might be too elaborate. Thus, the use of biochemical laboratory tests can give some indication of the degree of alteration in liver function, especially in patients with liver disease. Serum albumin and cholinesterase gave good correlations with the clearance of antipyrine ($p<0.01$) and obvious trends were seen with the clearance of lorcainide in our patients with alcoholic cirrhosis [9]. Also in other studies with different drugs (propranolol, antipyrine, amylobarbi-

tone) the value of albumin as a crude index of liver function was established. The same holds true for the prothrombin time (for review see 8, 17, 18).
In acute liver disease bilirubin and SGOT seem to have the highest predictive value for the characterisation of the elimination rate of drugs. In our own longitudinal studies with diazepam [7] a decline of the elevated $T_{1/2}$ (β) towards normal was observed, when normal values for SGOT and bilirubin indicated apparent

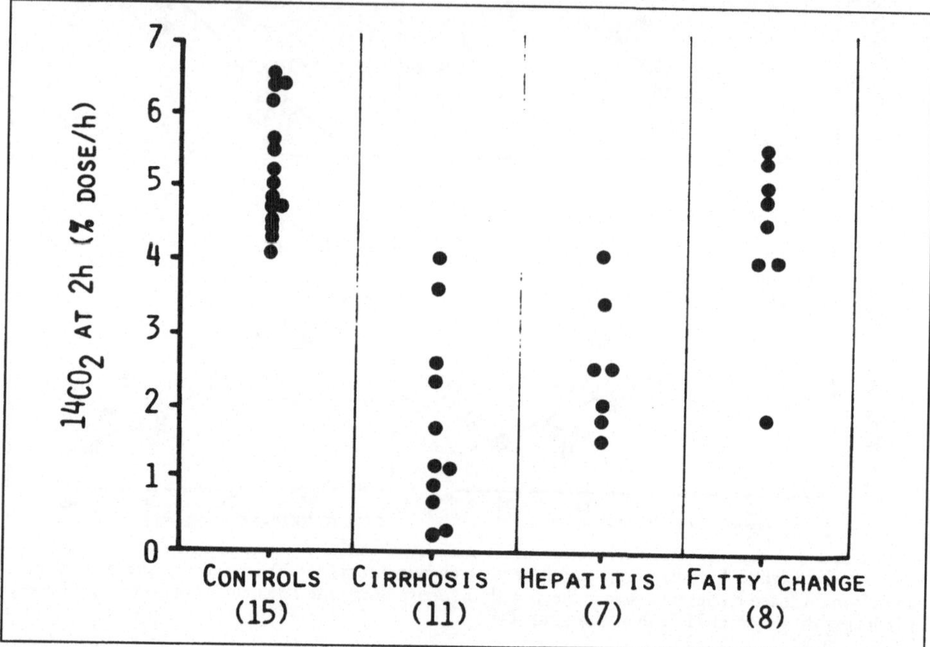

Figure 2: Two hour breath analysis in controls and alcoholic patients separated into 3 subgroups according to histological diagnosis (Data from J. Gallizzi et al.; 4)

Comparison of different liver function tests (mean values ± SD)

liver function test	controls	anticonvulsants	hepatocellular disease
diazepam breath test, %	14.0 ± 2.6	26.6 ± 7.1 ($p < 0.01$)	8.1 ± 2.3 ($p < 0.01$)
diazepam $T_{1/2(\beta)}$, h	53.1 ± 5.6	36.4 ± 4.9 ($p < 0.01$)	116.0 ± 9.8 ($p < 0.01$)
diazepam $\overline{Cl}$, ml/min	15.1 ± 1.8	18.7 ± 2.3 ($p < 0.05$)	9.8 ± 1.8 ($p < 0.05$)
aminopyrine breath test, %	6.4 ± 1.0	9.2 ± 3.0 ($p < 0.05$)	2.7 ± 1.6 ($p < 0.05$)
antipyrine $\overline{Cl}$, ml/min	50.0 ± 20.0	110.0 ± 40.0 ($p < 0.05$)	20.0 ± 13.0 ($p < 0.05$)
ICG elim. rate const., h^{-1}	0.24 ± 0.07	0.25 ± 0.04 (n.s.)	0.1 ± 0.05 ($p < 0.01$)

Figure 3: $^{14}CO_2$-breath analysis and pharmacokinetic parameters in control subjects, patients on anticonvulsants and patients with hepatocellular disease (Data from G. W. Hepner et al.; 6)

recovery from acute viral hepatitis. From the different liver function tests one could conclude that on one side indocyanine green and antipyrine clearance and on the other side albumin and bilirubin will give the best answers. However, in extensive studies with chemically closely related drugs, such as the benzodiazepines, no significant correlations between clinical laboraty tests and the elimination could be observed in patients with liver disease. This situation is additionally complicated by the fact, that benzodiazepines which are eliminated by conjugation with glucuronic acid (*e.g.* oxazepam and lorazepam) demonstrate a normal elimination, while derivatives which are hydroxylated or dealkylated (*e.g.* chlordiazepoxide, diazepam, desmethyldiazepam) exhibited an impaired elimination (Figure 6).
In conclusion, despite the possibility that some liver function tests might be qualitative or even semiquantitative markers for the metabolic capability of a particular patient's liver, the empiric relationship for each drug of interest has to be determined. There is a considerable overlap in any liver function parameter be-

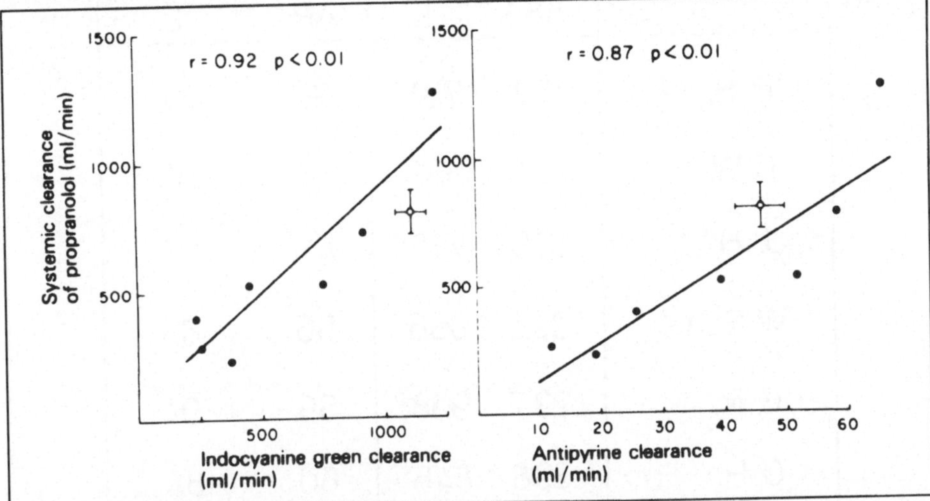

Figure 4: Relationships between the clearances of indocyanine green, antipyrine and propranolol in 9 normal subjects (○ ± SEM) and 7 patients with cirrhosis (•). Statistics are for the cirrhotic patients only (Data from A. J. J. Wood et al.; 19)

DISPOSITION OF BENZODIAZEPINES IN PATIENTS WITH LIVER DISEASE

BENZODIAZEPINES	$T_{1/2}$, h cirrhosis	controls	$\overline{Cl}$, ml/min cirrhosis	controls	Vd, l/kg cirrhosis	controls
CHLORDIAZEPOXIDE	62.7	23.8	7.7 (154)	15.3 (381)	0.48	0.33
DIAZEPAM	47	106	13.8 (294)	26.6 (1209)	1.74	1.13
DESMETHYLDIAZEPAM	108.2	50.9	4.6	11.3	0.63	0.64
OXAZEPAM	5.8	5.6	155.5	136.0	0.88	0.67
LORAZEPAM	31.9	22.1	0.81 (10.6) §	0.75 (11.7) §	2.0	1.3

§ ml/min/kg

numbers in parenthesis refer to free drug

Figure 6: Comparison of the pharmacokinetic profiles of different benzodiazepines in normal subjects and in patients with cirrhosis

Comparison of the clearance of antipyrine (AP) and lorcainide (L)

patients with cirrhosis	$\bar{Cl}$, ml/min		percent of control values	
	AP	L	AP	L
P. H.	11.9	721	30	72
O. W.	14.4	551	36	55
J. H.	16.5	719	41	72
W. Sch.	22.5	856	56	85
G. M.	23.7	938	59	94
O. H.	23.8	846	60	84
O. F.	25.0	1002	63	100
K. K.	37.3	877	93	88
control values	40	1002	p = 0.0003	

Figure 5: Comparison of the clearances of antipyrine and lorcainide in 8 patients with alcoholic cirrhosis (Data from U. Klotz et al.; 9)

tween different groups of patients, which necessitates individual and multifactorial analyses, especially for the many interfering extrahepatic factors. The benzodiazepines can be taken as an example that one cannot generalize from the results with one drug to another in respect to liver function and drug elimination. Since up to now no consistant pattern seems to exist, each drug of interest has to be investigated seperately.

Acknowledgements

These studies were supported by the Robert Bosch Foundation, Stuttgart/Germany

References

[1] Andreasen, P. B., Ranek, L., Statland, B. E., Tygstrup, N.: Clearance of antipyrine-dependence of quantitative liver function. Eur. J. Clin. Invest. *4*, 129—134 (1974)

[2] Fischer, C., Klotz, U.: High-performance liquid chromatographic determination of aminosalicylate, sulfapyridine and their metabolites: Its application for pharmacokinetic studies with salicylazosulfapyridine in man. J. Chromatogr. *162*, 237—243 (1979)

[3] Freundt, K. J.: Production of endogenous D-glucaric acid and oxidative N-demethylation of amidopyrine in man: lack of correlation. Internat. J. Clin. Pharmacol. Biopharm. *17*, 104—106 (1979)

[4] Galizzi, J., Long, R. G., Billing, B. H., Sherlock, S.: Assessment of the (^{14}C) aminopyrine breath test in liver disease. Gut *19*, 40—45 (1978)

[5] Hepner, G. W., Vesell, E. S.: Aminopyrine disposition: Studies on breath, saliva, and urine of normal subjects and patients with liver disease. Clin. Pharmacol. Ther. *20*, 654—660 (1977)

[6] Hepner, G. W., Vesell, E. S., Lipton, A., Harvey, H. A., Wilkinson, G. R., Schenker, S.: Disposition of aminopyrine, antipyrine, diazepam and indocyanine green in patients with liver disease or on anticonsulvant drug therapy: diazepam breath test and correlations in drug elimination. J. Lab. Clin. Med. *90*, 440—456 (1977)

[7] Klotz, U., Avant, G. R., Hoyumpa, A., Schenker, S., Wilkinson, G. R.: The effect of age and liver disease on the disposition and elimination of diazepam in adult man. J. Clin. Invest. *55*, 347—359 (1975)

[8] Klotz, U.: Influence of liver disease on the elimination of drugs. Eur. J. Drug Metab. Pharmacokin. *3*, 129—140 (1976)

[9] Klotz, U., Fischer, C., Müller-Seydlitz, P., Schulz, J., Müller, W. A.: Alterations in the disposition of differently cleared drugs in cirrhosis. Clin. Pharmacol. Ther. *26*, 221—227 (1979)

[10] Naranjo, C. A., Busto, U., Mardones, R.: Adverse drug reactions in liver cirrhosis. Eur. J. Clin. Pharmacol. *13*, 429—434 (1978)

[11] Nies, A. S., Shand, D. G., Wilkinson, G. R.: Altered hepatic blood flow and drug disposition. Clin. Pharmacokin. *1*, 135—155 (1976)

[12] Ohnhaus, E. E.: Methods of the assessment of the effect of drugs on liver blood flow in man. Brit. J. Clin. Pharmacol. *7*, 223—229 (1979)

[13] Ohnhaus, E. E., Park, B. K.: Measurement of urinary 6-β-hydroxycortisol excretion as an *in vivo* parameter in the clinical assesssment of the microsomal enzyme-inducing capacity of antipyrine, phenobarbitone and rifampicin. Eur. J. Clin. Pharmacol. *15*, 139—145 (1979)

[14] Pirttiaho, H. I., Sotaniemi, E. A., Pelkonen, R. O., Pitkänen, U.: Influence of liver size on the relationship between *in vivo* and *in vitro* studies of drug metabolism. Eur. J. Drug Metab. Pharmacokin. *4*, 217—222 (1978)

[15] Schöne, B., Fleischmann, R. A., Remmer, H., von Oldershausen, F.: Determination of drug metabolizing enzymes in needle biopsies of human liver. Eur. J. Clin. Pharmacol. *4*, 65—73 (1972)

[16] Wilkinson, G. R., Shand, D. G.: A physiological approach to hepatic drug clearance. Clin. Pharmacol. Therap. *18*, 377—390 (1975)

[17] Wilkinson, G. R., Schenker, S.: Drug disposition and liver disease. Drug Metab. Rev. *4*, 139—175 (1975)

[18] Wilkinson, G. R., Schenker, S.: Effects of liver disease on drug disposition in man. Biochem. Pharmacol. *25*, 2675—2681 (1976)

[19] Wood, A. J. J., Kornhauser, D. M., Wilkinson, G. R., Shand, D. G., Branch, R. A.: The influence of cirrhosis on steady state blood concentrations of unbound propranolol after oral administration. Clin. Pharmacokin. *3*, 478—487 (1978)

Urinary metabolite profile of antipyrine as a tool in the assessment of oxidative drug metabolizing capacity of man

M. Danhof and D. D. Breimer

Department of Pharmacology, Subfaculty of Pharmacy,
University of Leiden, Sylvius Laboratories, Leiden, The Netherlands.

Introduction

It is a well-established phenomenon that great differences in intensity and duration of drug response may arise between individual patients when the same dose of a drug is given to each patient. Such interindividual differences can often be related to differences in the rate of drug elimination. This is in particular the case for lipid soluble drugs that are hardly excreted unchanged into urine and which have to be inactivated through biotransformation (drug metabolism). One of the major routes of drug metabolism is oxidation which occurs predominantly in the liver by the mixed function oxidase system. There are great differences in the activity of this enzyme system between individuals, due to genetic, environmental, disease related and other factors. Antipyrine has been widely used as an *in vivo* model substrate to measure the influence and contribution of these factors on the rate of drug oxidation (VESELL 1972, 1978). Other substrates used for similar purposes include aminopyrine (HEPNER and VESELL 1974, 1975, BIRCHER *et al.* 1976), amobarbital (INABA and KALOW 1975) and hexobarbital (BREIMER *et al.* 1977). However, the elimination rate of neither antipyrine nor of the other substrates, is an absolute measure of an individual's capacity to metabolize drugs, since poor correlations have been observed between the elimination half-life or clearance of oxidatively metabolized drugs (VESELL and PAGE 1968; SJÖQVIST and VON BAHR 1973). A possible explanation for the observed lack of correlation between rates of drug metabolism *in vivo* is the qualitative and quantitative heterogeneity of the mixed function oxidase system. Multiple forms of cytochrome P-450 may exist that interact differently with drug substrates (THOMAS *et al.* 1976; VESELL 1978).
The metabolism of antipyrine is rather complicated: at least four primary metabolites, which are formed through oxidation, have been identified in urine of man and rats (BRODIE and AXELROD 1950; SCHÜPPEL 1966; BATY and PRICE-EVANS 1973; YOSHIMURA *et al.* 1968, 1971). Their chemical structures are given in Figure 1. Recently, evidence was obtained in rats that there may be a different regulatory control of oxidative enzymes for the formation of each of these metabolites (DANHOF *et al.* 1979 d). If this were also true in man, the urinary metabolite profile of antipyrine would be a tool not only to study total oxidative drug metabolizing capacity, but also to study changes in the activity of different forms of cytochrome P-450 in man.
In the following account a brief review will be given of the methodology developed for the quantitative determination of the four primary metabolites, as well as their conjugates, of antipyrine in urine. Subsequently data on the metabolite profile of antipyrine in healthy volunteers obtained at various

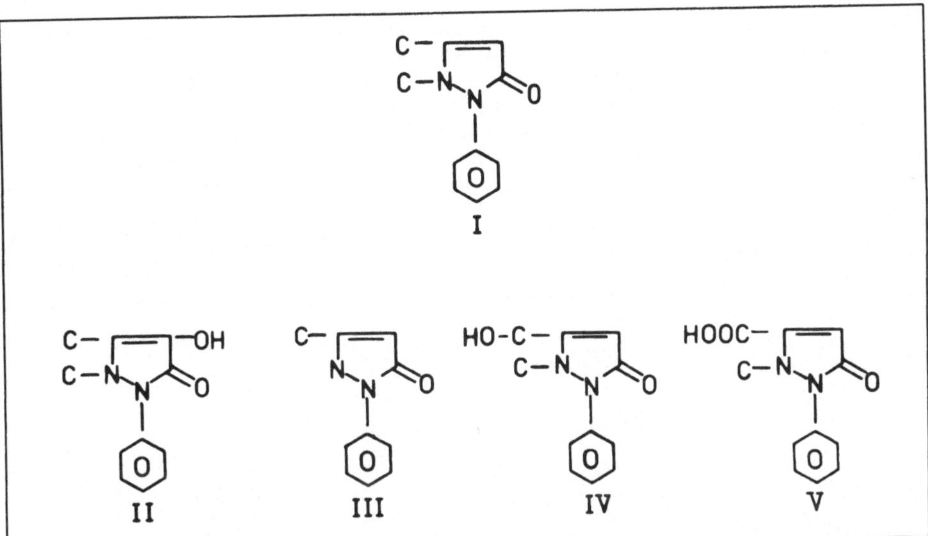

Figure 1: The chemical structures of antipyrine and its unconjugated metabolites I = antipyrine, II = 4-hydroxyantipyrine, III = norantipyrine, IV = 3-hydroxymethyl-antipyrine, V = 3-carboxy-antipyrine.

dose levels will be presented. In the next paragraph a brief account will be given of the evidence obtained in rats for the involvement of different types of cytochrome P-450 in the metabolism of antipyrine and finally some of the possible implications of these findings will be discussed.

1. Assay of antipyrine metabolites in urine

The assay of antipyrine, 4-hydroxyantipyrine, norantipyrine and 3-hydroxymethyl-antipyrine were performed by high perfomance liquid chromatography (HPLC) (Danhof *et al.* 1979 a). The columns used were 100 mm long and made of 2.8 mm I.D. and 6.35 mm O.D. precision bore stainless steel tubing. The column support was LiChrosorb RP-2 (Merck) with a mean particle size of 5 µm, and a solution of 5% acetonitrile in 0.05 M phosphate buffer pH = 6.5 was used as the mobile phase. 4-Hydroxyantipyrine and norantipyrine were assayed following extraction of 0.25 ml of urine at pH = 4.5, twice with a mixture of dichloromethane-pentane (3:7), using phenacetin as internal standard. The combined layers were evaporated to dryness, the residue was dissolved in 100 µl eluent of which 25 µl were injected into the chromatograph. An example of the chromatograms obtained is given in Figure 2. The concentrations were calculated with the aid of calibration curves, measuring peak height ratios. The coefficients of variation of these assays were found to be ±3.6% and ±7.0% for 4-hydroxyantipyrine and norantipyrine respectively in the concentration range 1—400 µg/ml ($n = 5$). In this assay the use of silanized glass-ware is of critical importance, since particularly norantipyrine, and to a lesser extent also 4-hydroxyantipyrine, tend to adsorb rather strongly to unsilanized glass.

Unchanged antipyrine and 3-hydroxymethyl-antipyrine were extracted from 0.25 ml of urine at pH = 11 with 10 ml of dichloromethane, using phenacetin as internal standard. The organic layer was evaporated to dryness, the residue redissolved in 100 µl eluent of which 25 µl were injected into the chromatograph, which resulted in chromatograms as shown in Figure 3. The coefficients of variation of these assays were found to be ±3.6% and ±5.0% for 3-hydroxymethyl-antipyrine and unchanged antipyrine in the concentration range 1—400 µg/ml and 1—40 µg/ml respectively ($n = 5$).

Using this HPLC system it appeared impossible to assay 3-carboxy-antipyrine, because of interference with endogenous compounds co-extracted from urine. Therefore a gas chromatographic method was developed for the determination of this compound, using a support-coated open tubular

(SCOT) capillary column (Carbowax 20M), a solid injection system and nitrogen selective detection (DANHOF *et al.* 1979b). 3-carboxy-antipyrine was extracted from 0.1 ml of urine at pH = 1 twice with 5 ml of a mixture of dichloromethane-pentane-isopropanol (50 : 50 : 3) using 4-bromo-antipyrine as internal standard. After evaporation of the organic layers 3-carboxy-antipyrine was methylated with a freshly prepared ethereal solution of diazomethane. Following evaporation of the ethereal layer the residue was redissolved in 100 µl of absolute ethanol and 1 µl of the obtained solution was injected into the gas chromatograph. The coefficient of variation of the method was found to be ±5.0% in the concentration range 1—50 µg/ml (n = 5).
Because the primary metabolites are mainly excreted into urine in conjugated from, hydrolysis of these conjugates is necessary to obtain data on total metabolite formation. Hydrolysis was per-

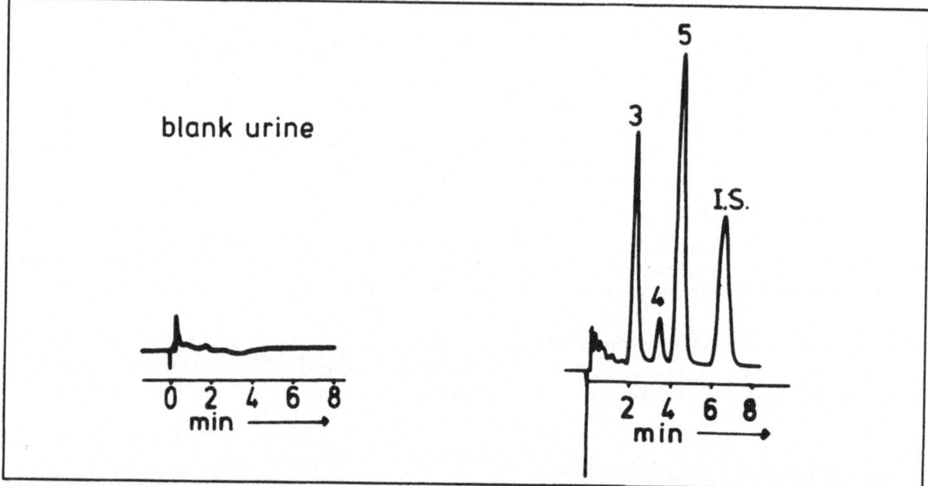

Figure 2 : Chromatograms obtained after extraction of blank hydrolyzed urine and of a 24 hours' urine sample obtained after intake of 500 mg antipyrine by a human volunteer; the concentrations were 55 µg norantipyrine/ml [3]; 105 µg 4-hydroxy-antipyrine/ml [5] and 40 µg phenacetin/ml internal standard (IS). Conditions: see text.

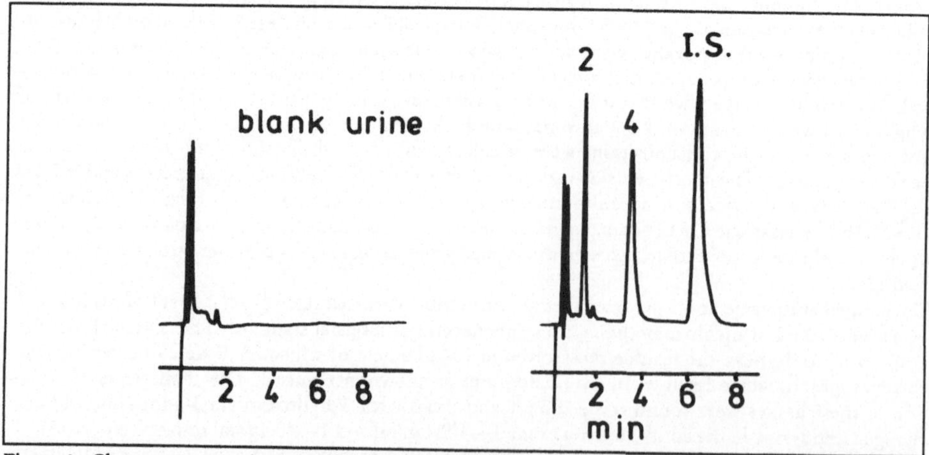

Figure 3: Chromatograms obtained after extraction of blank hydrolyzed urine and of a 24 hours' urine sample after intake of 500 mg by a human volunteer containing 60 µg 3-hydroxymethyl-antipyrine/ml [2]; 20 µg antipyrine/ml [4] and 40 µg phenacetin/ml internal standard (IS). Conditions: see text.

formed enzymatically with β-glucuronidase-sulphatase (Limpet Acetone Powder type I, Sigma) after dilution of the urine samples with acetate buffer 0.05 M (pH=4.5). However, since aqueous solutions of antipyrine metabolites are relatively unstable, precaution had to be taken to prevent decomposition during enzymic hydrolysis. It appeared for example that in a sample stored at 37° C for 24 hours, the concentrations of 4-hydroxyantipyrine decreased by 75% as a result of rapid oxidation (Figure 4). Stability could be highly improved by adding sodium-pyrosulphite ($Na_2S_2O_5$) in a concentration of 1 mg/ml to urine samples. By adding this anti-oxidant no decomposition of the metabolites was observed during a 3 hours' enzymic hydrolysis.

2. Salivary elimination rate and urinary metabolite profile of antipyrine in healthy volunteers

In five healthy volunteers salivary antipyrine eliminiation and urinary metabolite profile were studied (Danhof and Breimer 1979 c). Since antipyrine metabolite formation might possibly be dose dependent, this study was performed in a cross-over design in the same panel of volunteers following oral administration of three different dosages: 250, 500 and 1000 mg with an interval of at least 4 weeks. They took antipyrine dissolved in 100 ml water at 9.00 a. m. after an overnight fast. Saliva samples were collected at regular time intervals in order to establish some pharmacokinetic parameters of antipyrine: elimination half-life, apparent volume of distribution and clearance. Furthermore urine was collected at intervals up to 52 h after drug administration.
The mean antipyrine half-life was 11.5±2.3 h following 500 mg and almost equal values were found after 250 and 1000 mg. After 500 mg the apparent volume of distribution and metabolic clearance were 54.2±9.3 l and 3.4±0.9 l/h respectively. The values obtained for these parameters at 250 and 1000 mg antipyrine were not significantly different (paired t-test).
In Figure 5 an example is given of the cumulative excretion curves obtained for antipyrine and metabolites (conjugated + free) for one individual following 1000 mg antipyrine. The curves show that the urinary excretion of antipyrine and metabolites (conjugated + free) was complete in 52 hours. The amounts of antipyrine and metabolites excreted at the various dose levels are given in Table I. Following 500 mg, 3.3±1.2% of the dose was excreted into urine as unchanged antipyrine, 28.5±2.2% as 4-hydroxyantipyrine, 16.5±6.0% as norantipyrine, 35.1±7.2% as 3-hydroxymethyl-antipyrine and 3.3±0.8 as 3-carboxy-antipyrine. The values obtained at the other dose levels were not significantly different.
Since the metabolites of antipyrine are excreted into urine partly in a conjugated form, an attempt was made to determine the extent of conjugation and also to differentiate between glucuronides and sulphates. The urine samples were analyzed in three ways: treatment with β-glucuronidase-sulphatase, with sulphatase and without enzymic hydolysis. The findings of these experiments are given in

Compound	250 mg	500 mg	1000 mg
Antipyrine	2.6±0.5	3.3±1.2	2.1±0.7
4-Hydroxyantipyrine	26.3±3.8	28.5±2.2	27.7±2.8
Norantipyrine	16.7±5.3	16.5±6.0	17.3±2.5
3-Hydroxymethyl-antipyrine	31.3±2.7	35.1±7.2	31.0±7.3
3-Carboxy-antipyrine	3.4±0.9	3.3±0.8	3.0±1.3
Total	80.4±5.9	86.7±6.6	81.1±7.1

Table 1: Relative amounts (% dose) of antipyrine and metabolites excreted in 52 hours' urine of five healthy male volunteers after oral administration of 250, 500 and 1000 mg antipyrine (M±S.D.)

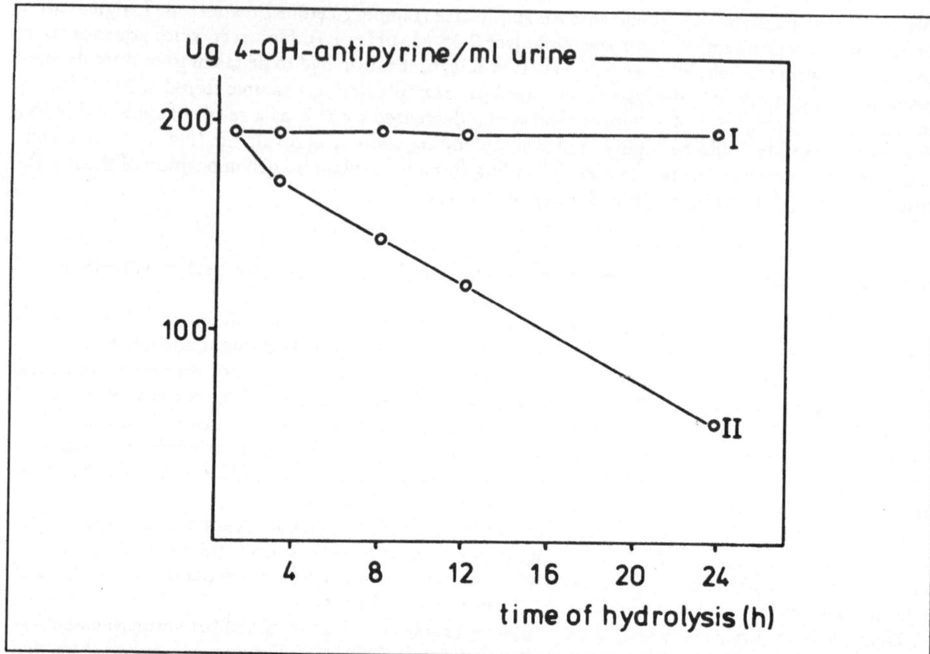

Figure 4: The stability of 4-hydroxy-antipyrine during simulated enzymic hydrolysis at 37° C after addition of 200 μg of this compound to blank urine with (I) and without (II) addition of sodiumpyrosulphite.

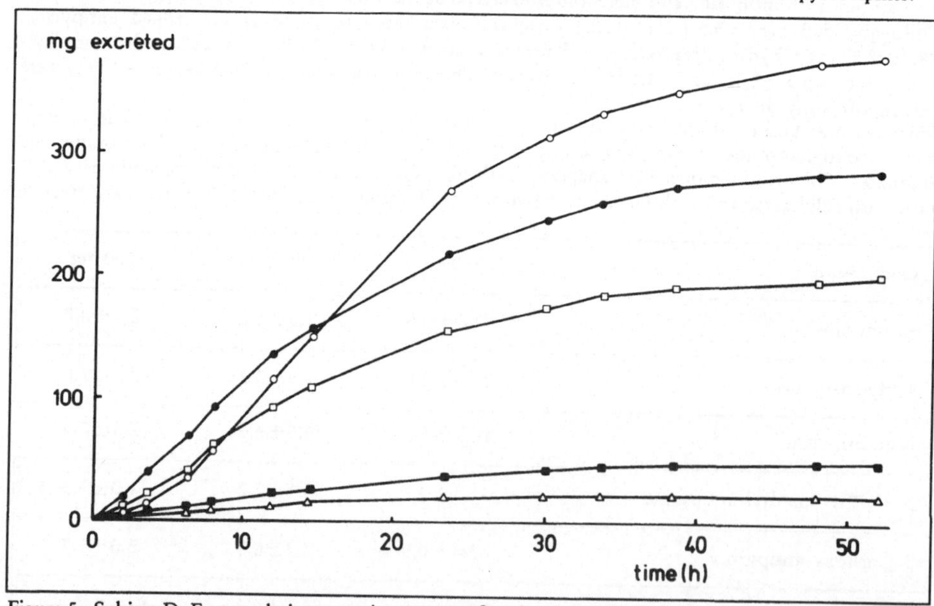

Figure 5: Subject D. E.: cumulative excretion curves of antipyrine and metabolites (conjugated + free) in urine following oral administration of 1000 mg.
Δ = antipyrine □ = norantipyrine ○ = 3-hydroxymethyl-antipyrine
■ = 3-carboxy-antipyrine ● = 4-hydroxyantipyrine

Table II. It appeared that antipyrine and 3-carboxy-antipyrine were excreted entirely in the free form. Following no enzymic treatment of the samples, the concentrations of 4-hydroxyantipyrine and norantipyrine were below the detection limit of the analytical procedure. Hence it can be concluded that these metabolites are excreted into urine in the free form only to a very minor extent. On the other hand, 42% of 3-hydroxymethyl-antipyrine was excreted unconjugated. Furthermore it can be concluded that sulphation is probably of minor importance in the conjugation of antipyrine metabolites, since the values found after treatment with sulphatase were not significantly different from those obtained without enzymic hydrolysis.

In Figure 6 the urinary excretion rates of antipyrine and metabolites (conjugated + free) are plotted as a function of time on a semi-logarithmic scale for one individual after intake of 1000 mg antipyrine. From 12 h onwards good linearity existed between excretion rate and time in particular for E-hydroxyantipyrine, norantipyrine and 3-hydroxymethyl-antipyrine. The half-lives calculated

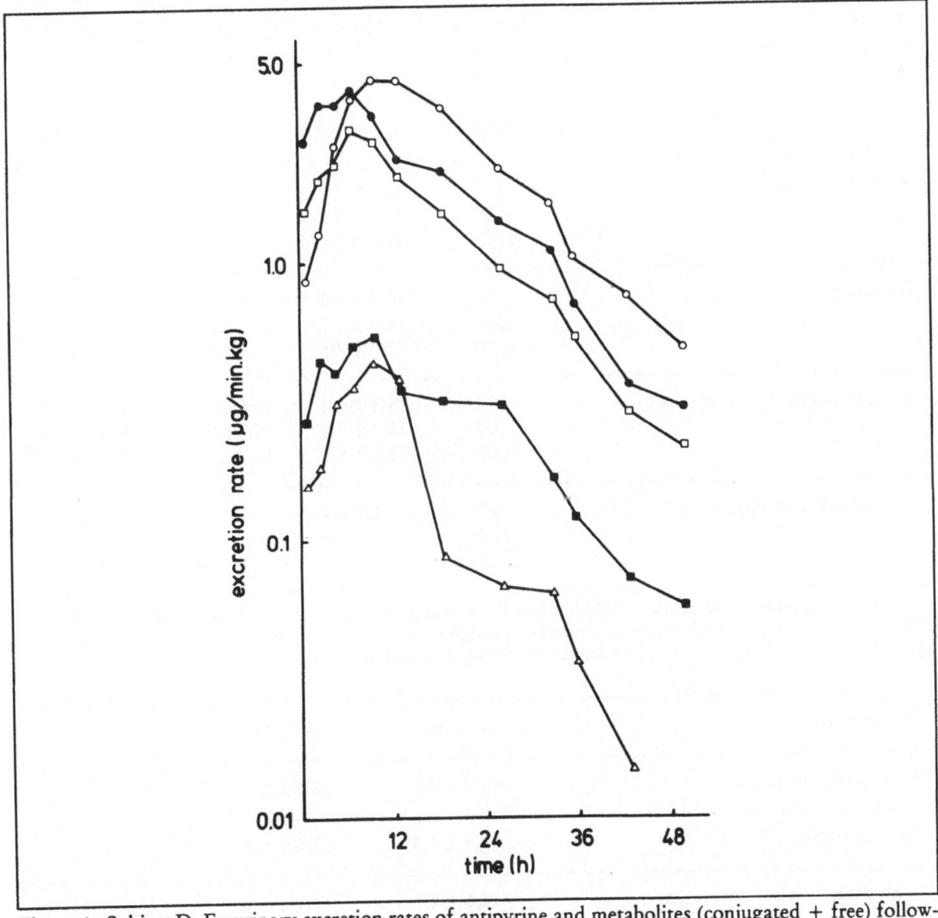

Figure 6: Subject D. E.: urinary excretion rates of antipyrine and metabolites (conjugated + free) following oral administration of 1000 mg.

Δ = antipyrine
■ = 3-carboxy-antipyrine
□ = norantipyrine
● = 4-hydroxyantipyrine
○ = 3-hydroxymethyl-antipyrine

from the linear part of these curves for 4-hydroxyantipyrine, norantipyrine and 3-hydroxymethyl-antipyrine were 12.2±2.8 h, 11.9±6.4 h and 12.5±4.2 h respectively following a 500 mg dose and these figures were not significantly different from the values found at the other dose levels (Table III). Furthermore it appeared that these values were in the same order of magnitude as the salivary half-lives, and that they correlated significantly. It can be concluded therefore that the rate limiting step in the excretion of antipyrine metabolites in urine is most probably their rate of formation by oxidation from the parent compound. It also became clear from these investigations that there is no dose dependency involved in the metabolism of antipyrine in healthy men in the dose range 250—1000 mg.

Compound	Dose (mg)	G+S	S	F
Antipyrine	250	2.6±0.5		2.6±0.5
	500	3.3±1.2		3.3±1.2
	1000	2.1±0.7		2.1±0.7
4-Hydroxyantipyrine	250	26.3±3.8	<1.0	
	500	28.5±2.2	<1.0	
	1000	27.7±2.8	<1.0	
Norantipyrine	250	16.7±5.3	<1.0	
	500	16.5±6.0	<1.0	
	1000	17.3±2.5	<1.0	
3-Hydroxymethyl-antipyrine	250	29.3±4.3	10.5±2.5	11.5±2.1
	500	35.1±7.2	15.2±1.8	14.6±3.9
	1000	31.0±5.6	14.5±2.1	14.4±2.6
3-Carboxy-antipyrine	250	3.4±0.9		3.3±0.8
	500	3.3±0.8		3.2±0.8
	1000	3.0±1.3		3.0±1.2

Table 2: Mean relative amounts ± S.D. (% Dose) of antipyrine and metabolites found after treatment of the 52 h urine samples with β-glucuronidase-arylsulphatase (G+S), arylsulphatase (S) and without enzymic hydrolysis (F) after oral administration of 250, 500 and 1000 mg.

Compound	250 mg	500 mg	1000 mg
4-Hydroxyantipyrine	12.3±2.7	12.2±2.8	11.4±1.1
Norantipyrine	13.4±4.0	12.5±4.2	14.3±4.6
3-Hydroxymethyl-antipyrine	11.5±2.1	11.9±6.4	11.0±2.7
Saliva	12.6±2.2	11.5±2.3	12.5±2.8

Table 3: Mean half-lives (h) ± S.D. deduced from the linear part of the urinary excretion rate curves of 4-hydroxyantipyrine, norantipyrine and 3-hydroxymethyl-antipyrine after oral administration of 250, 500 and 1000 mg antipyrine. The mean antipyrine saliva half-lives are given as well.

3. Effect of phenobarbital and 3-methylcholanthrene treatment on the metabolic disposition of antipyrine in rats.

The influence of phenobarbital and 3-methylcholanthrene treatment on the plasma elimination rate and the urinary metabolite profile of antipyrine were studied in *male Wistar rats* weighing 180—220 gram (DANHOF *et al.* 1979 d). The induction studies were performed in a longitudinal mode whereby the same rat received 10 mg of antipyrine prior to and after treatment with phenobarbital (100 mg/kg daily during 8 days) and 3-methylcholanthrene (18 mg/kg daily during 3 days). In order to establish the pharmacokinetic parameters of antipyrine, blood samples of 100 µl were taken at intervals up to 180 min from freely moving carotid artery cannulated rats. For the determination of the urinary metabolite profile 24 h urine samples were collected by placing the rats in individual metabolism cages.
Phenobarbital treatment resulted in a significant increase of antipyrine clearance from 10.4 ± 3.0 ml/min · kg to 26.0 ± 4.5 ml/min · kg (Figure 7). The influence of phenobarbital treatment on the urinary antipyrine metabolite profile is given in Figure 8a. There was a decrease in the amount of unchanged antipyrine from 2.4 ± 0.3% to 1.4 ± 0.4% of the dose. Furthermore, a small, but statistically significant, decrease in the amount of 4-hydroxyantipyrine also became apparent, however a similar

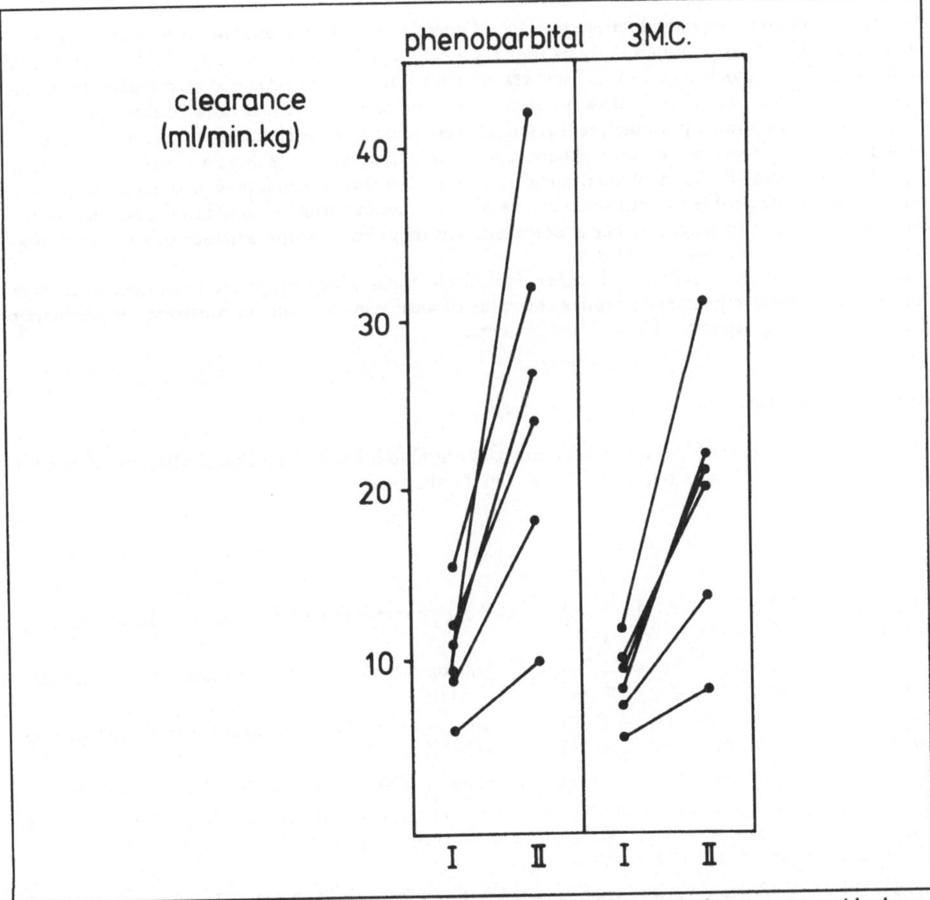

Figure 7: Clearance values of antipyrine found in individual rats before and after treatment with phenobarbital and 3-methylcholanthrene.

change was observed in control rats treated with saline. The urinary excretion of the other metabolites was essentially unchanged after phenobarbital. These findings indicate that at least in rats all the metabolic pathways of antipyrine are inducible by phenobarbital.
A different situation was encountered after 3-methylcholanthrene treatment. Now antipyrine clearance also had increased considerably from 8.7 ± 0.9 ml/min · kg to 20.7 ± 3.3 ml/min · kg (Figure 7), but interestingly, an almost twofold increase in the excreted amount of 4-hydroxyantipyrine occurred whereas the amount of 3-hydroxymethyl-antipyrine and 3-carboxy-antipyrine were decreased. The amount of norantipyrine remained unchanged (Figure 8b).
These results indicate that there is probably a different regulatory control for the 4-hydroxylation of antipyrine on the one hand and the formation 3-hydroxymethyl-antipyrine on the other. Most likely 4-hydroxyantipyrine is formed predominantly via the cytochrome P-448 system—which is known to be induced selectively by 3-methylcholanthrene—whereas another cytochrome system whose activity is not influenced by 3-methylcholanthrene is predominantly involved in the formation of 3-hydroxymethyl-antipyrine.

Conclusions

As was mentioned in the introduction, the lack of correlation between the rate of elimination of different drugs which are predominantly oxidatively metabolized, may partly be due to the existence of multiple forms of cytochrome P-450. The present investigations have provided quantitative information on the different metabolic pathways of antipyrine in man and the real value of these data lies in the fact that there probably is a different regulatory control for the formation of these metabolites as became apparent from the induction experiments in rats. In other words there are probably different types of cytochrome P-450 involved in their formation. For this reason it may be speculated that the urinary metabolite profile of antipyrine can be used as a tool to study changes in the activity of different cytochromes in man. Further experiments are required to show whether this extrapolation from rats to man is indeed justified.
Also further cross-over studies with other oxidatively metabolized drugs are indicated, since such studies are of great importance to judge the value of antipyrine as a model substrate for predicting drug metabolizing capacity of individual patients.

Acknowledgement

This work was supported in part by a grant from the Dutch Prevention Fund, Ministry of Health and Environmental Protection, The Hague, The Netherlands.

Literature

[1] Baty, J. D., Price-Evans, D. A.: Norphenazone, a new metabolite of phenazone in human urine. J. Pharm. Pharmac. 25, 83—84 (1973)

[2] Bircher, J., Küpfer, A., Gikalow, I., Preisig, R.: Aminopyrine demethylation measured by breath analysis in cirrhosis. Clin. Pharmacol. Ther. 20, 917—928 (1976).

[3] Breimer, D. D., Zilly, W., Richter E.: Pharmacokinetics of hexobarbital in acute hepatitis and after apparent recovery. Clin. Pharmacol. Ther. 18, 433—440 (1975).

[4] Brodie, B. B., Axelrod, J.: The fate of antipyrine in man. J. Pharmacol. exp. Ther. 98, 97—104 (1950).

[5] Danhof, M., de Groot-van der Vis, E., Breimer, D. D.: Assay of antipyrine and its primary metabolites in plasma, saliva and urine by high performance liquid chromatography and some preliminary results in man. Pharmacology 18, 210—224 (1979a).

[6] Danhof, M., de Boer, A. G., de Groot-van der Vis, E., Breimer, D. D.: Assay of 3-carboxy-antipyrine in urine by capillary gas chromatography with nitrogen selective detection, some preliminary results in man. Pharmacology, (1979b), 19, 215—220 (1979b).

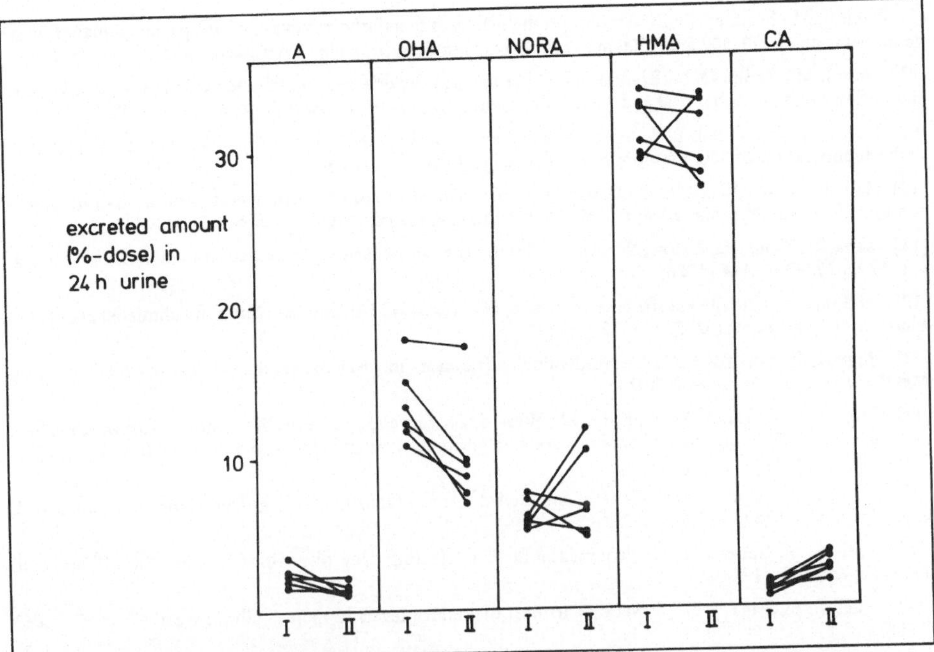

Figure 8a: Amounts of antipyrine and metabolites excreted in six individual rats in 24 h urine (% dose) before and after treatment with phenobarbital

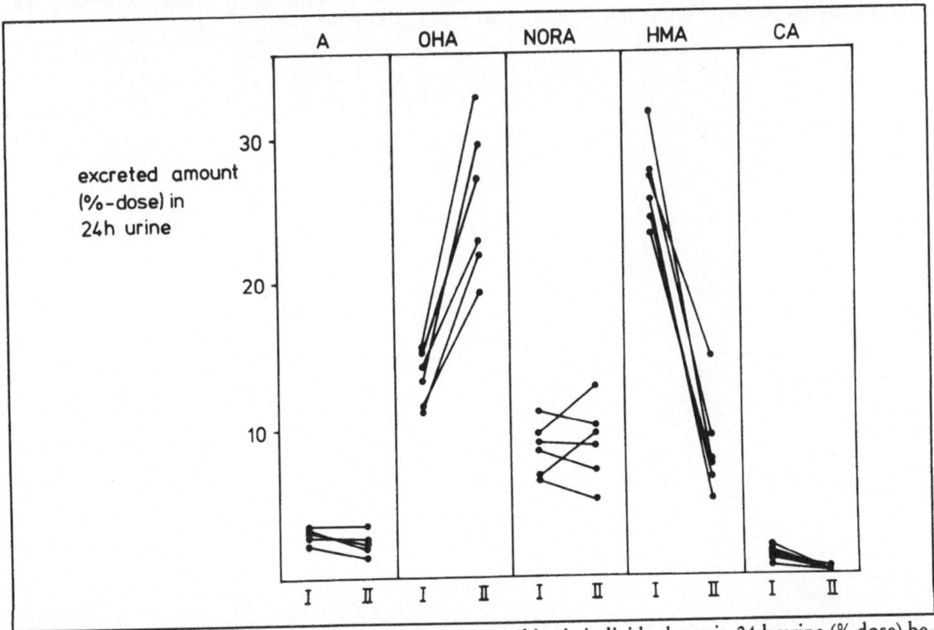

Figure 8b: Amounts of antipyrine and metabolites excreted in six individual rats in 24 h urine (% dose) before and after treatment with 3-methylcholanthrene.

[7] Danhof, M., Breimer, D. D.: Studies on the different metabolic pathways of antipyrine in man. I. Oral administration of 250, 500 and 1000 mg to healthy volunteers. Br. J. clin. Pharmacol., 8, 529—537 (1979c).

[8] Danhof, M., Krom, D. P., Breimer. D. D.: Studies on the different metabolic pathways of antipyrine in rats: influence of phenobarbital and 3-methylcholanthrene treatment. Xenobiotica, 9, 695—702 (1979d).

[9] Hepner, G. W., Vesell, E. S.: Assessment of aminopyrine metabolism in man by breath analysis after oral administration of ^{14}C-aminopyrine. New Engl. J. Med. 291, 1384-1388 (1974).

[10] Hepner, G. W., Vesell, E. S.: Quantitative assessment of aminopyrine metabolism in man by breath analysis after oral administration of ^{14}C-aminopyrine. Ann. Int. Med. 83, 632—638 (1975).

[11] Inaba, T., Tang, K., Kalow, W.: Amobarbital: probe of hepatic drug oxidation in man. Clin. Pharmacol. Ther. 20, 439—444 (1976).

[12] Schüppel, R.: Die Stickstoffdemethylierung am Phenazon (Antipyrin). Naunyn Schmiedebergs Arch. Pharmakol. Exp. Pathol. 255, 71—72 (1966).

[13] Sjöqvist, F., von Bahr, C.: Interindividual differences in drug oxidation: clinical importance. Drug Metab. Disposit. 1, 469—482 (1973).

[14] Thomas, P. E., Lu, A. Y. H., Ryan, D., West, S. B., Kawalek, J., Levin W.: Multiple forms of rat liver cytochrome P-450. Immunochemical evidence with antibody against cytochrome P-488. J. Biol. Chem. 251, 1385—1391 (1976).

[15] Vesell, E. S.: Introduction: Genetic and environmental factors affecting drug response in man. Fed. Proc. 31, 1253—1269 (1972).

[16] Vesell, E. S.: Genetic and environmental factors affecting drug disposition in man. Clin. Pharmacol. Ther. 22, 659-679 (1978).

[17] Vesell, E. S., Page, J. G.: Genetic control of dicumarol levels in man. J. Clin. Invest. 47, 2657—2663 (1968).

[18] Yoshimura, H., Shimeno, H., Tsukamoto, H.: Metabolism of drugs. LIX. A new metabolite of antipyrine. Biochem. Pharmac. 17, 1511—1516 (1968).

[19] Yoshimura, H., Shimeno, H., Tsukamoto, H.: Metabolism of drugs. LXX. Further study on antipyrine metabolism. Chem. Pharm. Bull. Tokyo 19, 41—51 (1971).

Elimination of drug metabolites in liver disease*

Richter, E., Heusler, H., Buschmann, J., Joeres, R., Epping, J., Zilly, W.
Department of Medicine, University of Würzburg, Würzburg, W. Germany

Vermeulen, N.P.E., Breimer, D. D.
Gorlaeus Laboratories, Leiden, The Netherlands

Introduction

In previous investigations of the pharmacokinetics of hexobarbital (HB) in patients with liver diseases a lack of correlation was found between the HB-plasma-clearance and the urinary excretion of the main HB-metabolite, 3'-Keto-HB (Figure 1) [2, 10, 11, 19].
In patients with cholestasis, for example, the HB-plasma-clearance was within the normal range, but the urinary excretion of 3'-Keto-HB was reduced to as low as one half to one third that of the control group [11].
Moreover, in rats with cholestasis induced by ANIT-treatment (1-naphthyl-isothiocyanate) or bile duct ligation the cytochrome p 450 in the liver and the activity of the HB-oxidase are unchanged. In spite of a corresponding normal HB-plasma-clearance the urinary excretion of 3'-Keto-HB was significantly reduced to about 50% of control [1, 5, 6].
In order to discuss the principles of biliary and urinary excretion of drug metabolites, data are presented containing
1) a retrospective analysis of urinary excretion of
   a) 3'-Keto-HB in volunteers induced by rifampicin
   b) 3'-Keto-HB in patients with hepatitis, cirrhosis or cholestasis.
2) Data of the "Epoxide-Diol" pathway in the metabolism of HB in patients with cirrhosis and cholestasis [15].
3) Biliary and urinary excretion of ^{14}C-HB-metabolites in one patient with cholestasis.
4) Biliary and urinary excretion of ^{14}C-HB-metabolites in rats during the early phase of cholestasis (ANIT).
The basic knowledge concerning the characteristics of drug molecules and their influence on biliary excretion have been reviewed recently by several authors [7, 8, 9, 13, 14].

* Supported by: Bundesministerium für Forschung und Technologie (BAM 11) and Deutsche-Forschungs Gemeinschaft (Ri 184/2)

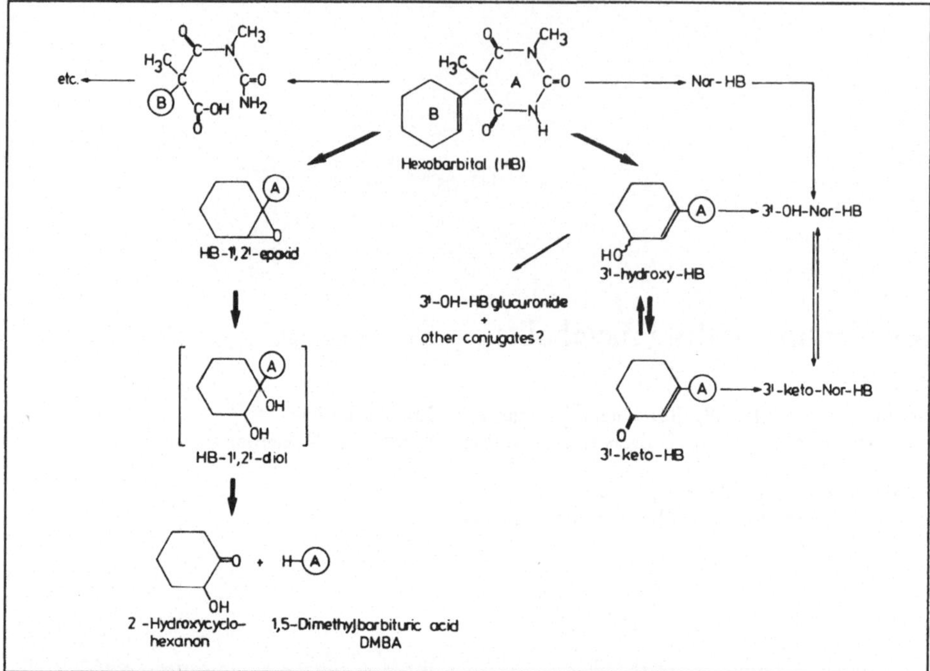

Figure 1: Pathways of hexobarbital-metabolism

Methods

Most of the analytical methods have been described in detail in corresponding papers [2, 3, 4, 10, 11, 12, 15, 16, 17, 18, 19].
With respect to the animal experiments the analytical procedure was as follows:
12 hrs after ANIT treatment (100 mg/kg bw) the bile duct and bladder were cannulated under light ether anaesthesia, and this was followed by the intraduodenal injection of 100 mg/kg bw ^{14}C-HB (5 micro Curies/animal). Bile and urine were collected for one hour in 15 minute fractions. All animals received an infusion of a solution containing 4 mg Furosemide (Lasix®), 160 mg glucose and 1.7 ml Ringer-solution at the rate of 5 ml/h. Lost bile acids were not substituted.
10 µl each of freshly collected bile or urine were placed on Silica-gel TLC plates (G25 Merck, Darmstadt, FRG) and developed for about eight hours at 4°C in a mixture of n-propanol/0.4 N NH_4OH (85:15 v/v).

Results

Retrospective analysis of urinary excretion of 3'-Keto-HB in volunteers and in patients with liver disease:
In Table 1 the tolbutamide and HB plasma clearances in healthy volunteers before and after rifampicin treatment are compared with the urinary excretion of the respective drug metabolites. The clearances of both model drugs are increased significantly after rifampicin induction and the urinary excretion of tolbutamide metabolites was also increased ($r = 0.85$).
On the other hand, the urinary excretion of 3'-Keto-HB was unchanged, although a marked reduction in the urinary excretion of unmetabolized hexobarbital is observed.
A comparison of HB plasma clearance and urinary excretion of 3'-Keto-HB in patients with various

		controls	Rifampicin
Tolbutamide			
Total-clearance	(ml · min^{-1} · kg^{-1})	0.21 ± 0.04 (5)	0.44 ± 0.07 (5)
2 hrs urinary excretion of metabolites	(mg)	257 ± 106 (5)	456 ± 168 (5)
Hexobarbital			
HB-clearance	(ml · min^{-1} · kg^{-1})	3.31 ± 1.03 (17)	9.31 ± 1.66 (11)
24 hrs urinary excretion of HB	(% dose)	0.29 ± 0.16 (11)	0.11 ± 0.05 (10)
24 hrs urinary excretion of 3'keto-HB	(% dose)	39 ± 18 (11)	41 ± 24 (10)

Table 1: Influence of rifampicin treatment (8 days, 1.2 g daily) on plasma clearance and urinary metabolite excretion of tolbutamide and hexobarbital in young healthy volunteers (data from [3, 4, 16, 18]).

	plasma clearance of hexobarbital (ml · min^{-1} · kg^{-1})	24 hrs urinary excretion of 3'keto-hexobarbital (% dose)
controls	3.41 ± 0.90 (21)	43 ± 14 (10)
acute hepatitis	2.18 ± 0.95 (16)	13 ± 6 (6)
liver cirrhosis	1.53 ± 0.66 (18)	5 ± 6 (6)
cholestasis	3.93 ± 1.90 (17)	17 ± 12 (15)

Table 2: Plasma clearance of hexobarbital and urinary excretion of 3'keto-hexobarbital in patients with various types of liver diseases in comparison to control subjects (data from [2, 10, 11, 17, 19]).

types of liver diseases is shown in Table 2. These figures show clearly that the reduction of urinary 3'-Keto-HB excretion was much more pronounced than would be expected from the plasma clearance.

A possible explanation for the discrepancy between the HB plasma clearance and the urinary excretion of 3'-Keto-HB may be the fact that considerable amounts of HB-metabolites are excreted into bile and possibly undergo enterohepatic circulation [12] (Figure 2).

Considering alternative transport pathways for HB-metabolites into bile or urine the following explanations for the reduced urinary excretion of 3'-Keto-HB in patients with liver diseases could be discussed:

1. Reduced enzyme activity in the diseased liver or decreased metabolite formation due to other factors (distribution, liver blood flow, extraction ratio, porto-systemic shunting, deranged liver architecture).
2. Alternative metabolic pathways for HB in liver disease.
3. Disturbance of biliary excretion of metabolites in cholestasis or in defect micelle formation.
4. Incomplete reabsorption of metabolites or breakdown products from the gut.
5. Decreased urinary excretion of metabolites due to functional renal failure or a hepato-renal syndrome.

"Epoxide-Diol" pathway of HB-Metabolism in patients with liver disease (Figure 1):

Vermeulen *et al.* identified the previously unknown metabolites 1,2-epoxide-HB and 1,5-dimethyl-barbituric acid (DMBA), thus demonstrating a epoxide-diol pathway in the metabolism of HB. This pathway accounts for 10—15% of HB-metabolism in man and rats as shown in Table 3.

However, neither in one patient with cholestasis investigated both before and after phenobarbital-treatment (Table 4) nor in five patients with cirrhosis of the liver, could a compensatory excretion of dimethyl-barbituric acid be demonstrated.

Biliary and urinary excretion of ^{14}C-hexobarbital metabolites in one patient with cholestasis:

With the methods currently available for the determination of HB-metabolites in urine, a total excretion of about 30% of the dose within 24 hrs was found in cholestasis (Table 4).
If ^{14}C-labelled HB is used as a test substance in a patient with a comparable degree of cholestasis, 85% of the label is recovered in a 24 hr urine (Table 5). As shown in Figure 3 about 50% of the label is present in a polar fraction which cannot be extracted by organic solvents.

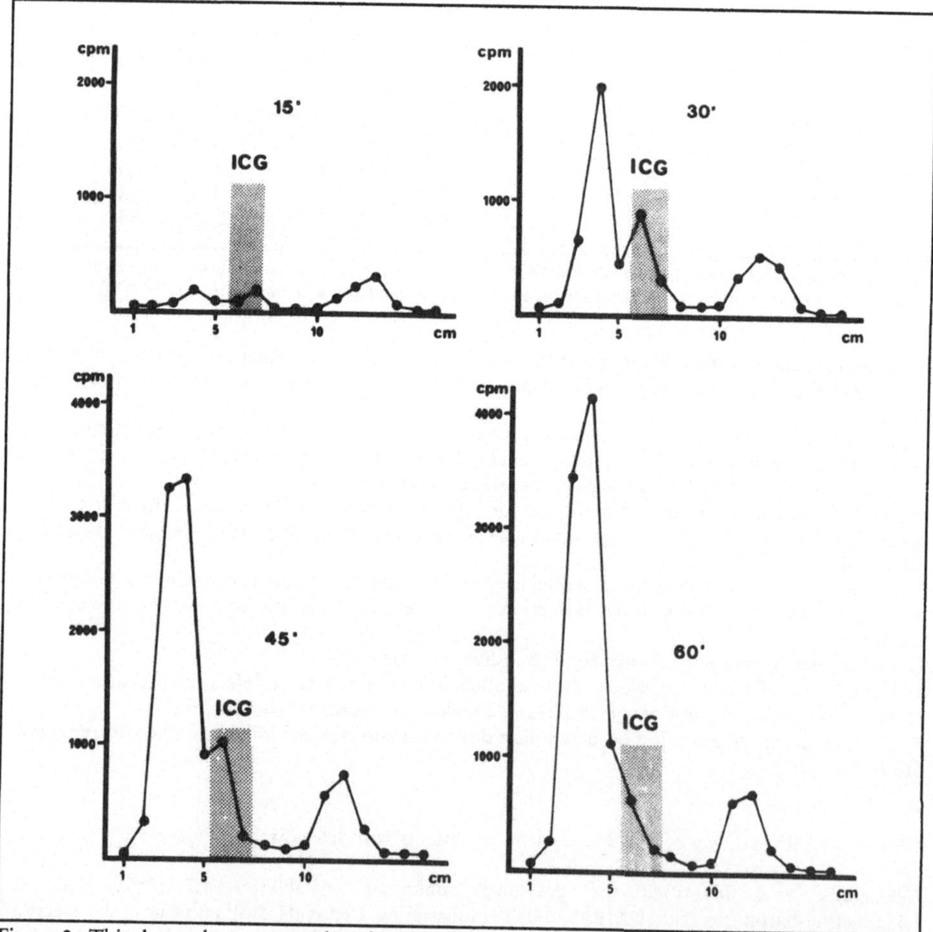

Figure 2: Thin-layer chromatography of rat bile fractions on silicagel Merck G 25 in propanol-ammonia

excretion products	man, 48 hrs % of dose	rats, 24 hrs % of dose
hexobarbital	< 1	< 1
3'-hydroxy-hexobarbital	10 ± 3	18 ± 4
3'-keto-hexobarbital	45 ± 12	58 ± 15
1',2'-epoxide-hexobarbital	—	p < 0.5
1,5-dimethyl-barbituric-acid	23 ± 4	15 ± 3

Table 3: Cumulative urinary excretion of hexobarbital and its metabolites in rats and man (data from [15]).

		before	after
plasma half-life	(h)	4.7	2.4
clearance	(ml/min)	524	1267
3'-hydroxy-HB	(% of dose excreted in 24 h urine)	1.9 (6%)	2.6 (8%)
3'-keto-HB		15.1 (49%)	15.7 (49%)
DMBA		13.8 (45%)	13.7 (43%)
total		30.8 (100%)	32.1 (100%)

Table 4: Cumulative urinary excretion of hexobarbital and its metabolites in a cholangitis patient before and after phenobarbital-treatment.

	micromoles	% dose	total micromoles	total (% dose)	polar metabolites (%)
0-4 hrs	113	5,7	113	5.7	51.3.
4-8 hrs	294	14.8	407	20.5	51.9
8-12 hrs	425	21.4	833	41.9	55.1
12-24 hrs	866	43.6	1699	85.5	57.5

Table 5: Urinary excretion of ^{14}C-hexobarbital-metabolites in one patient with cholestasis.

Biliary and urinary excretion of ^{14}C-hexobarbital-metabolites in rats with early-phase ANIT induced cholestasis:

In order to decide whether the urinary excretion of polar metabolites in patients with cholestasis can be regarded as a compensatory mechanism, investigations were carried out in a experimental model using rats with a mild form of cholestasis produced by aministration of ANIT (see methods).
In Figure 2 the TLC of HB-metabolites in bile, excreted via a biliary fistula in control rats over 60 min, in four 15 minute fractions, is demonstrated.
Polar metabolites are excreted in increasing amounts, so that at least 70% of total metabolite output consists of polar material.
In Table 6 (see methods) the excretion of HB-metabolites in bile and urine is quantitatively compared in bile- and bladder-fistula rats with and without cholestasis.
Treatment with ANIT induced significant changes in plasma bilirubin concentration and in the activity of alkaline phosphatase. The total bile acids showed an even higher increase (Table 6).
Bile flow was moderately decreased to about 50% of controls, but the biliary excretion of all ^{14}C-HB-metabolites was only 5%. The ratio of polar to non-polar metabolites in the treated group was reversed and the output of polar metabolites fell to 1—2% (Table 6).
The pronounced alteration in the biliary excretion of HB-metabolites in animals with cholestasis are

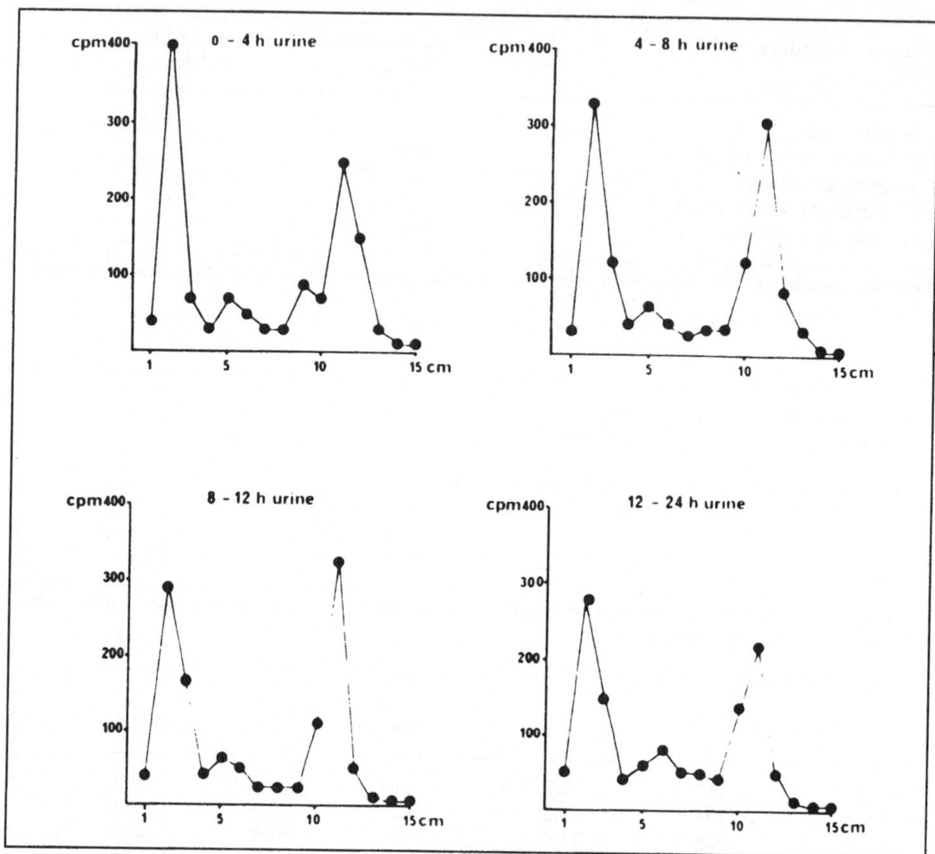

Figure 3: Thin-layer chromatography in one patient with cholestasis on silicagel Merck G 25 in propanol-ammonia

associated with corresponding changes in the urinary metabolite profile. Thus there is an increase of sixfold in the percentage of polar metabolites in this fraction (Table 6).

Conclusion and Summary

1. 3′-Keto-HB appearance in urine was independent of HB-clearance. This may indicate a considerable enterohepatic circulation of HB-metabolites.
2. Although patients with liver diseases—predominantly those with cholestasis—excreted far less 3′-Keto-HB into urine, HB-clearance was not impaired. On the other hand, considerable amounts of polar metabolites are found which normally appear in bile.
3. It is suggested that 3′-Keto-HB is not only a primarily formed HB-metabolite but that it may also arise as a secondary metabolite from degradation of polar metabolites in the intenstine.
4. Reduced urinary excretion of 3′-Keto-HB in patients with liver disease may be due to accompanying cholestasis. In patients with cirrhosis other important factors must be involved.
5. Bearing in mind the importance of the recently found "Epoxide-Diol" pathway, characteristics of the polar metabolite suggest the formation of a glutathione conjugate.

However, a precise characterization of the polar metabolites in bile and urine cannot be given at the present time.

		controls $n = 6$	ANIT $n = 6$
bilirubin	(mg/100 ml)	0.20 ± 0.001	0.85 ± 0.12
alc. phosphatasis	(U/l)	296 ± 15	454 ± 40
plasma bile acids	(μMol/l)	4.0 ± 0.5	23 ± 5
bile flow	(μl/100 g bw/hr)	406 ± 52	175 ± 79
total ^{14}C-excretion	(% dose/hr)	4.15 ± 1.20	0.21 ±0.12*
total polar metabolites	(μg/100 g bw/hr)	352 ± 113	5.3 ± 4.7*
total apolar metabolites	(μg/100 g bw/hr)	63 ± 10	16 ± 7*
urine flow	(μl/100 g bw/hr)	635 ± 188	415 ± 83
total ^{14}C-excretion	(% dose/hr)	0.93 ± 0.40	1.13 ± 0.20
total polar metabolites	(μg/100 g bw/hr)	4.7 ± 1.0	30.0 ± 6.0*
total apolar metbolites	(μg/100 g bw/hr)	89 ± 40	83 ± 16

Table 6: Liver function tests, biliary and urinary excretion of ^{14}C-hexobarbital metabolites in bile fistula rats with early-phase ANIT-cholestasis after intraduodenal application of 100 mg/kg bw ^{14}C-hexobarbital

* $p < 0.05$ in comparison to control group

Literature

[1] Brachtel, D., Gallenkamp, H., Richter, E.: Hexobarbital-Oxidation *in vivo* und *in vitro* bei Choledochusligatur und ANIT-Cholestase der Ratte. Z. Gastroenterologie *15*, 378—380 (1977).

[2] Breimer, D. D., Zilly, W., Richter, E.: Pharmacokinetics of hexobarbital in acute hepatitis and after apparent recovery. Clin. Pharmacol. Ther. *4*, 433 (1975).

[3] Breimer, D., D., Zilly, W., Richter, E.: Influence of rifampicin on drug metabolism: Differences between hexobarbital and antipyrine. Clin. Pharmacol. Ther. *4*, 470 (1977).

[4] Breimer, D. D., Zilly, W., Richter, E.: Influence of corticosteroid on hexobarbital and tolbutamide disposition. Clin. Pharmacol. Ther. *2*, 208 (1978).

[5] Gallenkamp, H., Richter, E.: Influence of Alpha-Naphthylisothiocyanate (ANIT) on microsomal cytochrome p 450, protein and phospholipid content in rat liver. Biochem. Pharm. *23*, 2431 (1974).

[6] Heynen, H. U.: Metabolit-Ausscheidung im Harn nach oraler Gabe von ^{3}H-Hexobarbital und ^{3}H-Paracetamol bei Ratten mit ANIT-Cholestase. Inaug. Diss. Würzburg (1978).

[7] Klaasen, C.: Bile excretion of xenobiotics. Crit. Rev. Toxicol. *4*, 1 (1975).

[8] Levine, W. G.: Biliary excretion of drugs and other xenobiotics. Ann. Rev. Pharmacol. Toxicol. *18*, 81 (1978).

[9] Millburn, P.: Excretion of xenobiotic compounds in bile. In: The hepatobiliary system. Fundamental and pathological mechanism. (Ed. W. Taylor) pp. 109, New York Plenum Press (1976).

[10] Richter, E., Gallenkamp, H., Keller, B., Brachtel, D., Zilly, W., Breimer, D. D.: Metabolismus von Hexobarbital bei Hepatitis und Zirrhose. Z. Gastroenterol. *15*, 381 (1977).

[11] Richter, E., Breimer, D. D., Zilly, W.: Disposition of hexobarbital in human intra- and extrahepatic cholestasis and the influence of drug-metabolism inducing agents. Europ. J. Clin. Pharmacol. *17*, 197 (1980).

[12] Richter, E., Joeres, R., Buschmann, J., Zilly, W.: Alternative transport pathways of cholephilic ^{14}C-hexobarbital metabolites in rats with experimental hepatitis and cholestasis. Acta hepato-gastrologica *26*, 429 (1979).

[13] Smith, R. L.: The excretory function of bile. New York: Wiley. p. 283 (1973).

[14] Stowe, C. M., Plaa, G. L.: Extrarenal excretion of drugs and chemicals. Ann. Rev. Pharmacol. *8*, 337 (1968).

[15] Vermeulen, N.P.E., Bakker, B. H., Schultin K. J., van der Gen, A., Breimer, D. D.: The epoxide-diol pathway in the metabolism of hexobarbital in rats and man. Xenobiotica *9*, 289 (1979).

[16] Zilly, W., Breimer, D. D., Richter, E.: Induction of drug metabolism in man after rifampicin treatment measured by increased hexobarbital and tolbutamide clearance. Europ. J. clin. Pharmacol. *9*, 219 (1975).

[17] Zilly, W., Breimer, D. D., Richter, E.: Stimulation of drug metabolism by rifampicin in patients with cirrhosis or cholestasis measured by increased hexobarbital and tolbutamide clearance. Europ. J. clin. Pharmacol. *11*, 287 (1977).

[18] Zilly, W., Breimer, D. D., Richter, E.: Pharmacokinetic interactions with rifampicin. Clin. Pharmacokinetics *2*, 61 (1977).

[19] Zilly, W., Breimer, D. D., Richter, E.: Hexobarbital disposition in compensated and decompensated cirrhosis of the liver. Clin. Pharmacol. Ther. *5*, 525 (1978).

Theophylline plasma pharmacokinetics and urinary metabolite pattern in patients with liver diseases

A. H. Staib, D. Schuppan, R. Lissner, W. Zilly, G. v. Bomhard, and E. Richter
Zentrum der Pharmakologie, Klinische Pharmakologie
der J. W. G.-Universität Frankfurt/M.
Medizinische Klinik der Universität Würzburg

Introduction

Clinically effective treatment of patients with bronchial asthma and obstructive airway diseases requires the control of theophylline (*T*) plasma levels: a range of 10 to 20 mg/l is considered optimal [6].

Metabolism of *T* occurs in the liver by demethylation and/or oxidation to 3-methylxanthin (3-MX), 1.3-dimethyl uric acid (1.3-DMU) and 1-methyl-uric acid (1-MU) [1, 5, 6, 7].

Only about 7—10% of the administered dose is excreted in the urine of healthy humans over 24 hour period as unchanged *T* [1, 2].

The functional state of the liver is considered to be an essential determining factor for the rate of elimination of T [4]. Several authors have reported a significant reduction of *T* plasma clearance in patients with liver cirrhosis as well as increase of toxic effect in patients with liver diseases (for review see [3]).

In this investigation we examined the extent and the kind of changes of *T* pharmacokinetics and metabolism in clinically defined groups of patients with liver diseases.

The plasma kinetics and the urinary metabolite pattern were determined and compared to those of healthy subjects.

Methods and Materials

1. Clinical Design

Patients with varying degrees of liver diseases (either sex; 19 to 75 years) were associated with the following diagnostic groups according to clinical, clinical-chemical and histological criteria (clinical-chemical data see Table 1):

Acute hepatitis — subdivided into cases without and with drug dependence.
Cholestasis — subdivided into cases without pretreatment and with pretreatment with phenobarbital or phenytoin (induction shown by hexobarbital kinetics [8]).
Liver cirrhosis — subdivided into cases with compensated and decompensated cirrhosis.

	n	Bilirubin mg/100 ml	GTP U/l	Quick %	Alk. P-Ase U/l
acute hepatitis	4	13.3 ± 5	1044 ± 532	61 ± 5	365 ± 123
acute hepatitis with heroin abuse	2	2.1	309	72.5	261
cholestasis	7	6.6 ± 7	105 ± 83	51 ± 23	710 ± 513
cholestasis with induction	3	3.9	93	44	621
liver cirrhosis (compensated)	5	1.3 ± 1	81 ± 75	54 ± 19	336 ± 236
liver cirrhosis (decompensated)	7	6.8 ± 10	52 ± 45	32 ± 7	240 ± 89
normal range		≤ 1.2	≤ 22	80—120	≤ 170

Table 1: Clinical-chemical parameters of the investigated diagnostic groups (Mean ± SD).

Healthy subjects — patients without liver diseases or volunteers.
(controls)
Following a 12-hour overnight fasting period 240 mg Euphyllin® (corresponding to 193 mg *T* monohydrate) was infused over a 5-minute period. Heparinized venous blood samples were obtained 1, 2, 3, 4, 5, 10, 20, 30 minutes and 1, 2, 4, 6, 8, 12, 24, 48 and 72 hours after injection.The 24-urine volume was collected at 4-hour intervals.

2. Analysis of theophylline and its metabolites

2.1 *Plasma levels of T:*

Plasma deproteinization and extraction with acetonitrile (proportion 1:1 or 1:2 v/v, containing the internal standard HPT = proxyphylline) preceded *T* quantitation by HPLC (LC 1082 A Hewlett Packard) with a reverse phase system (RP 8 column; mobile solvent 0.02 M KH_2PO_4/H_3PO_4 pH 3.5 and acetonitrile 95 : 5 v/v, or 0.004 M sodium acetate/acetic acid pH 0.4 and acetonitrile 95 : 5 v/v). Comparison was made with a plasma standard curve (2.5 to 40 mgT/l added; ISTD and ESTD program, respectively).

2.2 *Theophylline and metabolites in urine:*

An aliquot of every 4-hour sample was taken to dryness by evaporation and extracted with the same volume of methanol. The extract was divided into two parts, one of which was spiked with a mixture of *T* and its metabolites. This was followed by HPLC analysis according to the plasma analysis conditions (modification: control run for metabolites using eluent without acetonitrile). Quantitation was achieved using aqueous standard mixtures, ESTD program (Figure 1).

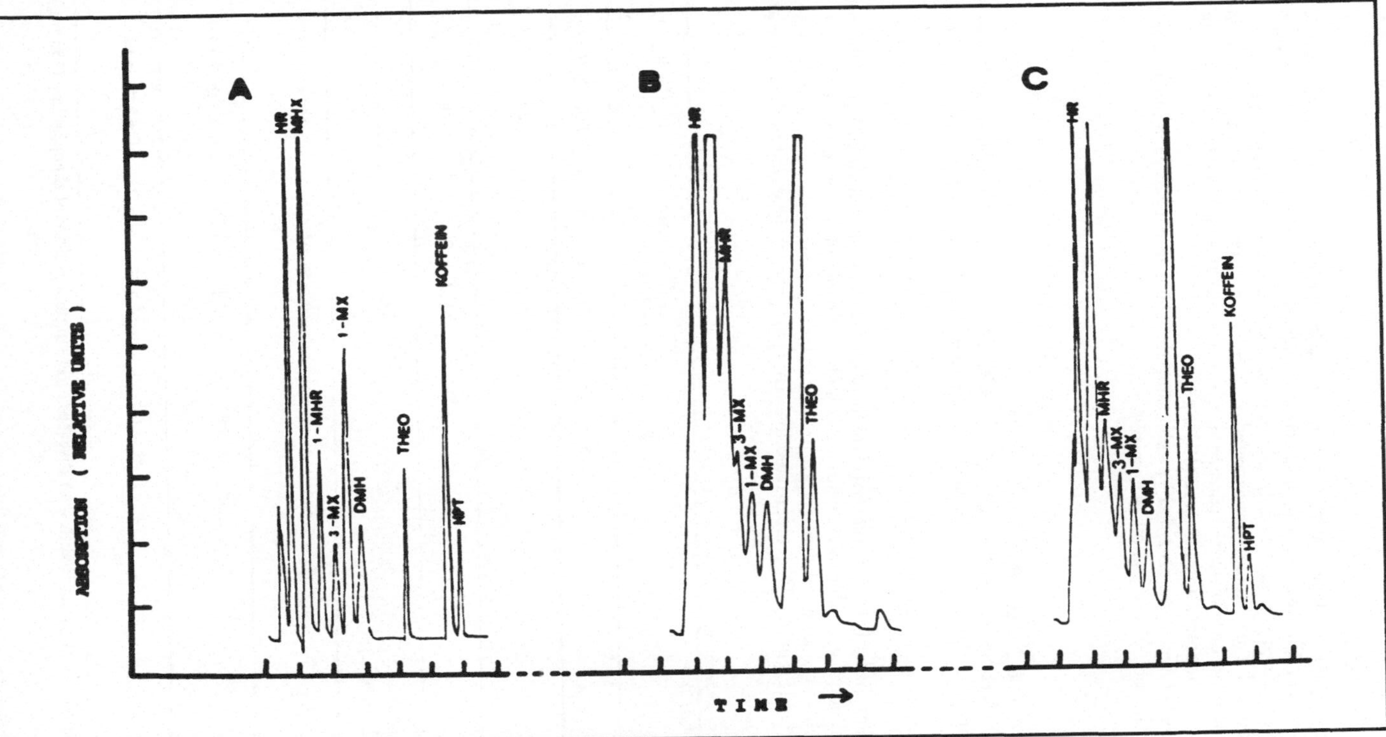

Figure 1: HPLC Analysis of theophylline and of theophylline metabolites in the urine of healthy subjects.
(HR = uric acid, 1-MHR = 1-methyl uric acid, 3-MX = 3-methyl xanthine, Theo = theophylline, DMH = 1.3-dimethyl uric acid, HPT = proxyphylline, MHX = 3-methyl hypoxanthine)
A: standard mixture containing (mg/l) uric acid (50), 3-methyl hypoxanthine (18.5), 1-methyl uric acid (25), 1.3-dimethyl uric acid (16.5), theophylline (30), 3-methyl xanthine (14), caffeine (104), proxyphylline (40).
B: methanolic urine extract.
C: urine extract spiked with the standard mixture (1:1) injection volume 10 µl.

3. Calculations

The measured plasma *T* levels were fitted to an open two compartment model (modified NONLIN program). Pharmacokinetic parameters ($t_{1/2}$, clearance = dose / AUC, $V_{D\,BETA}$) were averaged for each diagnostic group ($\bar{x} \pm SD$, individual values are listed separately).
The total amount of *T* and metabolites excreted over the 24-hour period was calculated from the measured urine concentrations after correction with a molecular weight factor. Results are expressed as percent of dose *T* administered (193 mg).
The metabolite "pattern" was obtained by expressing the urine content of each metabolite as a percentage of the total *T* + metabolites excreted.

Results

Pharmacokinetics (Table 2 A and B):
— In patients with decompensated liver cirrhosis or with acute hepatitis the plasma $t_{1/2}$ is significantly prolonged and the plasma clearance of *T* is decreased. No change in volume of distribution was observed.
— In two cases with acute hepatitis and heroin abuse no change in the half-life of theophylline or clearance was found (in comparison to control group without liver disease).
— A prolongation of the half-life in cholestasis is associated with a small increase of V_D. In the cholestasis group with induction, a "normal" value of $t_{1/2}$ and no change of V_D were found.
— When all patients were taken as a single group a correlation of plasma clearance with plasma half-life was observed (Figure 2). Decompensated liver cirrhosis patients appeared in the figure as a separate group.

	n	$t_{1/2}$ (h)	Clearance ($ml \cdot h^{-1} \cdot kg^{-1}$)	V_D ($l \cdot kg^{-1}$)
acute hepatitis	4	19.2 ± 1.3^x	21.0 ± 2.8^x	0.58 ± 0.1^x
acute hepatitis with heroin abuse	2	5.2*	73.7*	0.54*
cholestasis	7	14.4 ± 8.7^x	38.9 ± 24	0.58 ± 0.11^x
cholestasis with induction (phenobarbital, phenytoin)	3	7.4*	58.5*	0.48*
liver cirrhosis (compensated)	5	11.9 ± 7.4	39.1 ± 26.6	0.45 ± 0.05
liver cirrhosis (decompensated)	7	65.4 ± 29^x	7.1 ± 3.3^x	0.59 ± 0.14
healthy subjects (controls)	6	7.7 ± 1.3	37.9 ± 13.6	0.41 ± 0.12

Table 2A: Pharmacokinetics of patients with liver diseases after single *i. v.* dose of theophylline (193 mg), *n* ($\bar{x}$ ± SD)

^{x} t-test to controls $P \leq 0.05$; * $\bar{x}$ ± SD only for groups with $n \geq 4$, see Table 2B.

Subject	Age (y)	Weight (kg)	Sex	$t_{1/2}$(h)	Clearance (ml/h/kg)	V_D(l/kg)
acute hepatitis						
Wä.	47	79	m	18.8	19.4	0.52
La.	42	69	m	21.3	23.5	0.72
De.	63	45	m	19.0	17.8	0.49
Pa.	20	74.5	m	18.0	23.2	0.60
acute hepatitis (heroin abuse)						
Ech.	21	64	m	5.6	67.0	0.54
Bai.	19	75	m	4.7	80.3	0.54
cholestasis						
Sie.	57	76.9	m	24.1	14.0	0.49
Üb.	69	47.2	f	15.4	33.7	0.75
Va.I	61	68.3	f	27.9	12.3	0.50
Fl.	27	75	m	6.3	76.6	0.69
Wo.	76	58.1	m	6.8	54.6	0.54
We.	59	55.1	f	12.9	26.0	0.48
Ja. II	52	54.8	f	7.6	55.4	0.60
cholestasis with induction						
Ja. I	52	60.8	f	11.0	31.7	0.50
Pfü.	19	75.6	m	3.3	104.0	0.50
Va. II	61	71.1	f	7.74	39.9	0.45
liver cirrhosis (compensated)						
La.	60	74.8	m	8.3	36.4	0.43
Br.	62	70.2	f	3.8	77.5	0.42
Sa.	54	77	f	19.4	15.4	0.43
Tre.	40	77.6	m	8.1	45.5	0.53
Ba.	58	95	m	20.1	15.9	0.46
liver cirrhosis (decompensated)						
Str.	50	64.5	m	100.7	5.2	0.76
Sch.	44	72.1	m	82.2	4.6	0.54
Rö	31	58.6	f	32.8	12.4	0.59
Ko.	45	70.3	m	48.5	9.4	0.66
Ju.	63	83	f	39.8	5.2	0.30
Ja.	43	61.5	f	51.2	9.4	0.70
Eng.	44	91.2	m	102.3	3.7	0.55
healthy subjects (controls)						
Ra.	15	53	m	6.8	53.5	0.52
Pr.	75	80	f	10.0	24.7	0.36
Ho.	40	63	m	7.2	54.0	0.57
Bo.	30	74	f	8.4	36.6	0.45
Ri.	50	80	m	7.6	22.1	0.24
Zi.	42	68	m	6.4	36.2	0.34

Table 2B: Pharmacokinetics of patients with liver disease (single dose-kinetics following 193 mg theophylline *iv*, NONLIN-program), *individual values.*

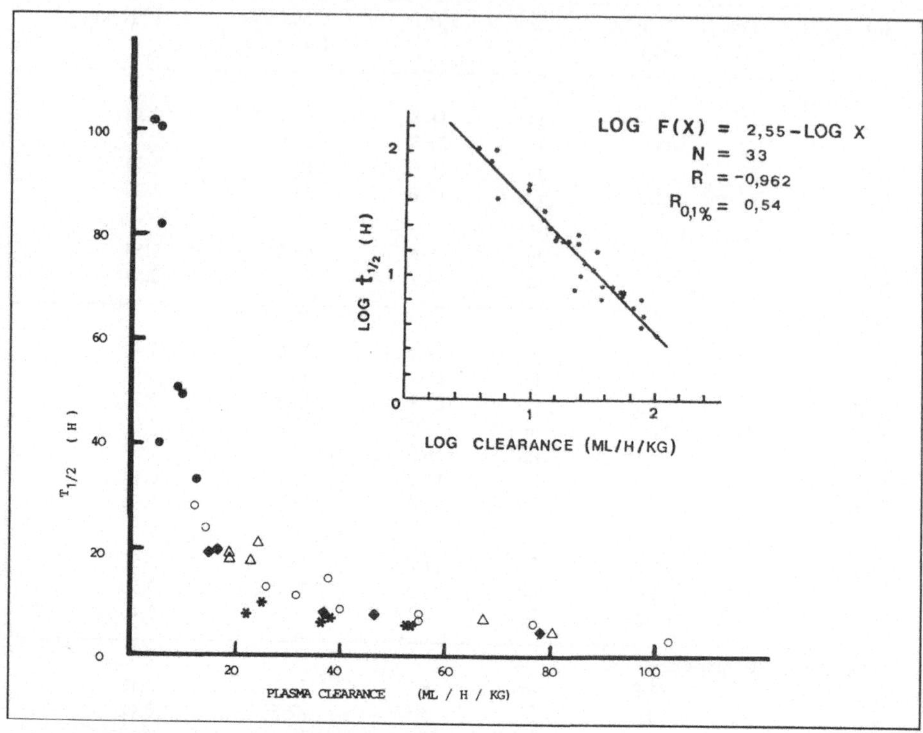

Figure 2: Correlation of theophylline plasma clearance and $t_{\frac{1}{2}}$ in patients with liver diseases (Δ acute hepatitis; ◆ compensated liver cirrhosis, O cholestasis, ● decompensated liver cirrhosis, ★ controls).

Urinary excretion of theophylline and metabolites (Table 3):

The relative proportion of *T* excreted unchanged in urine is similar in all groups and was not significantly different from that in healthy subjects [2].
— The observed metabolite pattern in urine of patients with liver diseases however is clearly different from that of healthy subjects. The proportion of 1-MU is increased, and the proportion of 3-MX and of 1.3-DMU decreased in liver disease.
— On the other hand no differences could be demonstrated between the various liver disease categories because of large inter-subject variations.

Conclusions

1. — Changes of *T* kinetics were most pronounced in patients with decompensated liver cirrhosis.
— Similar changes could be seen in acute hepatitis, when cases of heroin abuse were considered separately.
— The statistically significant elevation in volume of distribution in patients with acute hepatitis and cholestasis in this study is within the range reported for healthy subjects by other investigators.
— Cases with enhanced liver function (induction) show kinetics quite similar to those of healthy subjects.
— Our results differentiate findings [4] of an overall decrease of clearance of *T* in "hepatopathy" and non-differentiated cases of liver cirrhosis.

	n	1-MU	3-MX	1.3-DMU	theophylline unchanged	total amount excreted in 24 h as % of dose
acute hepatitis	2	81 (72—90)	0.1 (0.03—0.2)	16 (8—24)	3 (2—4)	86 (85—86)
acute hepatitis with heroin abuse	1	77	10	9	4	85
cholestasis	4	64 (15—85)	16 (1—55)	8 (2—3)	12 (7—21)	98 (58—128)
cholestasis with induction	2	79 (67—92)	1.5 (0—3.4)	14 (6—22)	6 (3—9)	110 (85—134)
liver cirrhosis (compensated)	3	63 (39—91)	14 (6—20)	19 (1.4—38)	4 (1—7)	86 (75—92)
liver cirrhosis (decompensated)	3	83 (71—96)	0.3 (0—1)	7 (3—10)	9 (1—19)	56 (30—79)
healthy subjects (own results)	2	24 (10—38)	36 (30—45)	30 (29—30)	9 (4—15)	77 (72—82)
healthy subjects (published by [2]	15	16.5 (9—23)	36.2 (21—44)	39.6 (32—47)	7.7 (2.3—23)	116 (62—190)

Table 3: Theophylline metabolite pattern in urine ($\bar{x}$ and range in percent of total excretion calculated as theophylline)

2. — The extent of excretion of *unchanged T* in 24-hour urine is not changed in patients with liver diseases in comparison with healthy subjects, and the two groups have a similar inter-subject variation. No correlation between severity or type of disease and extent of *T* excretion was observed.
— The *total amount* of *T and metabolites* excreted (percent of dose) is similar to values reported in the literature [2] for healthy subjects with the exception of patients with decompensated cirrhosis where a reduction was seen.
3. — Marked changes in *metabolite pattern* were found in all diagnostic groups, expressed by an increase in 1-MU and decrease of 3-MX resulting from a change in the metabolic pathway.
— The changes seem to be different between diagnostic groups. Decompensated cirrhosis for example is associated with very low 3-MX formation.
— These changes in metabolism may be one reason for the observed increased indicence of toxic effects in "liver diseases" when schematic dosage regimes are employed which have been derived from results in healthy subjects.
4. — In patients pretreated with "inducing drugs" (phenobarbital, phenytoin) or with drug abuse (heroin) a tendency to increased elimination rates whilst maintaining the same metabolite pattern was observed.
— The changed biochemical pathway of *T* metabolism in liver diseases seems to be associated with P_{450} dependent enzymes.

The possible explanations for observed changes of theophylline metabolism in liver diseases are:
1) inhibition of 1-demethylation *and* simultaneous increase of 3-demethylation *or*
2) increase of xanthine oxidation (Figure 3).
Our results are in agreement with those of PIAFSKY [4] and others who have also observed a decrease in clearance of theophylline in non-differentiated groups of liver disease patients. Our approach however suggests that decompensated liver cirrhosis patients can be regarded as a kinetically distinct group having an exceptionally low theophylline clearance.

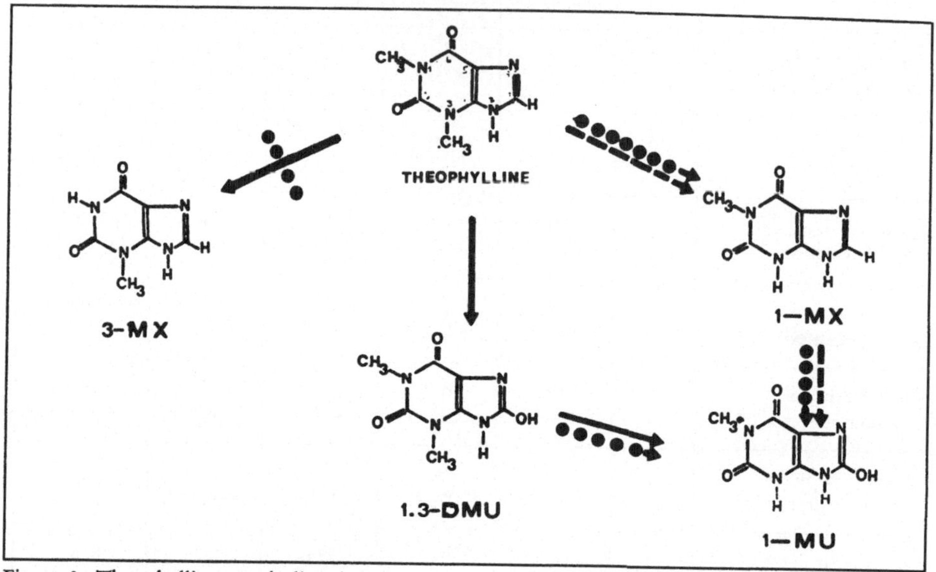

Figure 3: Theophylline metabolism in man.
———▶ metabolic pathway in healthy subjects; — — ▶ uncertain pathway; . . . . . .▶ suspected metabolic pathway in liver disease based upon study results.

Bibliography

[1] Brodie, B., Axelrod, J., and Reichenthal, J.: Metabolism of Theophylline in Man. J. Biol. Chem. *193*, 215—222 (1951)

[2] Jenne, J. W., Nagasawa, H. T., and Thompson, R. D.: Relationship of urinary metabolites of theophylline to serum theophylline levels.—Clin. Pharm. Ther. *19*, 375—381 (1976)

[3] Ogilivie, R. J.: Clinical Pharmacokinetics of Theophylline.—Clin. Pharmacokinetics *3*, 267—293 (1978)

[4] Piafsky, K. M., Sitar, D. S., Rangno, R. E., and Ogilivie, R. J.: Theophylline Disposition in Patients with Hepatitic Cirrhosis. N. Engl. J. Med. *296*, 1495—1497 (1977)

[5] Thompson, R. T., Nagasawa, H. T., and Jenne, J. W.: Determination of Theophylline and its metabolites in human urine and serum by high-pressure—liquid dromatography *84*, 584—593 (1974)

[6] Weinberger, M.: Theophylline for treatment of Asthma J. Ped. *92*, 1—7 (1978)

[7] Weinfeld, H., and Christman, A. A.: The metabolism of Caffeine and Theophylline. J. Biol. Chem. *200*, 345—355 (1953)

[8] Zilly, W., v. Bomhard, G., Richter, E., Staib, A. H., Lissner, R., and Schuppan, D.: Pharmakokinetik von Theophyllin und Hexobarbital bei Lebererkrankungen. 85. Tagung der Deutschen Gesellschaft für Innere Medizin 22.—26. April 1979 in Wiesbaden, Vortrag 367

First pass pharmacokinetics of methohexital in experimental liver disease of the rat*

Epping, J., Heusler, H., Brachtel, D., Richter, E.
Department of Medicine, University of Würzburg, Würzburg, W. Germany

Introduction

The hepatic first pass effect is defined as the elimination of a substance during its first passage of the liver. The systemic bioavailability is contingent on the route of administration. The hepatic first pass effect is dependent on the intrinsic hepatic clearance, liver blood flow and liver architecture (*e. g.* intra-hepatic shunts). Interestingly the phenomenon of the first-pass effect was alluded to as early as 1893, Figure 1.

Methohexital (1-methyl-5-allyl-5[1'-methyl-2'-pentynyl]barbituric acid)—extensively used for short term anesthesia [2, 4, 7], is a high clearance substance and is therefore suitable for investigating alterations of the first pass effect in liver disease.

Galactosamine (GalN) hepatitis [9] and ANIT (α-Naphthyl-Isothiocyanate) induced cholestasis [10] are both well established experimental models. We have used these models, inducing "minimal changes" (see methods), in order to examine alterations of the first pass effect.

Methods

a) Determination of methohexital and hydroxy-methohexital

Blood concentrations of methohexital and its hydroxy metabolite were analysed using gas-chromatography with a nitrogen selective detector. A Hewlett-Packard automation system (Model 3385 A) was calibrated with samples containing known amounts of methohexital and internal standard. A mixture of 0.1 ml rat whole blood and 0.3 ml dest. water was extracted four times with 2.5 ml of diethylether—light petroleum—propanol —2 (50:50:2); hexobarbital (0.5 µg) was used as the internal standard.

The extract was evaporated to dryness and the residue was dissolved in 50 µl abs. ethanol. About 2—3 µl of the solution were injected into a Hewlett-Packard gaschromatograph (Model 5711 A), equipped with a nitrogen detector (Model 18789 A). Column conditions: glass (6 ft × 2 mm I.D.), packed with 3% OV 17 on gaschrom Q 100—120 mesh, temp. 215° C. A typical chromatogram is shown in Figure 2. The identity of the metabolite was checked by gas chromatography—mass spectrometry [3].

* Supported by: Bundesministerium für Forschung und Technologie (BAM 11)

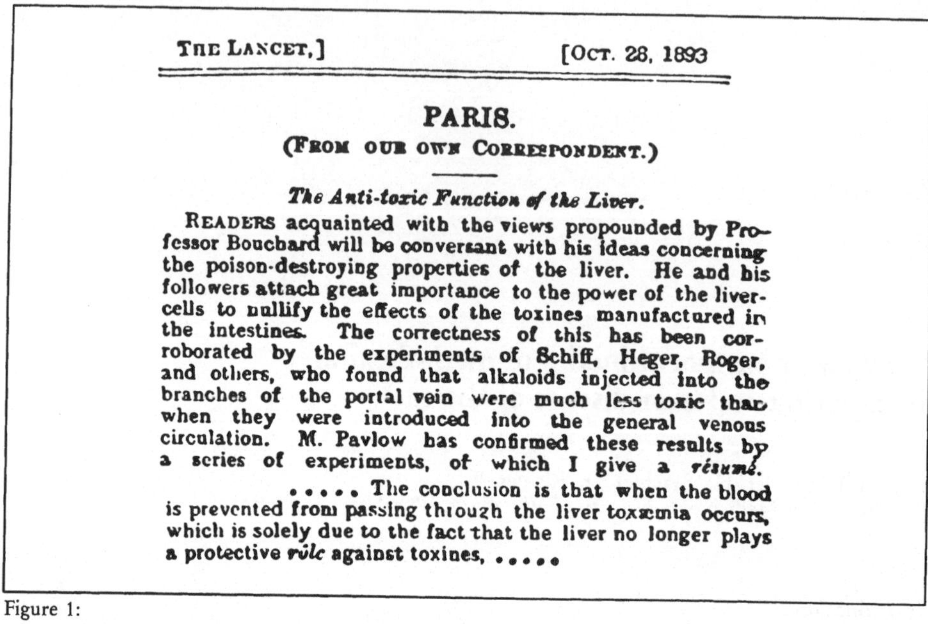

THE LANCET,] [OCT. 28, 1893

PARIS.

(FROM OUR OWN CORRESPONDENT.)

The Anti-toxic Function of the Liver.

READERS acquainted with the views propounded by Professor Bouchard will be conversant with his ideas concerning the poison-destroying properties of the liver. He and his followers attach great importance to the power of the liver-cells to nullify the effects of the toxines manufactured in the intestines. The correctness of this has been corroborated by the experiments of Schiff, Heger, Roger, and others, who found that alkaloids injected into the branches of the portal vein were much less toxic than when they were introduced into the general venous circulation. M. Pavlow has confirmed these results by a series of experiments, of which I give a *résumé*.

..... The conclusion is that when the blood is prevented from passing through the liver toxæmia occurs, which is solely due to the fact that the liver no longer plays a protective *rôle* against toxines, ...

Figure 1:

b) Determination of cytochrome p 450

Cytochrome p 450 was determined spectrophotometrically in the liver homogenate by the method of OMURA and SATO [8], modified by SCHOENE *et al.* [11].

c) Determination of methohexital oxidase

The 19000g supernatant of a rat liver homogenate was incubated with methohexital. After extraction of the incubation mixture the conversion of methohexital to its hydroxy-metabolite was measured with gas chromatography.

d) Methohexital administration protocol

200 mg Sprague-Drawly rats were used. Methohexital was given orally or intravenously (v. fem.). Blood was collected from a tail vein. Before the experiments all animals received phenobarbital in drinking water for seven days (ca. 30 mg/d).

e) Experimental liver disease ("minimal change")

GalN: rats received 350 mg/kg galactosamine i. p.
ANIT: rats received 20 mg/kg ANIT by intubation.
After the experiments all animals were investigated histologically and serologically (bilirubin, alkaline phosphatase, total protein and glycocheno-desoxycholic acid and glycocholic acid (RTA-Kit Nordiclab).

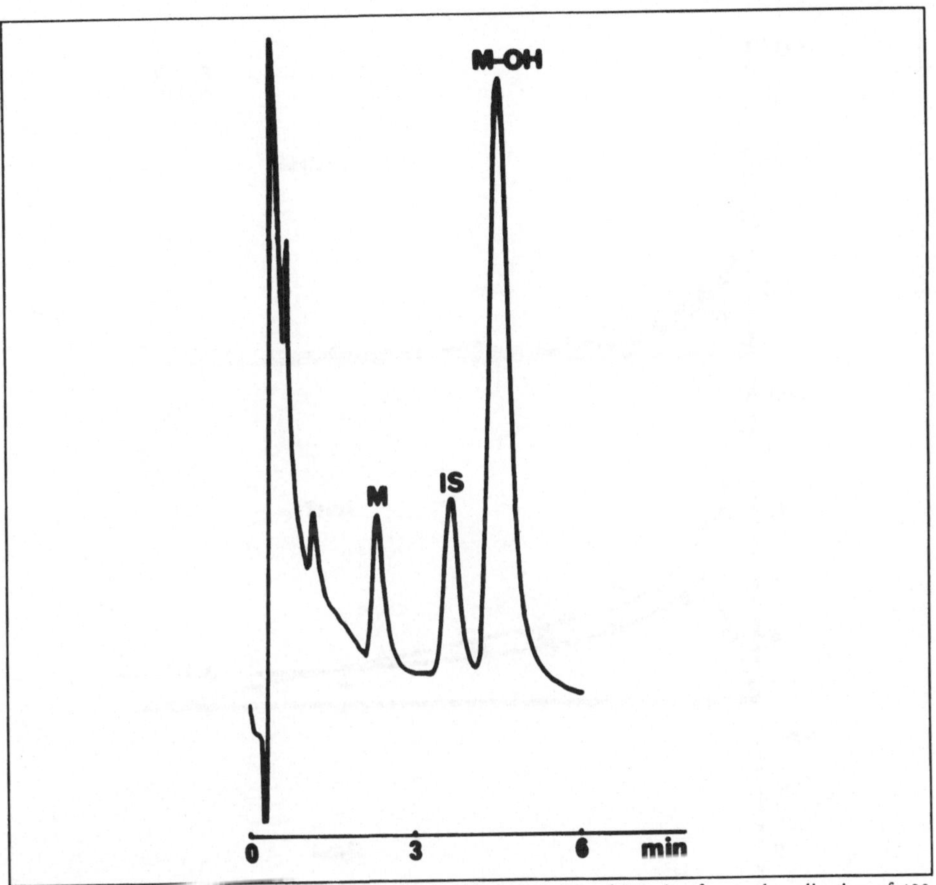

Figure 2: Gas chromatogram of an extract of 0.1 ml rat whole blood 15 min after oral application of 400 mg/kg methohexital (int. std. hexobarbital, 5.0 μg/ml; M = methohexital; M-OH = hydroxymethohexital).

Results

Figure 3 a) shows the blood concentration curve of methohexital in phenobarbital pretreated animals. The pharmacokinetic data have been computed using the two compartment model [1, 6]. The major metabolite 4'-hydroxymethohexital [7, 12] was identified by mass spectrometry [3] and its rapid formation and elimination from the blood was verified (Figure 3 b).

Taking into account the different dosage, a comparison of the methohexital concentrations after oral and *i. v.* application demonstrates the first pass effect. The rapid distribution and elimination is in keeping with the short term action of the drug.

Figure 4 shows the correlation between cytochrome p 450 content of the liver and the methohexital oxidase activity *in vitro* as well as the methohexital clearance *in vivo*. The correlation between cytochrome p 450 and the pharmacodynamic effect (using sleeping time as the parameter) was significant only when cytochrome p 450 was measured prior to methohexital application. Therefore, animals have been 2/3 partially hepatectomized and the cytochrome p 450 content determined in the excised tissue.

The lack of correlation between sleeping-time and cytochrome p 450 content measured after applica-

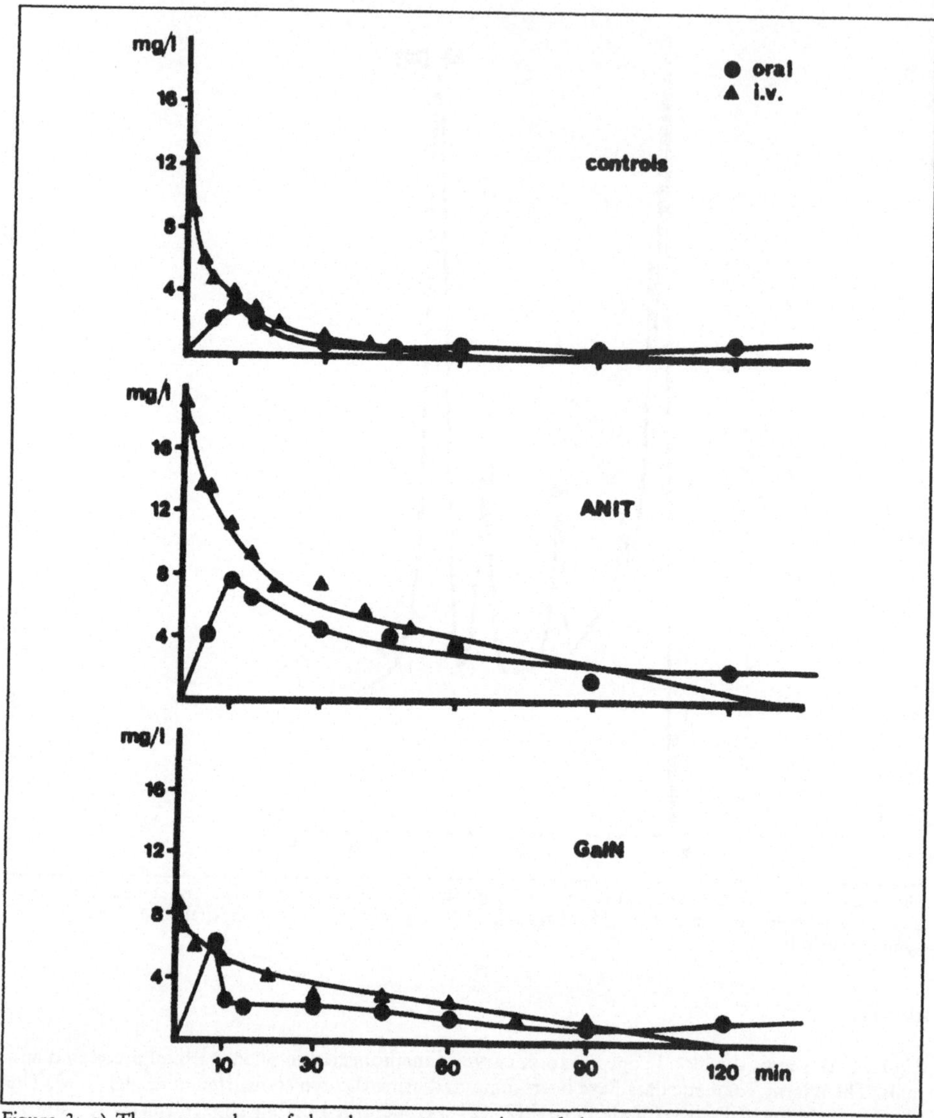

Figure 3: a) The mean values of the plasma concentrations of six animals are shown. All animals are pretreated with phenobarbital. Oral dose of methohexital: 400 mg/kg; *i. v.* dose: controls and ANIT 40 mg/kg; GalN 20 mg/kg (higher dosage is not tolerated).

tion of methohexital may be due to the rapid distribution and elimination of the drug or possibly to a direct action of methohexital on cytochrome p 450 itself. The destructive effects of secobarbital and other allylbarbiturates on cytochrome p 450 have previously been reported [5].

"Minimal change" experimental liver disease: The relatively low doses of galactosamine and ANIT, utilized in the experiments, cause only "minimal changes" in the liver; consequently, the morphological changes observed at high doses are not seen under the light-microscope. The common liver function tests (aspartate transaminase, bilirubin, total bile acids) are only slightly elevated (Figure 5).

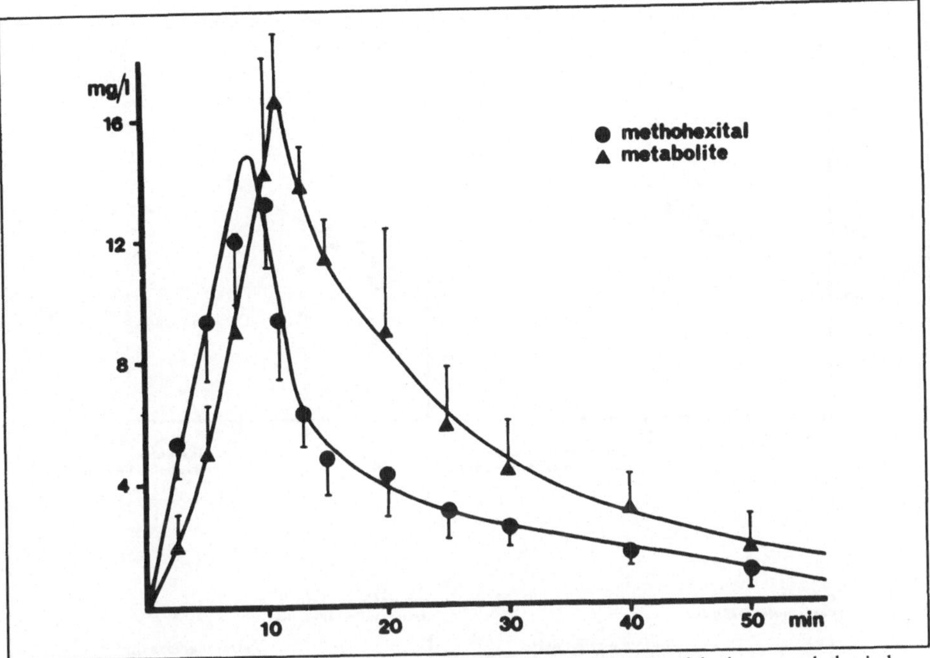

Figure 3: b) The mean values of plasma concentration of methohexital and hydroxy-methohexital are shown after *i. v.* application of methohexital in phenobarbital pretreated animals.

	controls	ANIT	GalN
AST (U/l)	9 ± 5	32 ± 26 $p < 0.0001$	56 ± 63 $p < 0.0001$
Bilirubin (µmoles/l)	3.5 ± 1.5	14.7 ± 15.2 $p < 0.0001$	5.1 ± 1.9 $p < 0.0001$
total bile acid (µmoles/l)	4.4 ± 2.6	9.5 ± 3.3 $p < 0.0005$	7.3 ± 4.2 $p < 0.025$
Methohexitaloxidase (µmoles/15 min/100 g bw)	123 ± 49	144 ± 51 n.s.	116 ± 51 n.s.
Cytochrome p 450 (nmoles / 100 g bw)	336 ± 65	379 ± 86 n.s.	350 ± 92 n.s.

Figure 5: Laboratory test on plasma, methohexital oxidase activity *in vitro* and cytochrome p 450 content in dissected liver. Rats of 200 g, $n = 13$ in controls, ANIT (20 mg/kg bw, 24 hrs before), GalN (250 mg/kg bw 12 hrs before). AST = aspartate transaminase.

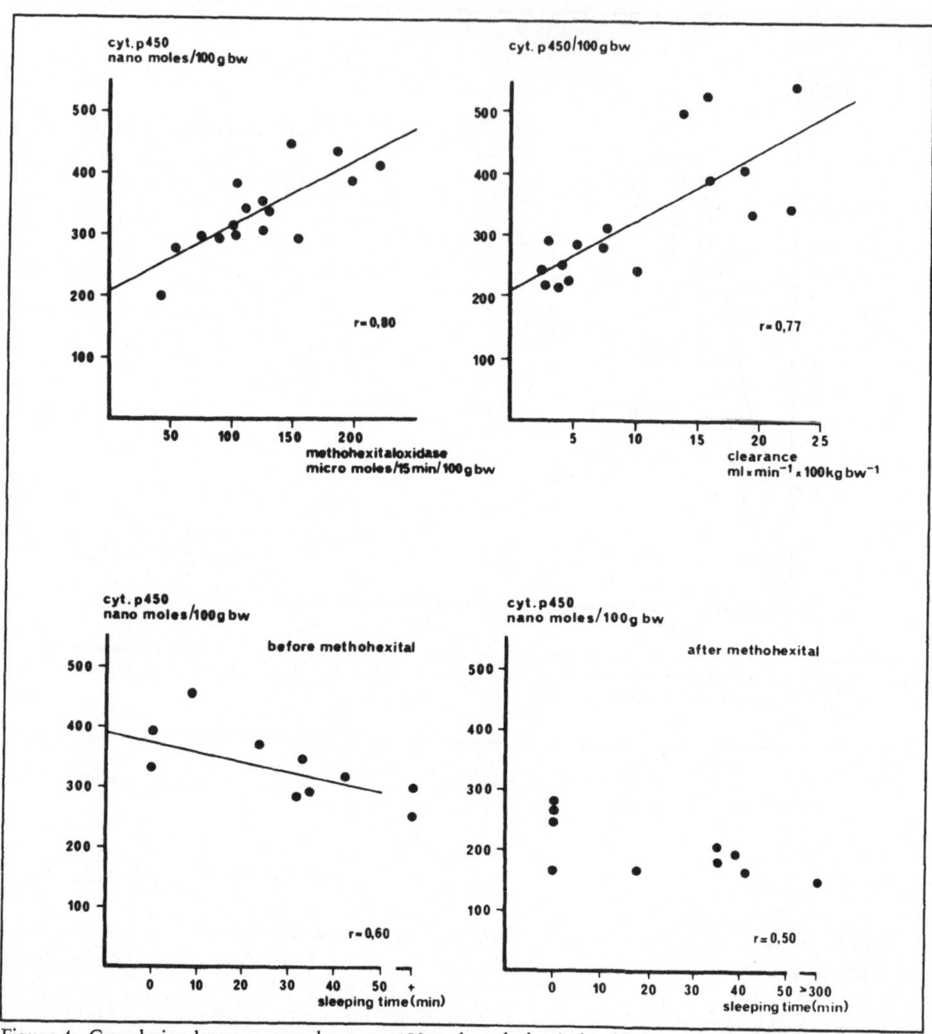

Figure 4: Correlation between cytochrome p 450 and methohexital oxidase, and sleeping time: Before application of methohexital the animals were hepatectomized.

The hepatic cytochrome p 450 content and methohexital oxidase activity which would be indicators of intrinsic hepatic clearance remain unchanged.
On the other hand however, a significant and biologically important decrease in the oral clearance and the first pass effect (expressed as $AUC_{oral}/AUC_{i.\,v.}$) was observed (Figure 6).
This corresponds to the pharmacodynamic effect expressed in a increased sleeping time and/or a decreased survival rate.

Conclusion and Summary

Methohexital—a short acting anesthetic—is a high clearance substance. The most important metabolism route in the rat is hydroxylation.

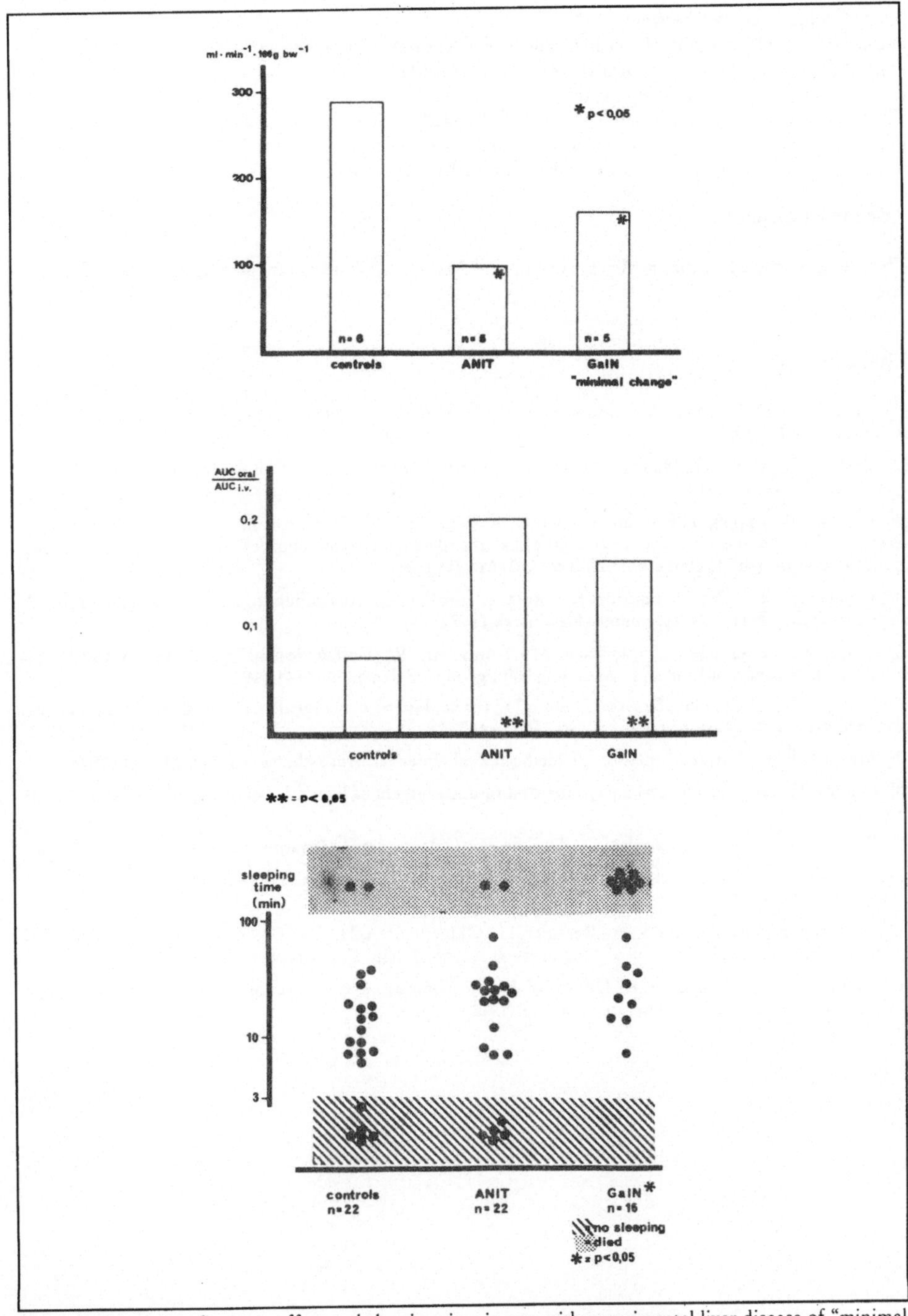

Figure 6: Clearance, first pass effect and sleeping time in rats with experimental liver disease of "minimal changes" character (ANIT 20 mg/kg bw, GalN 350 mg/kg bw).

A correlation is shown between:
cytochrome p 450 content of the liver and the methohexital oxidase *in vitro*;
methohexital oxidase *in vitro* and the clearance *in vivo*;
clearance *in vivo* and the sleeping time.
The first pass effect is diminished by "minimal change" experimental liver disease without alterations in the content of cytochrome p 450 or in the activity of methohexital oxidase. Thus, a change in the liver architecture may be the cause of the diminished first pass effect.

Acknowledgement

The authors wished to thank Ms. B. Albütz and Ms. M. Weisenberger for helpful technical assistance.

Literature

[1] Breimer, D. D.: Pharmacokinetics of methohexitone following intravenous infusion in humans. Brit. J. Anaesth. *48*, 643 (1976)

[2] Bush, M. T., Berry, G., Hume, A.: Ultra-short-acting barbiturates as oral hypnotic agents in man. Clin. Pharmac. Therap. 7, 373 (1966)

[3] Heusler, H., Epping, J., Heusler, S., Richter, E., Vermeulen, N. P. E., Breimer, D. D.: Simultaneous determination of blood concentrations of methohexital and its hydroxymetabolite by gaschromatography and identification of 4-hydroxymethohexital by GC-MS (in press)

[4] Lehmann, Ch.: Das Ultrakurznarkotikum Methohexital. Anaesthesiology and Resuscitation 57. Springer-Verlag-Berlin—Heidelberg—New York (1972)

[5] Levin, W., Sernatinger, E., Jacobsen, M., Kuntzman, R.: Destruction of cytochrome p 450 by secobarbital and other barbiturates containing allyl groups. Science *16*, 1341 (1972)

[6] Loo, J. C. K., Riegelman, S.: Assessment of pharmacokinetic constants from postinfusion blood curves obtained after *i. v.* infusion. J. Pharm. Sci. *59*, 53 (1970)

[7] Murphy, P. J.: Biotransformation of methohexital. Internat. Anaesthesol. Clinics *12*, 139 (1974)

[8] Omura, T., Sato, R.: The carban-monoxide-binding pigment of liver microsomes. J. biol. Chem. *239*, 23 (1964)

[9] Reutter, W., Lesch, R., Keppler, D., Decker, K.: Galactosamin-Hepatitis. Naturwiss. *55*, 497 (1968)

[10] Schaffner, H., Scharnbeck, H., Hutterer, F., Denk, H., Greim, H. A., Popper, H.: Mechanism of cholestasis: VII α-Naphtylisothiocyanate induced jaundice. Lab. Invest. *28*, 231 (1973)

[11] Schoene, B., Fleischmann, R. A., Remmer, H., Oldershausen, H. F. v.: Determination of drug metabolizing enzymes in needle biopsies of human liver. Europ. J. clin. Pharmacol. *4*, 565 (1972)

[12] Welles, J. S., Mc Mahan, R. E., Doran, W. J.: The metabolism and excretion of Methohexital in the rat and dog. J. Pharmacol. Exp. Therap. *139*, 166 (1962)

Chapter 7

Assessment of clinical importance of hepatic drug metabolism

Can lignocaine kinetics be predicted?

G. T. TUCKER, N. D. S. BAX, M. S. LENNARD, and H. F. WOODS
Department of Therapeutics, University of Sheffield
The Hallamshire Hospital, Sheffield U.K.

Introduction

The therapeutic value of lignocaine in acute myocardial infarction is still a subject of debate [1]. Some of the lack of success with this drug may arise from the use of inadequate dosage. Thus, several trials, such as those of BENNETT *et al* [2] and CHOPRA *et al* [3], failed to show benefit, whereas relatively higher doses were used by LIE *et al* [4] who did report success in preventing ventricular fibrillation. However, this was achieved at the expense of a 15% incidence of toxicity, underlining the fact that the therapeutic index of lignocaine is low.
With the recognition that therapeutic plasma concentrations of lignocaine range between 1.5—6 µg/ml, relatively sophisticated dosage regimens, such as that of APS *et al* [5] involving a step-down infusion rate, have been advocated to achieve a response rapidly and smoothly.
All of these regimens are general guidelines and no one regimen will be suitable for all post-myocardial infarct patients.
Studies by THOMSON *et al* [6] of lignocaine kinetics after *i. v.* bolus injections in patients with heart failure and liver cirrhosis have provided indications for further "fine-tuning" of the dosage. In these patients it was found that the plasma clearance of the drug is about 40% lower than in normals (6 ml/min/kg *vs* 10 ml/min/kg) suggesting, therefore, that usual infusion rates should be modified accordingly to achieve a similar therapeutic end-point. 'Terminal' elimination $t_{½}$ values of lignocaine were similar in both normals and in patients with heart failure and averaged just under 2h, but were considerably prolonged in patients with liver disease. Therefore, these studies lead to the prediction that, provided the patient does not have liver disease, a steady-state plasma concentration of drug would occur after about 8h of *i. v.* infusion at a constant rate.
Thus, if a method were available for predicting lignocaine kinetics in the individual patient a more effective control of blood drug concentration may be achieved.
A major cause of variability in the kinetics of lignocaine is alteration in hepatic blood flow since the hepatic extraction ratio of the drug is about 0.7 and non-hepatic routes of elimination are unimportant [7, 8]. Indocyanine green dye (ICG) is used to estimate liver blood flow and is a potentially useful marker of lignocaine clearance because the hepatic extraction ratio of this compound is similar to that of lignocaine [9]. It is easily measured by colorimetry either in neat plasma samples or non-invasively using an ear-piece densitometer, and it has a short plasma elimination half-life.
ZITO and REID [10] reported a strong correlation ($r = 0.95$; $p < 0.001$) between the plasma clearances of lignocaine and those of ICG in 26 patients with and without heart failure. On the basis of the ICG results, they suggested that this relationship allows the lignocaine infusion rate to be ad-

justed to achieve a desired steady-state plasma drug concentration in an individual patient. However, it has not been our experience, nor that of several other groups, that lignocaine kinetics are so straightforward. In the following discussion several issues are raised indicating that we still have more to learn about this drug before reliable kinetic models can be applied to its clinical use.

Effect of lignocaine on hepatic blood flow

Short *i. v.* infusions of lignocaine (4 mg/min over 150 min) in man have been shown to cause a 20—30% increase in hepatic blood flow [11]. This change is probably secondary to an increase in cardiac output mediated by a central effect evoked through the sympathetic nervous system [12]. Since lignocaine clearance is dependent upon liver blood flow, the haemodynamic effects of the drug could, therefore, exert a positive feedback influence on its own elimination. For this reason, kinetic parameters derived from *i. v.* bolus data might overestimate steady-state blood concentrations of the drug during continuous *i. v.* infusion [8].

Relationship between lignocaine clearance and ICG kinetics

Like Zito and Reid [10], we were also intrigued by the possibility that ICG might be a good predictor of lignocaine kinetics. A similar study to theirs was carried out using 18 post-myocardial infarct patients, half with heart failure and half without, and matched for age and weight*.
Each patient received a 100 mg i. v. injection of lignocaine HCl in 3 min and an infusion was started at a rate of 4 mg $\cdot$ min^{-1}. The rate was lowered to 2 mg $\cdot$ min^{-1} after 30 min. Serial blood samples were taken between 8 and 36h after the start of therapy for estimation of lignocaine and its N-deethylated metabolite (MEGX) by gas chromatography.
Mean values of lignocaine concentration over the sampling period were divided into the infusion rate to obtain estimates of clearance.
During the infusions, a bolus dose of ICG (0.5 mg $\cdot$ kg^{-1}) was injected into an antecubital vein and the elimination of the dye over the next 20 min was followed by assay of plasma samples taken from the opposite arm. Monoexponential decay of dye concentrations beyond 6 min allowed calculation of $t_{½}$ values, volumes of distribution and clearance in the usual manner.
Unlike Zito and Reid [10], we did not find a significant relationship between lignocaine and ICG clearances ($r_s = 0.31$; $p > 0.05$; $n = 18$). Although mean lignocaine clearance was significantly lower in the heart failure sub-group compared to the non-heart failure sub-group, none of the ICG parameters discriminated between the two clinical sub-groups (Table 1).

	Lignocaine CL_B (ml $\cdot$ min^{-1} $\cdot$ kg^{-1})	ICG CL_B (ml $\cdot$ min^{-1} $\cdot$ kg^{-1})	ICG Plasma $t_{½}$ (min)	ICG Vd_B (ml $\cdot$ kg^{-1})
No heart failure ($n = 9$)	11.8 ± 2.5	13.3 ± 5.3	3.9 ± 0.9	73 ± 23
Heart failure ($n = 9$)	7.2 ± 2.0	11.0 ± 2.8	4.7 ± 0.9	83 ± 30
	$p<0.002$	N. S.	N. S.	N. S.

Table 1: Lignocaine and indocyanine green—pharmacokinetic parameters in post-myocardial infarct patients with and without heart failure (mean values ± *s. d.*)
Cl_B = whole blood clearance; Vd_B = volume of distribution determined with reference to blood concentration-mean value between 8—36 h of infusion.

* Bax, N. D. S., Tucker, G. T., Woods, H. F.: Lignocaine and indocyanine green kinetics in patients following myocardial infarction. Brit. J. Clin. Pharmacol. (In press).

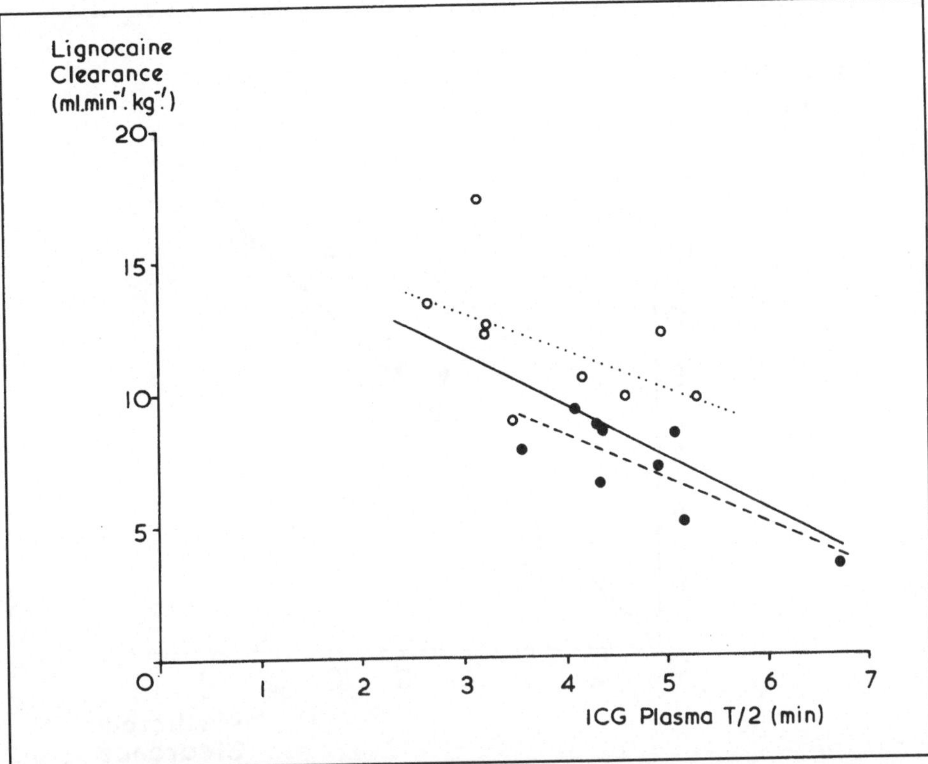

Figure 1: Relationship between lignocaine clearance and ICG half-life in post-myocardial infarct patients with (closed circles) and without (open circles) heart failure.
(Regression lines are shown for data from all patients and from each clinical sub-group).

There was a significant overall linear correlation between blood lignocaine clearance and ICG $t_{½}$ ($r_s = 0.67$; $p < 0.01$; $n = 18$), but, because of considerable overlap between ICG $t_{½}$ values in the clinical subgroups patients with and without heart failure can be viewed as separate populations with separate regression lines (Figure 1). Therefore, a better description of the data is based upon multiple linear regression analysis with both ICG $t_{½}$ and the presence or absence of heart failure as predictor variables. Using this approach it was possible to account for 75% of the variance between observed and predicted lignocaine clearance (Figure 2).
In contrast then to the findings of ZITO and REID [10], who observed that the clearances of lignocaine and ICG declined in parallel with increasing severity of heart failure, our results are consistent with a greater influence of heart failure on the hepatic elimination of lignocaine. The effects of heart failure on lignocaine kinetics may be more a function of changes in hepatic microsomal enzyme activity [13, 14] than of changes in hepatic blood flow marked by the ICG.

Rising blood concentrations of lignocaine during prolonged *i. v.* infusion

An assumption implied in the calculation of lignocaine clearance from data obtained during constant rate *i. v.* infusion is that blood concentrations of the drug have reached a steady-state. As indicated previously, bolus data would predict this to occur within 8h. However, in common with other groups [15, 16], we observed a significant rise (in our case 25%) in the blood drug concentration, and hence a fall in the 'apparent clearance' of lignocaine, between 8 and 36h of continuous infusion (Table 2).

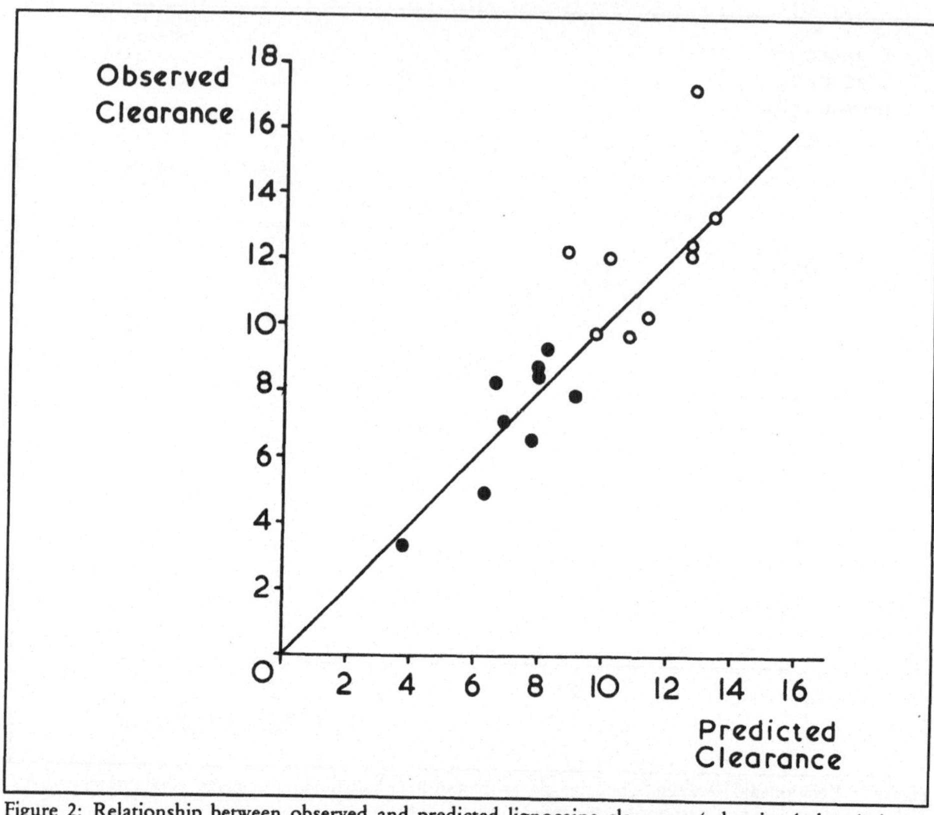

Figure 2: Relationship between observed and predicted lignocaine clearance (ml · min^{-1} · kg^{-1}) in 18 post-myocardial infarct patients with (closed circles) and without (open circles) heart failure. (Predicted values were derived by multiple linear regression analysis using the equation: $CL_B = 14.9 - 1.64\ X_1 - 0.765\ X_2 - 0.088(X_2)^2$; where CL = predicted clearance, $X_1 = -1$ (no heart failure) or $+1$ (heart failure) and X_2 = ICG half-life.)

Lignocaine Cl_B(ml · min^{-1} · kg^{-1})	8—12 h	24—28 h	Δ Cl_B (%)
No heart failure	13.4 ± 1.9	10.1 ± 2.2	24.4 ($p<0.05$)
Heart failure	10.1 ± 1.8	7.7 ± 0.9	24.2 ($p<0.05$)
Δ Cl_B (%)	24.7 ($p<0.05$)	24.5 ($p<0.01$)	

Table 2: Change in the apparent clearance of lignocaine during prolonged *i. v.* infusion in post-myocardial infarct patients with and without heart failure.

There was no clinical evidence of any progressive decrease in liver perfusion in these patients and, as mentioned already, lignocaine itself would be expected to cause an increase in hepatic blood flow.
Not only do blood lignocaine levels rise progressively during long infusions, but $t_{1/2}$ values on stopping such infusions are considerably longer than those reported following bolus injections, an observation made originally by Prescott, Adjepon-Yamoah, and Talbot [15] and which we have confirmed. Measurement of $t_{1/2}$ values in 4 patients between 5 and 28h after stopping 36h+ infusions gave a mean value of 7.2h (range 4.7—9.8h), nearly 4 times greater than the mean 'terminal' $t_{1/2}$ measured by Thomson *et al* [6] up to 4—6h after bolus injections of 50—100 mg lignocaine. Values of 'apparent' lignocaine clearance in our 4 patients calculated from 36h blood drug concentration averaged 36% less than the mean clearance value quoted by Thomson *et al* [6].
At least two possibilities could explain the discrepancy between bolus and infusion data.
Firstly, blood sampling during the original bolus studies may not have been continued for long enough to disclose the presence of an additional tissue compartment. We have measured blood lignocaine concentrations after 100 mg *i. v.* bolus injections in two volunteers and found that the 'terminal' $t_{1/2}$ remains at 2h even when sampling is continued for up to 14h. However, theoretical calculations showed that the addition of a hypothetical slower elimination phase beyond 14h might indeed account for some of the discrepancy between bolus and infusion kinetics.
The second possibility is a time-dependent change in lignocaine kinetics resulting from a decrease in the intrinsic hepatic clearance of the drug. Evidence in favour of this possibility comes from studies in animals. Le Lorier *et al* [17] observed that continuous *i. v.* infusion of lignocaine in dogs is associated with a progressive lowering of its hepatic extraction ratio from a mean value of 0.79 at 1.5h to 0.26 at 24h. Also in dogs, Vicuna *et al* [18] showed that an initial high infusion rate of lignocaine decreases clearance of the drug during a subsequent low infusion rate period. We have found a progressive decrease in the clearance of lignocaine following successive bolus injections in an isolated perfused rat liver preparation [20] (Figure 3).
One explanation of changes in kinetics consistent with all of these animal data is an effect due to accumulating lignocaine metabolites on the hepatic metabolism and/or uptake of the parent drug. The three main routes of lignocaine metabolism are amide-hydrolysis, N-dealkylation and aromatic hydroxylation [19]. On adding each of the known end-product metabolites to the perfusion medium in the isolated liver system, only MEGX was found to cause a consistent impairment of lignocaine elimination, suggesting that N-dealkylation may be the affected pathway. However, this does not necessarily prove that MEGX is the causative compound and there are several further reasons for believing that it is not. Firstly, in our experience, plasma MEGX levels in patients during lignocaine infusion are generally much lower (less than 30%) than those of the parent drug. Secondly, in the perfused rat liver system both perfusate and liver levels of MEGX require to be much higher to cause inhibition of lignocaine metabolism when the MEGX is added exogenously than when it is formed endogenously from lignocaine [20].

Conclusions

Can lignocaine kinetics be predicted?
The use of kinetic data obtained from *i. v.* bolus studies to predict lignocaine concentrations during and after *i. v.* infusions is complicated by a drug-induced increase in hepatic blood flow and, during prolonged administration, by the possibility of a time-dependent decrease in hepatic clearance. Although there is evidence for the latter phenomenon in animals, an alternative explanation for continuously rising lignocaine concentrations during infusion in man is that bolus data were not collected for long enough to detect a deep tissue compartment. To clarify this point further studies of the kinetics of lignocaine after *i. v.* bolus administration are required using very sensitive methods of drug assay.
Although ICG $t_{1/2}$ and lignocaine clearance are correlated, at least in our experience ICG appears to be of less direct value in predicting lignocaine dosage in the individual patient than suggested by other workers. We would suggest that the handling of these two compounds may be significantly different, with respect to each other, in patients with heart failure.

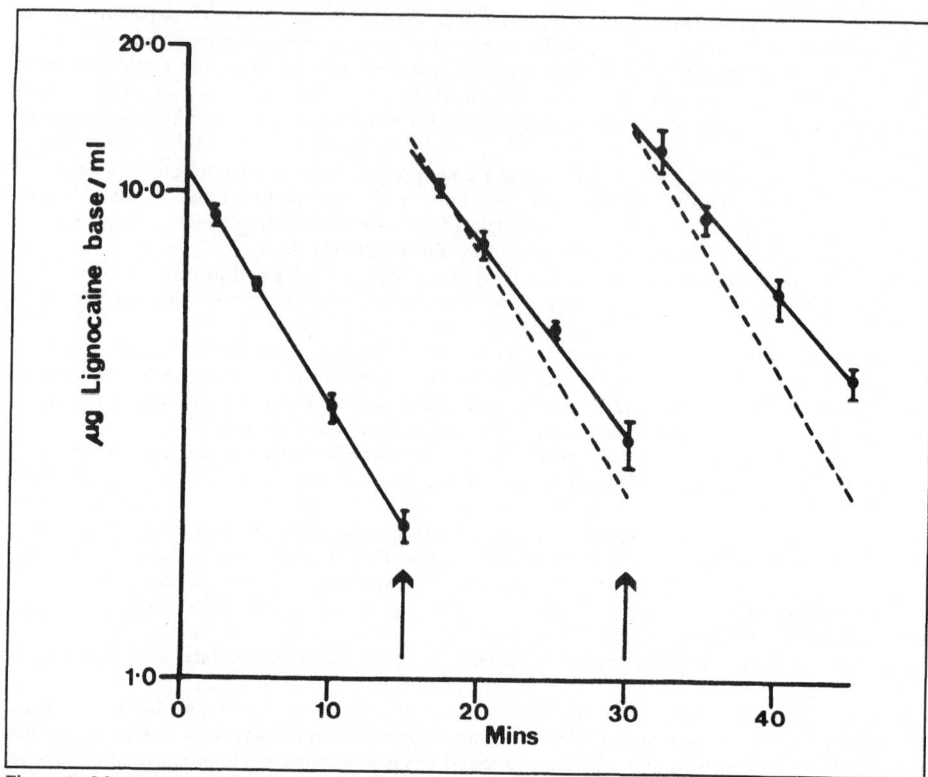

Figure 3: Mean concentrations of lignocaine (± *s. d.*) in the perfusate of a recirculating isolated perfused rat liver preparation ($n = 4$) after three successive bolus injections of 1.5 mg.
(Broken lines indicate concentrations predicted from initial dose data.)

The kinetics of lignocaine, one of the most extensively studied drugs in clinical pharmacology, appear to be more complex than was originally thought.
Note added in proof: A progressive increase in the plasma binding of lignocaine during prolonged infusion in post-myocardial infarction patients has been reported by Routledge *et al.* (Clin. Pharmacol. Ther. *27*, 282, 1980).

References

[1] Anonymous: Doubts about lignocaine.—Brit. Med. J. 1, 473—474 (1975).

[2] Bennett, M. A., Wilner, J. M., Pentecost, B. L.: Controlled trial of lignocaine in prophylaxis of ventricular arrhythmias complicating myocardial infarction. Lancet 2, 909—911 (1970).

[3] Chopra, M. P., Thadani, U., Portal, R. W., Aber, C. P.: Lignocaine therapy for ventricular ectopic activity after acute myocardial infarction: a double-blind trial. Brit. Med. J. 3, 668—670 (1971).

[4] Lie, K. I., Wellens, H. J., van Capele, F. J., Durrer, D.: Lidocaine in the prevention of primary ventricular fibrillation. A double-blind, randomized study of 212 consecutive patients. New Eng. J. Med. 291, 1234—1326 (1974).

[5] Aps, C., Bell, J. A., Jenkins, B. S., Poole-Wilson, P. A., Reynolds, F.: Logical approach to lignocaine therapy. Brit. Med. J. 1, 13—15 (1976).

[6] Thomson, P. D., Melmon, K. L., Richardson, J. A., Cohn, K., Steinbrunn, W., Cudihee, R., Rowland,

M.: Lidocaine pharmacokinetics in advanced heart failure, liver disease and renal failure in humans. Ann. Int. Med. 78, 499—508 (1973).

[7] Stenson, R. E., Constantino, R. T., Harrison, D. C.: Interrelationships of hepatic blood flow, cardiac output, and blood levels of lidocaine in man. Circulation 43, 205—211 (1971).

[8] Tucker, G. T., Wiklund, L., Berlin-Wahlen, A., Mather, L. E.: Hepatic clearance of local anesthetics in man. J. Pharmacokin. Biopharm. 5, 111—122 (1977).

[9] Caesar, J., Shaldon, S., Chiandussi, L., Guevara, L., Sherlock, S.: The use of indocyanine green in the measurement of hepatic-blood flow and as a test of hepatic function. Clin. Sci. 21, 43—57 (1961).

[10] Zito, R. A., Reid, P. R.: Lidocaine kinetics predicted by indocyanine green clearance. New Eng. J. Med. 298, 1160—1163 (1978).

[11] Wiklund, L.: Human hepatic blood flow and its relation to systemic circulation during intravenous infusion of lidocaine. Acta Anaesth. Scand. 21, 148—160 (1977).

[12] Blair, M. R.: Cardiovascular pharmacology of local anaesthetics. Brit. J. Anaesth. 47, 247—252 (1975).

[13] Benowitz, N. L., Meister, W.: Pharmacokinetics in patients with cardiac failure. Clin. Pharmacokin. 1, 389—405 (1976).

[14] Renton, K. W., Baker, J. C., Bailey, L. E.: Cytochrome P-450 and hepatic drug biotransformation during progressive cardiac disease in cardiomyopathic hamsters. Can. J. Physiol. Pharmacol. 57, 302—304 (1979).

[15] Prescott, L. F., Adjepon-Yamoah, K. K., Talbot, R. G.: Impaired lignocaine metabolism in patients with myocardial infarction and cardiac failure. Brit. Med. J. 1, 939—941 (1976).

[16] Le Lorier, J., Grenon, D., Latour, Y., Caille, G., Dumont, G., Brosseau, A., Solignac, A.: Pharmacokinetics of lidocaine after prolonged intravenous infusions in uncomplicated myocardial infarction. Ann. Int. Med. 87, 700—702 (1977).

[17] Le Lorier, J., Moisan, R., Gagne, J., Caille, G.: Effect of the duration of infusion on the disposition of lidocaine in dogs. J. Pharmacol. Exp. Therap. 203, 507—511 (1977).

[18] Vicuna, N., Lalka, D., Burrow, S. R., McLean, A. J., du Souich, P., McNay, J. L: Dose-dependent pharmacokinetic behaviour of lidocaine in the conscious dog. Res. Comm. Chem. Path. Pharmacol. 22, 485—491 (1978).

[19] Keenaghan, J. B., Boyes, R. N: The tissue distribution, metabolism and excretion of lidocaine in rats, guinea pigs, dogs and man. J. Pharmacol. Exp. Therap. 180, 454—463 (1972).

[20] Lennard, M. S., Tucker, G. T., Woods, H. F.: Dose-, time- and sex-dependent metabolism of lignocaine in the isolated perfused rat liver. Abstract. 7th Internat. Congr. Pharmacol., Paris, July 1978.

Evaluation of the clinical significance of the first-pass effect of verapamil in patients

Barry George Woodcock
Department of Clinical Pharmacology
University Clinic, Frankfurt a. M.

Hans Friedrich Vöhringer
Schloßparkklinik, Berlin

It has long been known that the hepatic clearance of drugs with high hepatic extraction ratios is largely determined by liver blood flow. Indeed, several such compounds, including bromosulphthalein and indocyanine green, were intensively investigated as indicators for measuring liver blood flow. Interest in this type of compound has been rekindled with the introduction of several therapeutic agents which are also avidly extracted by the liver, notable examples being lidocaine and propranolol. In addition to their elimination being effected by liver blood flow, it is now recognised that highly extracted drugs must undergo significant presystemic (or first pass) metabolism during their passage from the gut to the systemic circulation as a result of the anatomic arrangement of the hepatic portal circulation, even when gastrointestinal absorption is complete [11].

Introduction

The calcium antagonist verapamil can be described as an old drug with novel clinical applications. It has gained prominence as a significant agent in cardiovascular therapeutics and exhibits anti-anginal, anti-arrhythmic and anti-hypertrophic activity [9, 23, 31]. In 1971 McIlhenny [14] reported "the rapid disappearance of verapamil . . . and the rapid emergence and slow elimination of metabolites" following the intramuscular injection of ^{14}C-verapamil in dogs. The same author in studies on dogs and rats showed that verapamil was rapidly and well absorbed since following an oral dose peak plasma concentrations were attained within 1 to 2 hours and were comparable to those attained after parenteral (intramuscular) verapamil administration. Feces contained only metabolites of verapamil and urine contained less than 0.5% unchanged verapamil. The relative abundance of metabolites in feces after both oral and parenteral verapamil were similar to those found in fistula bile after enzymic hydrolysis of conjugates. These studies suggested the presence of a first pass effect for verapamil associated with hepatic biotransformation following drug absorption. Similar studies have recently been carried out in healthy volunteers [24]. After oral administration of ^{14}C-D,L-verapamil, absorption was almost complete as judged from the area under the plasma concentration time curve of ^{14}C-radioactivity and cumulative urinary excretion of ^{14}C. Considerable biotransformation occurred as only a small percentage (10 to 20%) of the radioactivity in plasma corresponded to unchanged verapamil after both intravenous and oral administration. Thus verapamil after oral administration in man undergoes extensive pre-systemic or first-pass metabolism in the same way as propranolol [25] and lignocaine [2] following oral administration. In this paper the first-pass effect of verapamil has been investigated in patients. Variation in verapamil bioavailability and the effect of hepatic blood flow on verapamil clearance has received particular attention.

Methods

Informed consent was obtained from all patients before commencement of verapamil administration. In the case of liver disease patients, diagnosis was based on clinical signs, biochemical function tests and was confirmed by liver biopsy. The much lower blood levels obtained after oral verapamil made it necessary to administer an oral dose (usually 80 mg) several times greater than the intravenous dose (usually 5 mg). The intravenous dose was administered over a 5 minute period by slow infusion so as to avoid the possibility of unwanted pharmacological effects that may result from a rapid infusion. Blood samples were collected at 5, 10, 15, 30 minutes and at 1, 2, 3, 4, 5, 6, 8, 12, 24 and 48 hours after the intravenous dose and at 30 minutes, 1, 1½, 2, 3, 4, 5, 6, 8, 10, 12, 24 and 48 hours after an oral dose. Because of the 5 minute infusion time a correction for the intercept of the slope of the α-phase with the y-axis was carried out [13]. Area under the concentration-time curve was determined using the trapezoidal method with extrapolation to infinity.

Determination of verapamil plasma concentration

Plasma was separated and stored at $-16°$ in glass tubes until assayed, usually within one week. Verapamil was determined by gas chromatography, after pH-controlled extraction with heptane, using a procedure similar to that developed by HEGE [6]. The practicality and specificity of gas chromatographic estimation of verapamil in plasma after oral dosage has been established by GC-MS studies [28]. Verapamil is strongly adsorbed onto untreated glass surfaces which has an effect on recovery. All glassware was therefore silanised by brief treatment with a 5% solution of trimethylchlorosilane in toluene, heated 1 hour at 120°, and finally rinsed in methanol. To 1 ml plasma in a 11 ml glass centrifuge tube was added 20 µl of 1 µg/ml solution in methanol of D-517, a verapamil analogue, as internal standard. Phosphate buffer (1/15 M, pH 7.4), 1 ml; 1 N sodium hydroxide, 0.2 ml; heptane, 3 ml were added and the tubes stoppered and gently rotated for 30 minutes. The organic layer after centrifugation was decanted and the extraction repeated. To the combined organic phases was added 2 ml 1 N hydrochloric acid and after 10 minutes rotation the tubes were centrifuged and the organic layer discarded. Heptane extraction, 2 × 3 ml was repeated as before after addition of 1 ml 10 N sodium hydroxide to the acidic phase. The heptane supernatants were pooled and evaporated to about 10 µl with a stream of air in a conical base vial. The vial walls were rinsed with 0.5 µl methanol and the volume reduced to about 10 µl in the conical tip. Injections of 4—8 µl were made into the gas chromatograph.

Gas chromatography was performed using a Hewlett-Packard model 5840 A fitted with a nitrogen detector and a 1 m × 0.2 cm internal diameter glass column packed with 5% OV 17/3% SE-30 on Gas Chrom Q 100/120 mesh. The carrier gas was helium (35 ml/min) and the separation of verapamil (retention time 3.6 minutes), D-517 (rentention time 2.9 minutes) and norverapamil (rentention time 4.3 minutes) was obtained with isothermal conditions at 300°.

The limit of detection of verapamil is approximately 1 ng/ml plasma and the between-batch coefficient of variation in our laboratory was 9.6% to 12% for the range 30—300 ng/ml on means of duplicate determinations. At 30 ng/ml and 300 ng/ml average recovery was 72.6 ± 8.7% and 73 ± 7.0% (Mean ± S.D.) respectively. Quality control specimens of plasma containing known quantities of verapamil were included in each assay batch. (A modification of the assay procedure providing savings in costs and time has recently been reported [16].)

Calculations. The equation for calculation of liver blood flow is basically that derived by GIBALDI, BOYES, and FELDMAN [5] for a perfusion limited model which has been further developed by others [23, 30] and verified by liver perfusion studies in experimental animals [18]. The equations for calculation of oral or intrinsic clearance, systemic clearance and hepatic blood flow are given. Their application to drugs having similar kinetic properties to verapamil has been previously reported [11, 19]. It has been assumed that no elimination takes place into the gastrointestinal tract or by the pulmonary route.

$$\text{Systemic clearance} = \frac{\text{Dose}_{i.\,v.}}{\text{AUC}_{i.\,v.\,(\text{blood})}}$$

$$\text{Intrinsic or oral clearance} = \frac{\text{Dose}_{\text{oral}}}{\text{AUC}_{\text{oral (blood)}}}$$

$$\text{Bioavailability} = \frac{\text{Dose}_{i.\,v.} \cdot \text{AUC}_{\text{oral}}}{\text{Dose}_{\text{oral}} \cdot \text{AUC}_{i.\,v.}} = 1 - \text{first pass extraction}$$

$$\text{Apparent hepatic blood flow} = \frac{\text{Dose}_{\text{oral}} \cdot \text{Dose}_{i.\,v.}}{\text{Dose}_{\text{oral}} \cdot \text{AUC}_{i.\,v.\,(\text{blood})} - \text{Dose}_{i.\,v.} \cdot \text{AUC}_{\text{oral (blood)}}}$$

Results and discussion

A diagram illustrating the first-pass effect and disposition of verapamil after oral administration is shown (Figure 1). Verapamil is mainly metabolised by cleavage of the dimethoxyphenylethyl mioety to products with apparently much lower cardiovascular activity than verapamil and demethylation to norverapamil, a metabolite having approximately one fifth the cardiovascular activity of verapamil [17, 24]. Thus verapamil, like lignocaine [7, 10] and propranolol [4], is probably metabolised by an enzymatic system in the liver which involves mixed function oxidases.

Preliminary results presenting a summary of verapamil bioavailability in man is shown (Table 1). Included are 4 patients with liver disease (3 cirrhosis, 1 fatty-liver), 2 patients with cardiac disease (1 insufficiency, 1 hypertrophic non-obstructive cardiomyopathy) and 2 normal subjects. One of the normal subjects N_2, has been taken from the literature [24] and represents apparently the only data available at this time for comparison.

The oral clearance of verapamil seems to be about double that for propranolol [11] and the systemic clearance is also appreciably higher. Intrinsic or oral clearance is a function of hepatic drug metabolising activity. Thus as might be expected there was no obvious relationship between oral clearance and hepatic blood flow or between oral clearance and systemic clearance. In contrast, in Figure 2 the relationship between systemic clearance and hepatic blood flow for verapamil shows excellent linearity as would be predicted for high hepatic clearance drugs (M. Gibaldi, personal communication). The systemic extraction ratio given by the slope 0.88 (Figure 2), is higher than that estimated for propranol, approximately 0.6 [11] although a higher value than this for propranolol has been reported for the dog [3]; for lignocaine, 0.61 [20]; and for indocyanine green, 0.74 [29].

The high oral clearance of verapamil leads to a minimal verapamil bioavailability, 0.2 or less (Figure 3 and Figure 4). In one patient L_3, the very low oral clearance and near normal systemic clearance supports the diagnoses of hepatic shunts and the hepatic blood flow in this patient is probably overestimated (Table 1 and Figure 4). As would be expected the bioavailability in this patient is high and the first-pass extraction is low (36%).

In the absence of shunts the first-pass extraction by patients with liver disease can be extremely high. The highest value is observed in the patient with fatty-liver disease L_4 where the apparent hepatic blood flow and systemic clearance were extremely low.

An illustration of the relationships between hepatic blood flow, protein-binding and extraction ratio for drugs cleared mainly by hepatic processes has been described [1]. It takes the form of a triangle (Figure 5). With a systemic extraction ratio of 90%, verapamil represents an extreme or near classic case of the flow limited drug whose clearance will be independent of changes in protein-binding. In the treatment of hypertrophic obstructive cardiomyopathy, the oral dose of verapamil is large

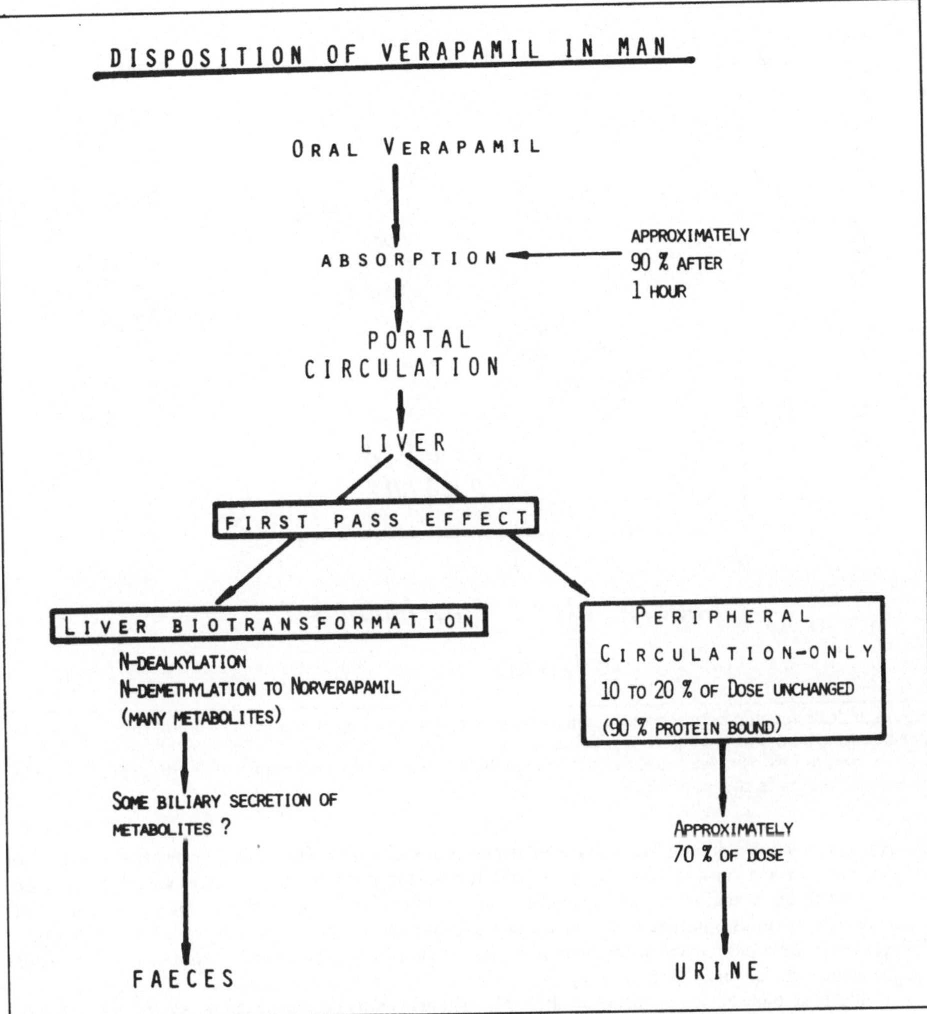

Figure 1: The disposition of orally administered verapamil in man.

(360—480 mg daily) [8] in comparison to the intravenous dose (5—10 mg) recommended for producing significant changes in hemodynamic responses, such as systemic vascular resistance [27]. The need for high oral doses of verapamil has also been reported for the treatment of arrhythmias where 10 to 20 times the recommended intravenous dose had to be given in order to observe antiarrhythmic effects [12]. Thus the presence of a first-pass effect leads to a difference between the required oral and intravenous dose and a considerable reduction in the bioavailability of verapamil in patients. In addition to reducing the bioavailability, when the fraction of dose reaching the systemic circulation is small, relatively small changes in the first-pass effect eg from 90% to 80%, will lead to large changes in plasma concentration in the systemic circulation. A change from 90% to 80% would double the quantity of drug reaching the heart and peripheral tissues and would necessitate a corresponding reduction in dosage.

A variable first-pass effect for verapamil may be the cause of widely different plasma verapamil concentrations in patients with hypertrophic obstructive cardiomyopathy [31]. Verapamil plasma con-

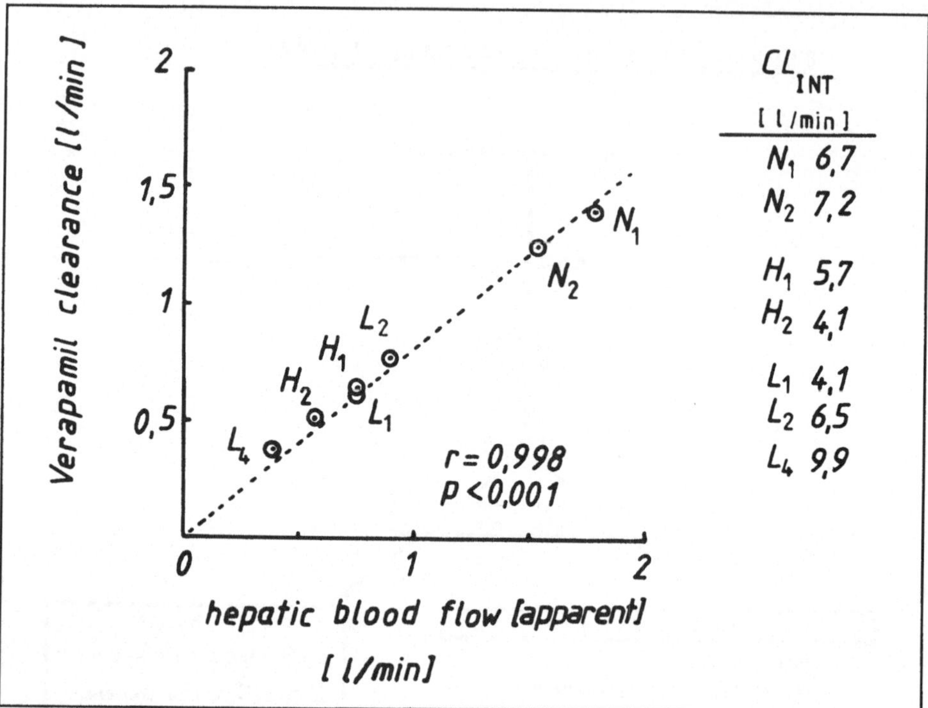

Figure 2: Relationship between verapamil systemic clearance and apparent hepatic blood flow in patients. For key to symbols in the figure see Table 1.
Cl_{int} = oral or intrinsic clearance. Patient L_3 is excluded from the figure because of the diagnosed presence of hepatic shunts in this patient.

centrations measured during maintenance therapy, immediately before and 1 hour after a test dose of verapamil show a variation of at least 10 fold at both sampling times (Figure 6) and this variation is too great to be explained by differences in body-weight. Differences in distribution volume and systemic extraction as opposed to first-pass extraction may also partly be involved. Inter-individual differences in first-pass metabolism seem to be the cause of the greater variation in plasma levels of propranolol after an oral dose in comparison to those after an intravenous dose [11].

A variable first-pass effect could arise through differences in enzyme activity in the liver parenchyma, rate of liver verapamil binding or uptake, or through differences in the flow of hepatic portal blood where rate of flow through liver sinosoids and/or the presence of a hepatic shunt would be important. The occurrence of hepatic shunts has been demonstrated anatomically and are not infrequently encountered in patients with liver disease [21, 22]. Hepatic shunts permit portal blood to pass by a short-circuit route into the systemic circulation. In such patients, verapamil would cease to be a high oral clearance drug and a particularly high bioavailability would be observed as seen for patient L_3, Table 1. A non-invasive method for the measurement of the amount of shunted blood has recently been reported [15].

In conclusion these preliminary studies are consistant with the view that the first-pass effect of verapamil is due to metabolism in the liver rather than metabolism in the gastrointestinal tract or in the intestinal wall after absorption. The first-pass extraction in subjects with normal liver vascular anatomy is considerable and at least 80% of the oral dose. The bioavailability is correspondingly low and much interpatient variation is likely to be present. Liver disease patients represent a group where interpatient variation is found in the extreme. Very low first-pass extraction can occur, probably due to the presence of hepatic shunts.

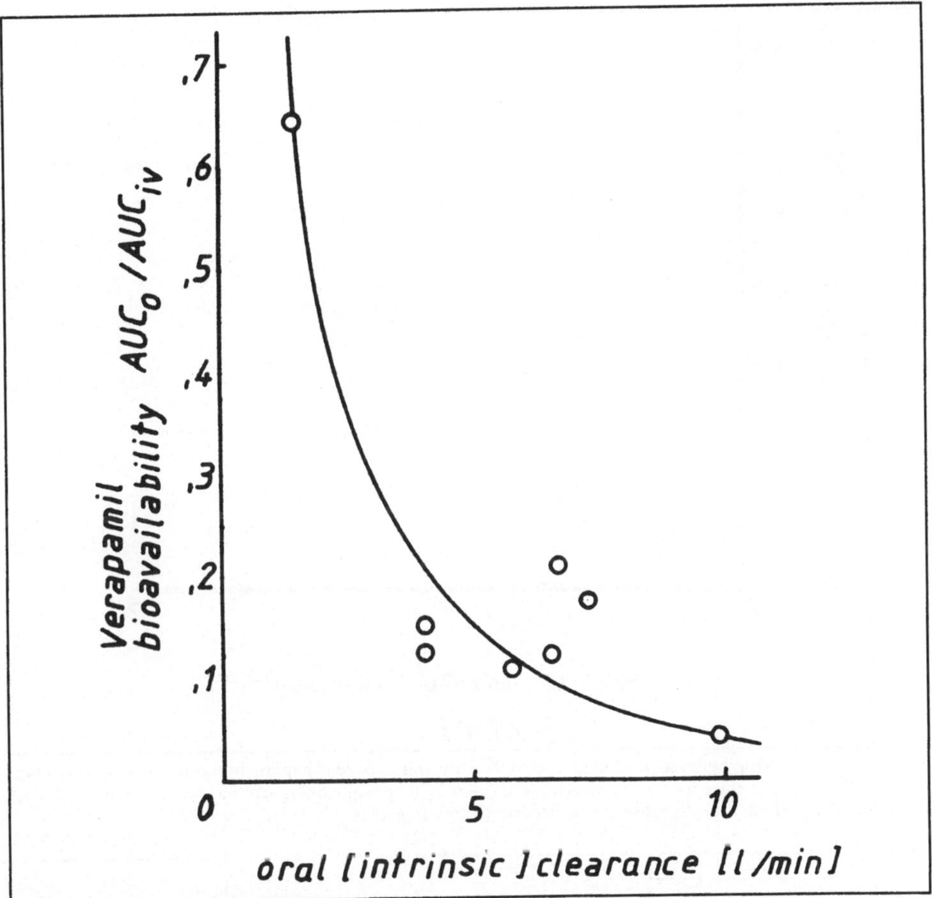

Figure 3: Relationship of verapamil oral clearance and bioavailability for the subjects shown in Table 1. The line drawn through the points is an approximation to the theoretical relationship.

Whilst the first-pass extraction and quantity of drug entering the systemic circulation is dependent on the liver metabolic enzyme activity and degree of shunted blood, the removal of verapamil from the systemic circulation is dependent on hepatic blood flow where the extraction ratio is estimated in this study at 0.88.

Variations in verapamil bioavailability are sufficiently great to require dosage adjustment. A proportion of the cardiac hypertrophy patients (Figure 6) may be undertreated because of a high first pass effect. Liver patients will usually require a reduced dose, even when the first-pass extraction is high, because the systemic clearance of verapamil was reduced in all liver patients examined. To control the plasma level of verapamil in patients, measurement of plasma verapamil concentration would be essential.

Acknowledgements

The authors wish to thank Prof. N. Rietbrock, University Clinic Frankfurt, for his encouragement and valuable advice generously given during the course of this study.

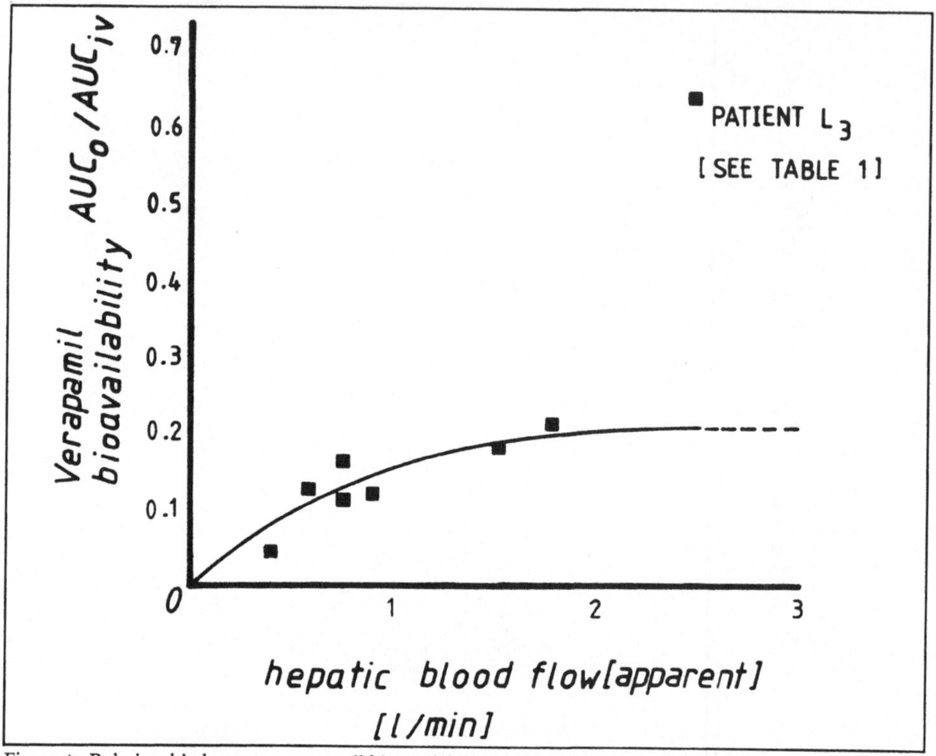

0.7
0.6
0.5
0.4
0.3
0.2
0.1
0
1
2
3

Verapamil bioavailability AUC_o/AUC_{iv}

PATIENT L_3
[SEE TABLE 1]

hepatic blood flow[apparent]
[l/min]

Figure 4: Relationship between verapamil bioavailability and apparent hepatic blood flow. The line drawn through the points is the expected relationship. Patient L3 (top right of figure) has an unusually high oral biovailability, perhaps due to presence of hepatic shunts (see text).

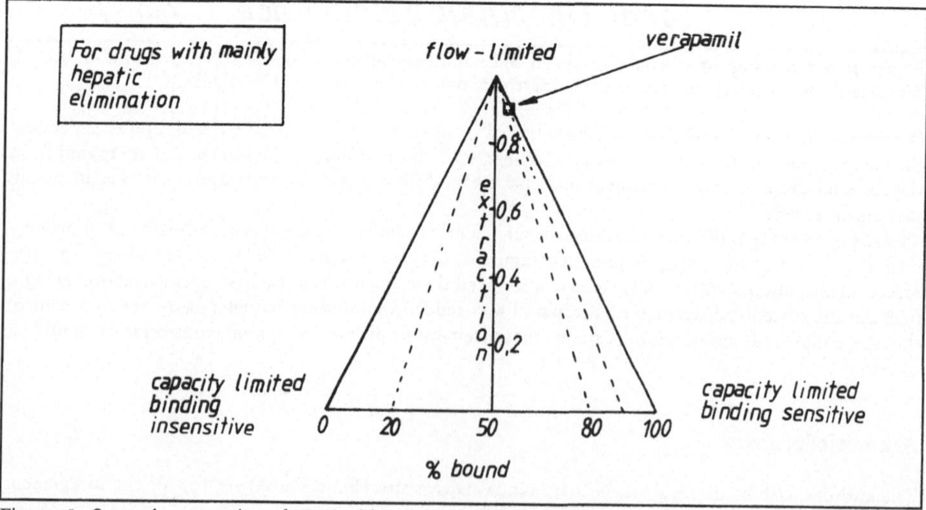

Figure 5: Systemic extraction, hepatic blood flow and proteinbinding relationships. Adapted from Blaschke (1977) [1].

Patient number	Diagnosis	Route	Dose (mg)	$AUC_{(blood)}$[a] ($ng \cdot ml^{-1} \cdot min$)	Systemic clearance (L/min)	Oral or instrinsic clearance (L/min)	Apparent hepatic blood flow (L/min)	Bioavailability (1 = 100%)	First pass extraction
L_1	Liver cirrhosis	iv po	5 80	6384 12336	0.783	6.485	0.891	0.121	0.878
L_2	Liver cirrhosis	iv po	5 80	7958 19584	0.628	4.085	0.743	0.154	0.845
L_3	Liver cirrhosis	iv po	5 80	5602 57168	0.892	1.399	(2.464)[d]	0.638	0.362
L_4	Fatty liver disease	iv po	5 80	13200 8064	0.379	9.92	0.394	0.038	0.962
H_1	Cardiac insufficiency	iv po	5 80	9888 19728[b]	0.506	4.055	0.578	0.125	0.875
H_2	Cardiac hypertrophy	iv po	10 160	15317 28032	0.653	5.708	0.737	0.114	0.886
N_1	Control	iv po	5 80	3979 11040	1.257	7.246	1.52	0.175	0.823
N_2	Control	iv po	10 80	7142[c] 11970	1.4	6.683	1.771	0.21	0.79

Table 1: Verapamil first pass extraction and clearance data from AUC in patients and control subjects

a) Blood/plasma ratio = 0.8, determined by adding verapamil to plasma and whole blood.; b) Corrected post-infusion data; c) AUC data taken from SCHOMERUS *et al.* Cardiovasc. Res. *10*, 605, 1976; d) The presence of hepatic shunts was diagnosed in this patient (see text).

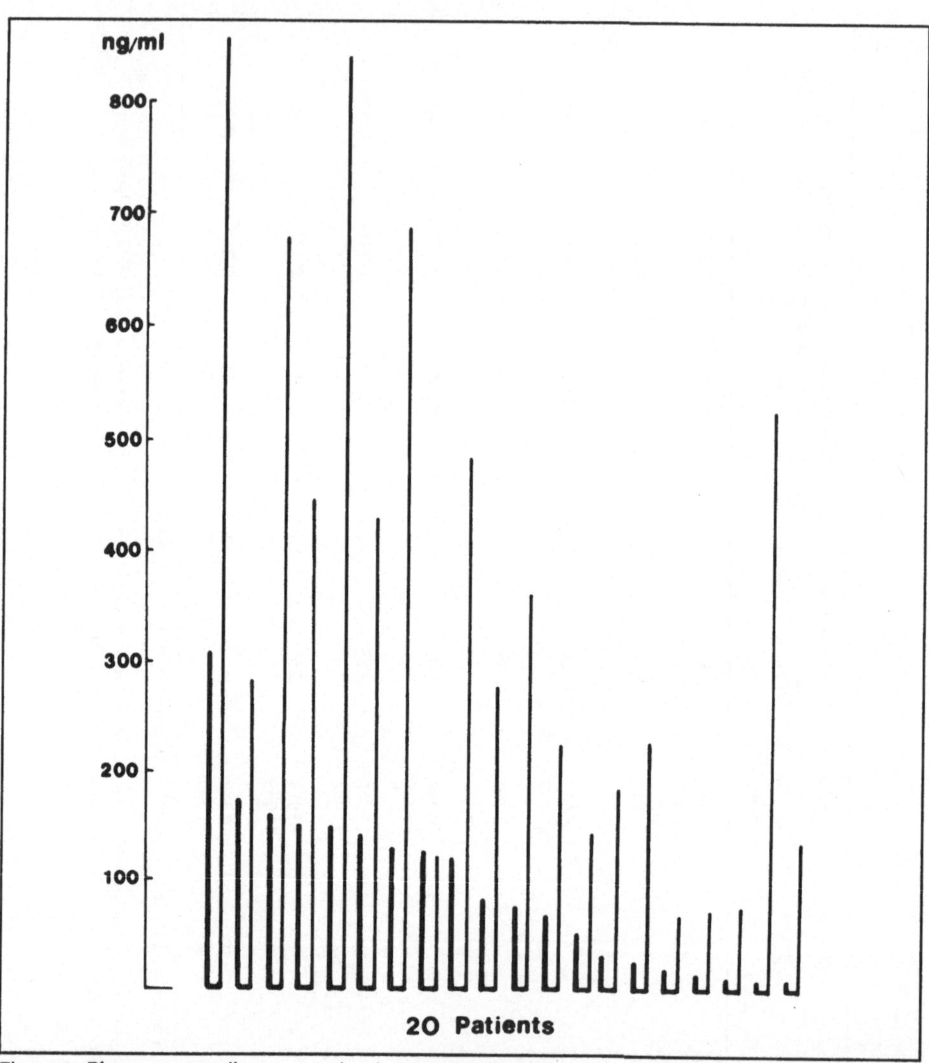

Figure 6: Plasma verapamil concentration in 20 patients with hypertrophic obstructive cardiomyopathy. Pre-dose (bold bars) and 1 hour after test dose of 160 mg orally (thin bars). Measurements were made after an overnight fast, approximately 12 hours after the last regular dose during maintenance therapy with 480 mg verapamil given as three equally divided doses daily. Patients are ranked in order of their pre-dose verapamil concentration.

Literature

[1] Blaschke, T. F.: Protein binding and kinetics of drugs in liver diseases.—Clin. Pharmacokinetics, *2*, 32—44 (1977).

[2] Boyes, R. N., Adams, H. J., and Once, B. R.: Oral absorption and disposition kinetics of lignocaine hydrochloride in dogs.—J. Pharmac. exp. Ther., *174*, 1—8 (1970).

[3] Branch, R. A., and Shand, D. G.: Propranolol disposition in chronic liver disease: A physiological approach.—Clin. Pharmacokinetics, *1*, 264—279 (1976).

[4] Dollery, C. T., Davies, D. S., Conolly M. E.: Differences in the metabolism of drugs depending upon their routes of administration.—Ann. N. Y. Acad. Sci. *179,* 108—144 (1971).

[5] Gibaldi, M., Boyes, R. N., and Feldman, S.: Influence of first-pass effect on availability of drugs on oral administration.—J. Pharm. Sci., *60,* 1338—1340 (1971).

[6] Hege, H. G.: Gas chromatographic determination of verapamil in plasma and urine.—Arzneimittel Forsch., *29,* 1681—1684 (1979).

[7] Hollunger, G.: On the metabolism of lignocaine: ii The biotransformation of lignocaine.—Acta Pharmac. Tox., *17,* 356—365 (1960).

[8] Kaltenbach, M., Hopf, R., Kober, G., Bussmann, W.-D., Keller, M., and Petersen, Y.: Treatment of hypertrophic obstructive cardiomyopathy with verapamil.—Br. Heart J., *42,* 35—42 (1979).

[9] Kaltenbach, M., Hopf, R., and Keller, M.: Calcium antagonistische Therapie bei hypertrophobstructiver Kardiomyopathie.—Dtsch. Med. Wochenschr., *100,* 590—593 (1976).

[10] Keenaghan, J. B., and Boyes, R. N.: The tissue distribution, metabolism and excretion of lignocaine in rats, guinea pigs, dogs and man.—J. Pharmac. exp. Ther., *180,* 454—463 (1972).

[11] Kornhauser, D. M., Wood, A. J. J., Vestal, R. E., Wilkinson, G. R., Branch, R. A., and Shand, D. G.: Biological determinants of propranolol disposition in Man.—Clin. Pharmac. Ther., *23,* 165—174 (1978).

[12] Krikler, D.: Verapamil in cardiology. — Eur. J. Cardiol., 2, 3—10 (1974).

[13] Loo, J. C. K., and Riegelman, S.: Assessment of pharmacokinetic constant from postinfusion blood curves obtained after *iv* infusion.—J. Pharm. Sci., *59,* 53—55 (1970).

[14] McIlhenny, H. M.: Metabolism of ^{14}C-verapamil.—J. Med. Chem., *14,* 1178—1184 (1971).

[15] McLean, A., du Souich, P., Gibaldi, M.: Non-invasive kinetic approach to the estimation of total hepatic blood flow and shunting in chronic liver disease—a hypothesis.—Clin. Pharmac. Ther., *25,* 161—166 (1979).

[16] Nelson, K., Woodcock, B. G., and Kirsten, R.: Improvement of the quantitative determination of verapamil in human plasma.—Int. J. Clin. Pharmacol., *17,* 375—379 (1979).

[17] Neugebauer, G.: Comparative cardiovascular actions of verapamil and its major metabolities in the anaesthetised dog.—Cardiovasc Res., *12*: 247—254 (1978).

[18] Nies, A. S., Evans, G. H., Shand, D. G.: The hemodynamic effects of beta adrenergic blockade on the flow dependent hepatic clearance of propranolol.—J. Pharmacol. Exp. Ther., *184,* 716—720 (1973).

[19] Nies, A. S., Shand, D. G., Wilkinson, G. R.: Altered Hepatic Blood Flow and Drug Disposition.—Clin. Pharmacokinetics, *1,* 135—155 (1976).

[20] Perucca, E., and Richens, A.: Paracetamol disposition in normal subjects and in patients treated with antiepileptic drugs.—Br. J. clin. Pharmac., 7, 201—206 (1979).

[21] Popper, H.: Pathologic aspects of cirrhosis.—Am. J. Pathol., *87,* 228—258 (1977).

[22] Popper, H., Elias, H., and Petty, D. E.: Vascular pattern of the cirrhotic Liver.—Am. J. Clin. Pathol., 22, 717—729 (1952).

[23] Rowland, M.: Influence of route of administration on drug availability.—J. pharm. Sci., *61,* 70—74 (1972).

[24] Schomerus, M., Spiegelhalder, B., Stieren, B., and Eichelbaum, M.: Physiological disposition of verapamil in man.—Cardiovasc. Res., *10,* 605—612 (1976).

[25] Shand, D. G., Rangno, R. E.: The disposition of propranolol. 1. Elimination during oral absorption in man.—Pharmacology 7: 159—168 (1972).

[26] Singh, B. N., Ellrodt, G., and Peter, C. T.: Verapamil: A review of its pharmacological properties and therapeutic use.—Drugs., *15,* 169—197 (1978).

[27] Singh, B. N., and Roche, A. H. G.: Effects of intravenous verapamil on hemodynamics in patients with heart disease.—Am. Heart J., *94,* 593—599 (1977).

[28] Spiegelhalder, B., Eichelbaum, M.: Determination of verapamil in human plasma by mass fragmentography using stable labelled verapamil as internal standard.—Arzneim. Forsch., *27,* 94—97 (1977).

[29] Wiegand, B. D., Ketterer, S. G., Rapaport, E.: The Use of Indocyanine Green for the Evaluation of Hepatic Function and Blood Flow in Man.—Am. J. Digest. Dis., *5*, 427—436 (1960).

[30] Wilkinson, G. R., Shand, D. G.: A physiological approach to hepatic drug clearance.—Clin. Pharmac. Ther., *18*, 377—390 (1975).

[31] Woodcock, B. G., Hopf, R., and Kaltenbach, M.: Verapamil and norverapamil plasma concentrations during long-term therapy in patients with hypertrophic obstructive cardiomyopathy.—J. Cardiovasc. Pharmac. *2*, 17—23 (1980).

Evaluation of altered pharmacokinetics in intensive-care patients

A Clinical Approach

Ingrid Rietbrock and Günter Lazarus
Department of Anaesthesiology, University of Würzburg
Würzburg, W. Germany

In recent years there has been increasing interest in factors which modify drug disposition. Variations in drug absorption, distribution, metabolism and excretion are factors which contribute to wide variations in drug response in man. Since the liver is the major site of drug metabolism many studies have measured plasma or blood concentration-time profiles in patients with liver disease in an attempt to individualise drug dosage regimens and to provide a desired clinical effect without dose related toxicity. In the literature however, there exists little information on the altered pharmacokinetic behaviour of drugs in intensive-care patients. This communication presents some of the difficulties of drug dosage selection in severe disease that result from adaptative changes of the liver to multiple supportive medication and from the actual disease process itself. In addition, it demonstrates the problems in drawing direct conclusions from kinetic data when confrontated with biological changes. Lastly initial steps are pointed out to illuminate the problem of interaction between drug disposition and disease.

I. Drug consumption and adaptative changes of the liver in intensive-care patients.

a) Drug consumption in relation to the treatment period.
It is generally known in clinical practice that with increasingly severe disease the duration of stay in hospital and the use of medication increase not arithmetrically but rather exponentially [16, 22]. This is especially true for various types of respiratory failure, where an abundance of single preparations are used daily during the respiratory support period. Table 1 illustrates the multiple drug therapy required by patients in an anaesthesiological care unit. In addition to disease-specific drugs which are used usually in chronic situations, muscle relaxants, neuroleptics, analgesics, hypnotics and other psychoactive drugs in their different combinations are regularly employed; for example during controlled ventilation in order to maintain constant physiological conditions such as sedation and muscular relaxation. Additionally, it is becoming more and more usual to treat patients who have suffered skull fractures and brain damage with high doses of barbiturates. Many of these patients require nutrition through high-caloric parenteral infusions.

How the body in severe illness, handles these drugs when given one after the other, is far from being understood. What is known is that in the case of drugs whose action can be readily monitored, the dose must be constantly raised, as the duration of controlled ventilation increases, in order to achieve the same therapeutic effect.

DRUGS RECEIVED BY IC-PATIENTS

I. Drugs applied regularly

sedatives and neuroleptics
analgesics (morphine derivates)
antipyretics
muscle relaxants
antibiotics (one or two combined)
diuretics and carboanhydrase inhibitors
secrolytics
cardiovascular drugs (glycosides, α-inhibitors dopamine)

others:
- acetylcholine esterase inhibitors
- H_2-antagonists
- vitamins
- heparin

II. Drugs applied in special cases

anticonvulsants
antiarrhythmics
β-mimetics and β-antagonists
hormones and hormone antagonists (insulin prednisolone spironolactone)
antimycotics
antiemetics

III. Intravenous solutions

electrolytes and buffer solutions
carbohydrates (40 %)
amino acids and human proteins (albumin, γ-globulin)
lipids

Table 1: Multiple drug therapy required by patients in an anaesthesiological care unit.

Table 2 shows that the average consumption of muscle relaxants, analgesics, neuroleptics and hypnotics is dependent on the duration of the mechanical controlled respiratory period. Over a two day respiratory support period the average total quantity administered for example of the three drugs: imbretil, dehydrobenzperidol and fentanyl is 53 mg, 36 mg and 65 mg, respectively. With a respiratory support period six times longer, the quantity of imbretil used rises twelve times and that for dehydrobenzperidol and fentanyl rises nine times. Noticeable is the large variation in dosage for these drugs between patients, indicated by the high standard deviation and pointing to considerable interindividual variation in the pharmacokinetics in these patients (Table 2).

b) Adaptative changes of the liver size and behaviour of gamma GT activity in proportion to the duration of therapy.

The liver has a central place in drug metabolism where enzyme systems exist which are capable of catalysing the biotransformation of foreign compounds. Our attention is now directed to the way in which adaptative changes in the liver in intensive-care patients are dependent on the length of the treatment. It is for example quite striking the extent to which, even in the absence of cardiac disturbances, the liver size increases under these conditions. This is true not only for patients with septicaemia but also for example those with tetanus stage 3 under complication-free respiratory support. Not infrequently a liver weight of three kilogram is found on death. Evaluation of fifty-four adult respiratory patients who died in the Anaesthesiology Intensive-care Unit, University of Würzburg 1976, shows that the liver weight increases rapidly during the first week of intensive-care treatment, on average by almost 100 per cent ($p<0.001$; Figure 1).
Of the conventional liver function tests, analysis shows that only serum gamma GT-activity increases in proportion to the duration of therapy [16]. The rise in gamma GT in patients with preserved spontaneous breathing and limited medication is smaller than in patients with controlled ven-

Jntensive-Care-Patients		
Male 8, Female 3	age (y) 41 ± 17	
Jntensive-Care-Treatment (days)	7 ± 3 (4)	37 ± 16 (7)
Controlled Ventilation (days)	2 ± 1 (4)	13 ± 7 (7)
Drugs		
Jmbretil^R mg	53 ± 61 (4)	648 ± 570 (7)
Dehydrobenzperidol^R mg	36 ± 49 (4)	319 ± 288 (7)
Fentanyl^R mg	65 ± 87 (4)	574 ± 518 (7)
Nembutal^R g	1,5 (1)	12 or 6 (2)
Valium^R / Psyquil^R mg	37 ± 25 (3)	105 ± 49 (5)
Ozothin^R/Bisolvon^R Amp.	20 ± 13 (4)	126 ± 78 (7)

Table 2: Average consumption (Mean ± S. D.) of muscle relaxants, analgesics, neuroleptics and hypnotics for example in dependence on the duration of the mechanical controlled respiratory period. Figures in parentheses are numbers of intensive-care patients (from Ingrid Rietbrock and E. Richter, 1978).

tilation (Figure 2). The significance of changes in gamma GT is open to various interpretations. One of these is that the activity in serum is an expression of microsomal enzyme induction (drug metabolising enzyme induction; [3, 8, 9, 26]), whilst another is that the activity is attributable to the overall action of disease on the liver and biliary tract [6, 19, 11, 20].

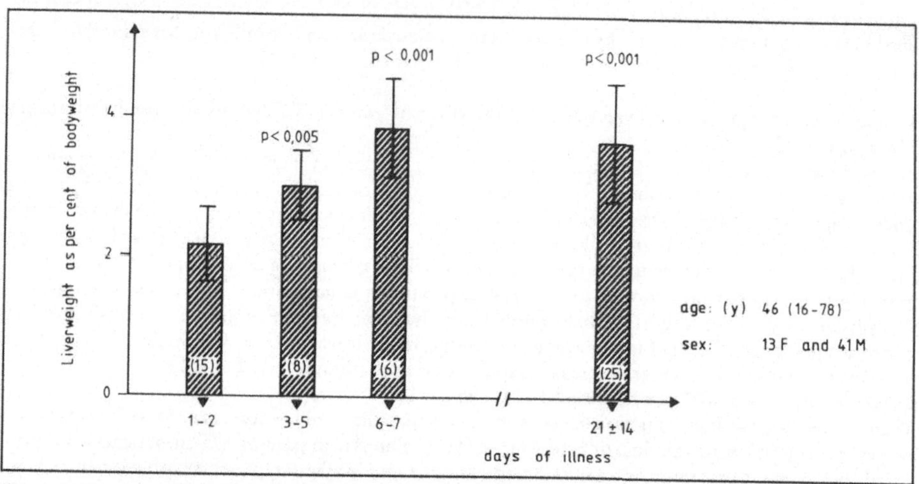

Figure 1: Average values of the liver weight as per cent of body weight (Mean ± S. D.) of adult intensive-care patients *v.* duration of intensive-care treatment. An evaluation of 54 mechanically ventilated patiens who died in the Anaesthesiology Intensive-care Unit, University of Würzburg, 1976).

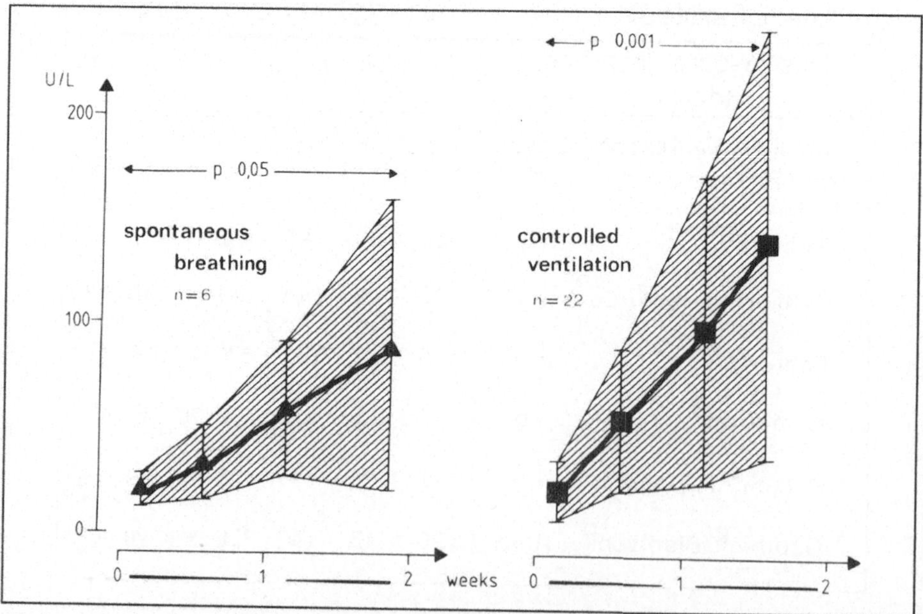

Figure 2: Average values of serum gamma glutamyltranspeptidase activity (gamma GT; Mean ± S.D.) of intensive-care patients with preserved spontaneous breathing and limited medication (on the left) and patients with controlled ventilation (on the right) (from Ingrid Rietbrock and E. Richter, 1978).

In order to clarify the question of the cause of liver enlargement we have carried out a systemic investigation of the liver in intensive-care patients, in collaboration with W. Romen of the Pathology Institute, University of Würzburg (Figure 3).
The studies, where $n = 4$ or 5, included controls without liver enlargement (column 1), patients with hepatic hypertrophy as a consequence of cardiac disease (column 2), and patients from the intensive-care unit without and with fatty liver (column 3 and 4). The morphometric findings show that liver

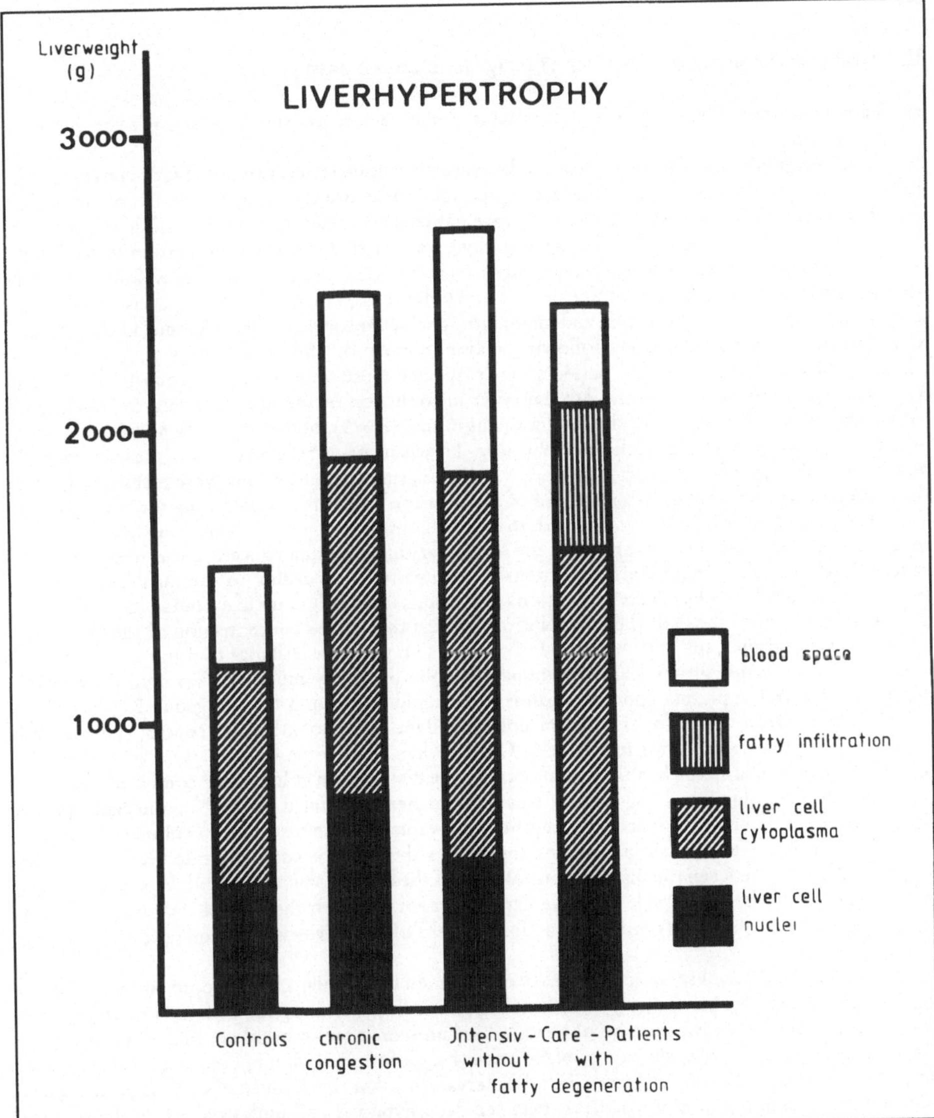

Figure 3: Morphometric studies of the liver at autopsy in controls, without liver enlargement (column 1), in patients with hepatic hypertrophy as a consequence of cardiac disease (column 2) and in intensive-care patients without and with fatty liver (column 3 and 4). $n = 4$ or 5 patients in each group; mean values of liver cell cytoplasma, blood space, fatty infiltration and liver cell nuclei.

growth in these patients is a genuine liver hypertrophy. The liver enlargement is essentially due to a hypertrophy of the hepatocytes, more specifically, an increase in cytoplasmic volume (hatched area). Accompanying this, there is an increase in liver weight due to enlargement of the blood space (light area) and occassionally as a result of fatty infiltration (long hatched area), whilst the volume of nuclei remains unchanged. Detailed investigations of the extent to which pharmacotherapy, the disease itself and the high-caloric paranteral nutrition are involved in the liver enlargement process are however still in progress.

II. Effects on the pharmacokinetics of drugs in intensive-care patients

a) Pharmacokinetic behaviour of hexobarbital in intensive-care patients in relation to the duration of treatment.

In view of the possibility that the increase in hepatocyte volume reflects an increase in activity of the endoplasmic reticular enzyme systems leading to higher drug dosage requirement, the pharmacokinetic behaviour of hexobarbital in intensive-care patients was examined for a possible dependence on the duration of treatment [18]. The investigations were carried out on a total of twenty-two intensive-care patients (sixteen male, six female) aged 20 to 75 years and average body weight 77 kg. All patients received treatment on a respirator. They included 9 cases of severe trauma, 6 cases of tetanus stage 3 one of them with pericarditis and meningitis, one patient with viral pneumonia, and 6 patients with post-operative complications following major thoracic or abdominal surgery. According to clinical and bacteriological signs, 8 patients were suspected septicaemia cases. In group 1 ($n = 7$), the test was carried out on the 3rd and 4th day after introduction of the intensive-care treatment and following control of the primary shock phase; in group 2 ($n = 9$), between the 5th and 8th day, and in group 3 ($n = 6$), between 13th and 29th day. Hexobarbital was given as an infusion over 60 minutes at a dosage of 7.32 mg per kg body weight. Plasma concentrations were measured by gas chromatography immediately after the end of the infusion and at intervals during the following 24 hours [18]. The results were compared with those of a control group of 13 volunteers having a similar age range [18]. Figure 4 demonstrates the semilogarithmic plasma concentration-time cürves of hexobarbital in healthy volunteers and intensive-care patients according to the duration of treatment. The hexobarbital plasma concentrations of group 1, initially and up to 4 hours after the end of the infusion, lie above those of the control group, whilst the plasma concentration of the intensive-care patients in group 2 and 3 after the end of the infusion period are similar to those of the control group. At a later stage, group 2 and 3 eliminate hexobarbital very much quicker than the control group, and the fall in plasma concentration is more rapid in group 3 than in group 2.

The calculated mean values for the pharmacokinetic data for hexobarbital in control subjects and intensive-care patients is shown in Figure 5. Group 1 has a half-time for the β-phase closely similar to the healthy volunteers but the distribution volumes for compartment 1 and 2 are smaller in group 1 and the hepatic clearance of hexobarbital is slightly diminished. As the course of stay in the intensive-care unit lengthens the values for the distribution volume of the central compartment at steady state of patients approaches those of the control group until there is no longer a difference between the distribution volumes of the healthy volunteers and the intensive-care patients, group 3. After one week intensive-care treatment however, the plasma clearance increases to approximately 87 per cent (group 2) and after 2 weeks of intensive-care treatment to 143 per cent (group 3).

Corresponding to these observations, it has been observed that patients at the commencement of intensive-care therapy are particularly sensitive to hypnotic drugs. During the course of treatment the acceleration in the biotransformation of hexobarbital presents a major problem. In the extreme case, for patients in group 3 it may be impossible to achieve a uniform sedation by repeated bolus application of drug. It can be deduced from clinical observations, that the frequency of dosage increases, and that the patient's condition oscillates between deep hypnosis and undesired wakefulness. Disturbances of heart rhythm and reduced peripheral circulation, probably arising from elvated catecholamine output, are additional and frequently observed consequences. An accelerated biotransformation in intensive-care patients can be demonstrated not only for hexobarbital, but also for tolbutamide, antipyrine and digitoxin [16, 17]. However in the example described here there is a

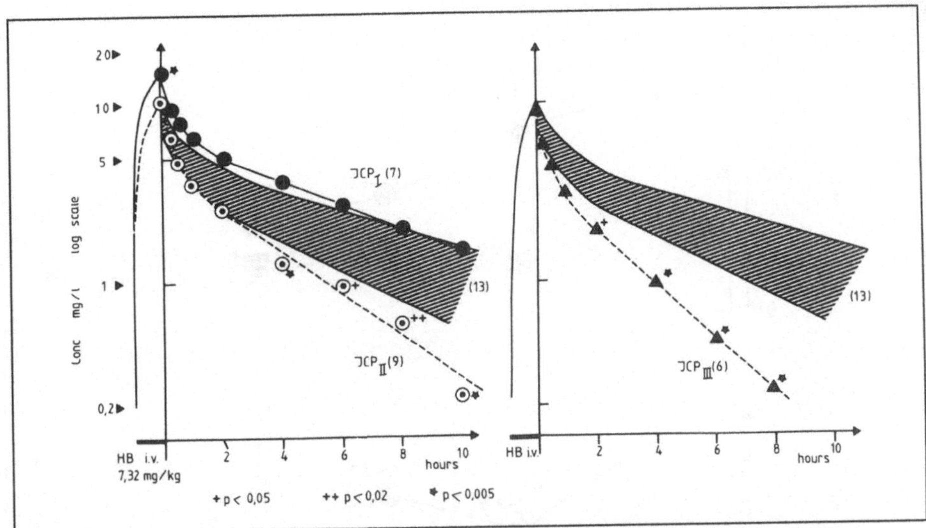

Figure 4: Semilogarithmic plasma concentration-time curves of hexobarbital of healthy volunteers (Mean ± S. D., shaded area, $n = 13$) and intensive-care patients (see text) after a 60-min linear infusion of 7.32 mg per kg body weight. Each point is mean for the group. The p values are against the controls. (The test was carried out in group 1 ($n = 7$) on the 3rd and 4th day, in group 2 between the 5th and 8th day and in group 3 between the 13th and 29th day after introduction of the intensive-care treatment) (from Ingrid RIETBROCK *et al.*, Br. J. Anaesthesiol. In press).

large inter-individual variation in plasma clearance of hexobarbital and it is uncertain whether or not the patient has become induced by frequent medication during intensive-care treatment.

b) Pharmacokinetic behaviour of drugs in intensive-care patients in relation to cardiac insufficiancy and septicaemia.

In the literature there is little information on they way in which disease or drug therapy in intensive-care patients can change the various processes which define the pharmacokinetic profile of a drug [4, 5, 15, 16, 21, 23]. The extent to which various pathophysiological conditions change pharmacokinetic parameters such as distribution volume, and plasma clearance in particular, depends it seems, on the characteristics of the drug [1, 13, 27].

Cardiac insufficiency

The distribution of drugs in the tissues is facilitated by the pumping action of the heart. Patients with "Low output syndrome" show a relatively uniform situation. For drugs with clearance dependent on hepatic blood flow, the reduced heart minute volume leads not only to reduction in the distribution volume but also to a drop in hepatic clearance so that an elevation in pharmacological effect must be taken into account [10, 12, 13, 14, 25]. Information on the practical importance of the size of calculated pharmacokinetic parameters on the actual pharmacological effect of a drug can be learned by direct observation and judgement in the same way as one obtains other knowledge by clinical experience. Thus the management of for example lidocaine treatment after cardio-pulmonary resuscitation in patients with heart rhythm disturbances does not present too great a problem.

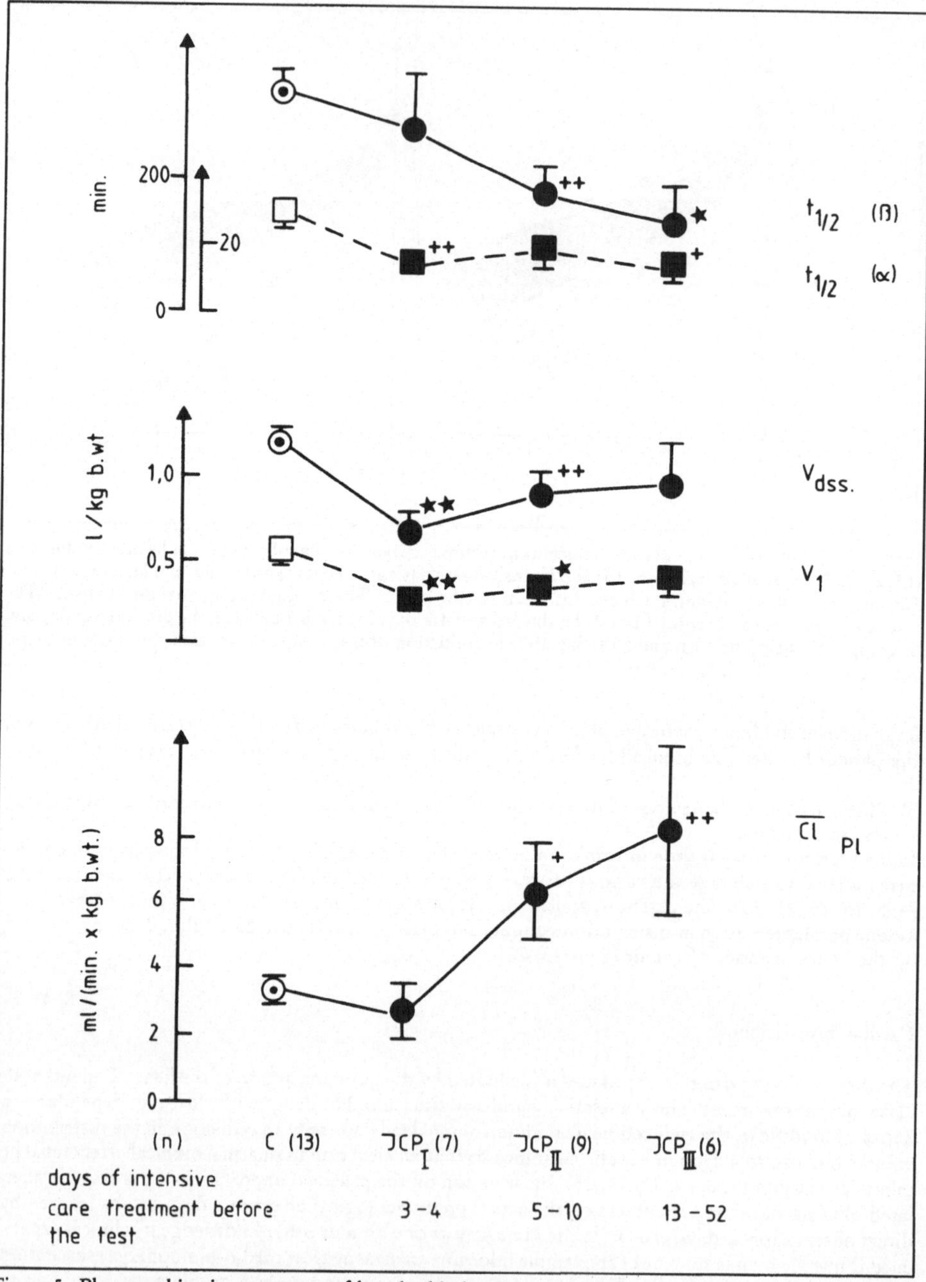

Figure 5: Pharmacokinetic parameters of hexobarbital (Mean ± S. E.) for healthy volunteers (open symbols) and intensive-care patients in the different groups (closed symbols).
The p values are against the controls
$+ p < 0.05$; $+ + p < 0.02$; $* p < 0.001$
(from Ingrid Rietbrock *et al.*, Br. J. Anasthesiol. In press).

Septicaemia

Special problems are presented to the clinician by patients with septic-toxaemia. This is particularly so in the case of patients who are prone to decrease in peripheral resistance and where the cardiac output has risen to 12 litres/min and higher. In these patients, the extent of pharmacokinetic changes for lipid soluble substances is even more difficult to predict than for example in the case of patients with liver disease. This is probably due to the fact that the hepatic clearance and distribution volume can increase or decrease independently of one another, so that the resulting pharmacological effect may be elevated, unchanged or diminished. Up to now only scanty information has been available.
For tolbutamide in intensive-care patients with septicaemia, and similarly also for liver cirrhosis patients, a diminution in the protein-binding of the sulfonylurea derivates can be demonstrated [7, 16, 24, 28]. The free fraction rises and the distribution volume grows larger. A significant correlation exists between albumin content, binding capacity and distribution volume [16]. As the result of these changes, the compounds are transported to, and concentrated at, the site of biotransformation in adequate amounts. An elevation of tolbutamide plasma clearance can already be seen at the beginning of the intensive-care treatment [16]. Of course, for drugs which are bound in tissues or concentrated in peripheral compartments, like tolbutamide, estimates of V_d are estimates of apparent volume of distribution, and are virtual rather than real. Increases in V_d thus can arise through a decrease in total or plasma drug concentration as a result of the lowered albumin level. Thus an increase in V_d can be calculated arising solely from a diminution in the albumin bound fraction, and in the absence of a real increase in distribution. Therefore the calculated increase in distribution volume in patients with septicaemia may be due to an increase in permeability of the blood vessels with extravasation of fluid and albumin [15, 16]. This effect could explain the 3 fold increase in the distribution space from 8L to 24L in patients with septic shock.
In contrast, antipyrine in the same patients has an unchanged distribution volume and a reduced plasma clearance that continues to decrease with progressive worsening of the patient's condition [16]. A diminished oxygen partial pressure is correlated with the diminution in the clearance at this stage and a causal relationship may exist between the two [2, 15].

III. Changes in liver uptake and liver intrinsic metabolic activity for methohexital
(preliminary results)

Evidence as to what extent, sepsis for example, influences liver uptake and intrinsic metabolic activity in the liver for a particular drug, is not satisfactorily obtained by calculation of pharmacokinetic data from plasma concentrations alone.
In severely ill patients an unexplained drop in tolerance to sedatives is becoming more and more apparent. In order to achieve a better control of therapy we examined the possible causes of changed pharmacokinetics under clinical conditions in collaboration with E. Richter, H. Heusler and coworkers, Department of Internal Medicine and G. Viehweger, Department of Surgical Roentgenology of the University Würzburg. In addition to a pulmonary catheter for monitoring of pulmonary circulation and cardiac output, a cava catheter, routinely used for high caloric parenteral nutrition, was placed for a short time in a hepatic vein in order to determine the liver extraction rate of drugs. The test substance used up to the present has been methohexital which was infused at constant rate over a 60 minute period at a dosage of 3 mg/kg body weight. During the infusion and decay phase, arterial, venous and hepatic venous blood specimens were collected for estimation of unchanged drug and its metabolite hydroxy-methohexitol, by gas chomatography. Preliminary results obtained on two intensive-care patients are presented in Figure 6. Both patients showed a severe trauma (polytrauma stage 3 and blunt chest trauma with bilateral rib fractures) and were treated on a respirator. One of them developed septic-toxaemia and a corresponding hyperdynamic circulation syndrome (CI: 6.0 l/min · m^2) whilst the other had complication-free respiratory support.
In the upper part of Figure 6 the methohexital plasma concentration-time curves are shown for the two patients compared with a healthy control subject. In the lower part of the figure their corresponding liver extraction rate measurements for methohexital are illustrated. Higher concentrations

Semilogarithmic Plasma Concentration-Time Curves of Methohexitone

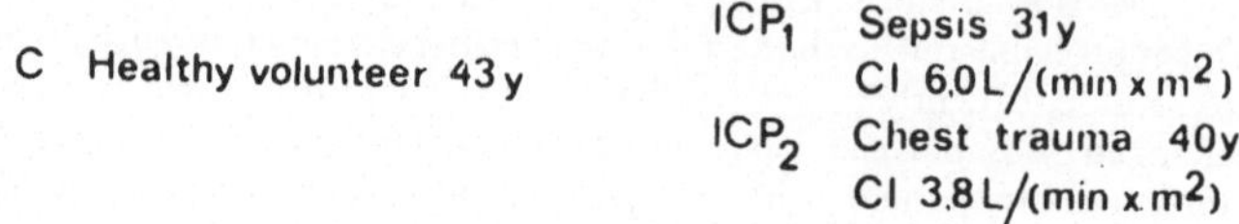

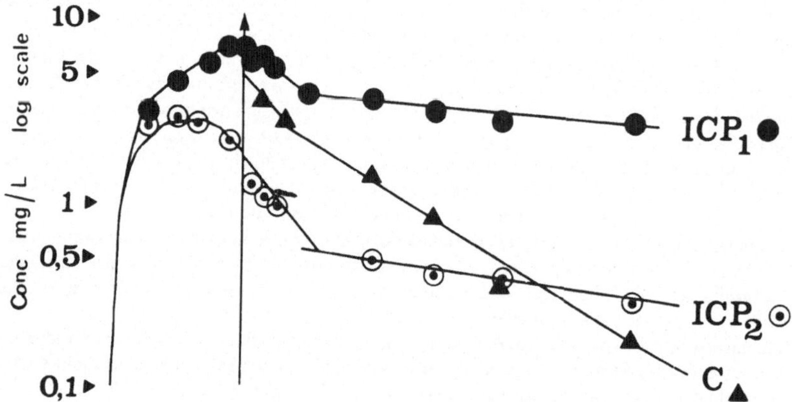

Liver Extraction Ratio of Methohexitone

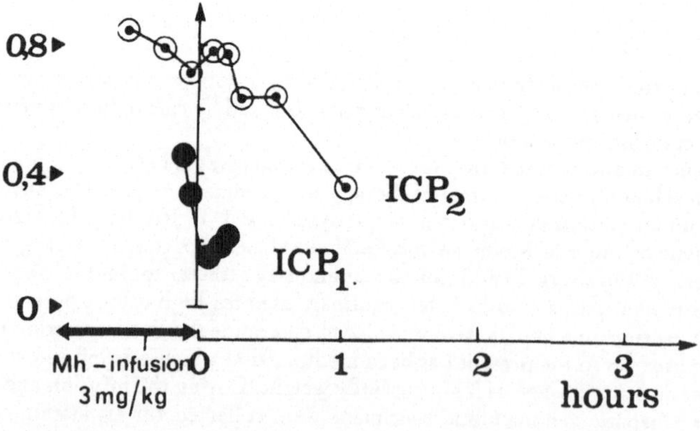

Figure 6: Semilogarithmic plasma concentration-time curves of methohexital of a healthy volunteer (C) and two intensive care patients (ICP_1 and ICP_2) during and after a 60 min linear intravenous infusion of 3 mg/kg b. wt. (upper part) and the corresponding liver extraction rate measurements for methohexital of the intensive-care patients (lower part).

(ICP_1: polytrauma stage 3 with septic toxaemia and accompanying hyperdynamic circulation syndrome. ICP_2: blunt chest trauma with bilateral rib fractures and complication-free respiratory support).

are present in the patient with septic-toxaemia during the infusion, and also during the decay phase. The liver extraction rate is accordingly low. The second intensive-care patient on the other hand, when compared to the healthy subject, has initially lower plasma concentrations during the infusion phase and also during the first hour of the decay phase. The fall in concentration then proceeds more slowly. The liver extraction rate for this patient was not constant, being higher in the early stages. Corresponding results for metabolite concentrations in these patients have been discussed in detail by E. Richter, elsewhere in these proceedings.
The diminished extraction rate and the prolongation of the drug in the circulation of the patient with sepsis leads to an increased duration of effect, but the clinical implication of the fall-off in extraction rate of methohexital seen in the other patient is more difficult to interpret.

Summary

In intensive-care patients, marked alterations in pharmacokinetics of drugs (protein-binding, distribution volume and elimination) result from adaptative changes of the liver to multiple supportive medication and to the actual disease process itself, and lead to difficulties of drug dosage selection.
1. Patients under intensive-care conditions show an increase in liver weight in relation to the number of days of treatment, which is a genuine liver hypertrophy. Of the conventional liver function tests only the gamma GT activity in plasma rises continuously in proportion to the duration of therapy.
2. At the beginning of intensive-care treatment the pharmacokinetic behaviour of hexobarbital in man indicated a decreased volume of distribution and a reduced total clearance of the drug. Due to the liver enlargement and multiple drug therapy, 8—14 days later an enhanced total clearance of hexobarbital was noticed, frequently associated with an induced microsomal enzyme activity.
3. However a large interindividual variation in plasma clearance was noticed, indicating that the disease by itself can change the pharmacokinetic profile of a drug.
In patients with low cardiac output there exists a relatively uniform situation in pharmacokinetic behaviour of drugs, particularly of those with clearance dependent on hepatic blood flow. Not only a reduced distribution volume but also a drop in hepatic clearance was observed. There are however no general guidelines for the disposition of drugs in patients with septic toxaemia. For instance in intensive-care patients with septicaemia the protein-binding of tolbutamide is diminished and the distribution volume and elimination rate of this drug are enhanced, whilst in contrast antipyrine in the same patients has an unchanged distribution volume and a reduced plasma clearance, that continues to decrease with progressive worsening of the patients condition.
4. Preliminary results for methohexital indicated that, due to an increase in the half-life and corresponding increase in duration of pharmacological effect, the liver extraction rate is diminished in patients with septic toxaemia.
These results point out that especially in severe septicaemia, independently or simultaneously, the volume of distribution and the hepatic clearance of a drug is affected. We stand at the beginning in understanding the cellular changes that may occur through disease or drug therapy and indeed we are daily overwhelmed with new drug preparations for which the available basic information for use in intensive-care patients is inadequate. Thus it appears essential in the future to discover the causes and extent of these changes for the different drugs used in intensive-care treatment in order to reduce the incidence of adverse reactions or undertreatment resulting form too high or low doses.

References:

[1] Blaschke, T. F., Protein binding and kinetics of drugs in liver diseases. Clinical Pharmacokinetics *2*, 32 (1977)

[2] Cumming, J. F., The effect of arterial oxygen tension on antipyrine half-time in plasma. Clin. Pharmacol. Ther. *19*, 468 (1976)

[3] Davidson, D. C., McIntosh, W. B., Ford, B. A., Assessment of plasma glutamyltranspeptidase activity and urinary D-glucaric acid excretion as indices of enzyme induction. Clin. Sci. Mol. Med. *47*, 279 (1974)

[4] Elfström, J., Johansson, H., Lindgren, S., Postoperative disappearance of phenazone from plasma in man. Europ. J. Clin. Pharmacol. *10*, 63 (1976)

[5] Forrest, J. A. H., Roscoe, P., Prescott, L. F. Stevenson, I. H., Abnormal drug metabolism after barbiturate and paracetamol overdose. Br. Med. J. *4*, 499 (1974)

[6] Goldberg, D. M., Martin, J. V., Role of γ-glutamyl-transpeptidase activity in the diagnosis of hepatobiliary disease. Digestion *12*, 232 (1975)

[7] Held, V. H., Eisert, R., von Oldershausen, H. F., Pharmakokinetik von Glymidine (Glycodiazin) und Tolbutamid bei akuten und chronischen Leberschäden. Arzneim.-Forsch. *23*, 1801 (1973)

[8] Hildebrandt, H. G., Roots, I., Speck, M., Saalfrank, K., Kewitz, H., Evalution of *in vivo* parameters of drug metabolizing enzyme activity in man after administration of clemastine, phenobarbital or placebo. Europ. J. clin. Pharmacol. *8*, 327 (1975)

[9] Ivanov, E., Krustev, L., Adjarov, D., Chernev, K., Apostolov, I., Dimitrov, P., Drenska, E., Stefanova, M., Pramatarova, V., Studies on the mechanism of the changes in serum and liver γ-glutamyl transpeptidase activity. Enzyme *21*, 8 (1976)

[10] Koch-Weser, J., Klein, S. W., Procainamide dosage schedules, plasma concentrations, and clinical effects. JAMA *215*, 1454 (1971)

[11] Kokot, F., Sledzinski, Z., Die γ-Glutamyltransferase (γ-GT). Z. Klin. Chem. Klin. Biochem. *12*, 374 (1974)

[12] Mather, L. E., Tucker, G. T., Pflug, A. E., Lindop, M. J., Wilkerson, C., Meperidine kinetics in man. Intravenous injection in surgical patients and volunteers. Clin. Pharmacol. Ther. *17*, 21 (1975)

[13] Nies, A. S., Shand, D. G., Wilkinson, G. R., Altered hepatic blood flow and drug disposition. Clinical Pharmacokinetics *1*, 135 (1976)

[14] Prescott, L. F., Nimmo, J., Plasma lidocaine concentrations during and after prolonged infusion in patients with myocardial infarction, in: O. B. Scott, D. G. Julian (edit): Lidocaine Treatment of Ventricular Arrhythmias, p. 168. Edinburgh, EaS. Livingstone, Ltd. (1971)

[15] Rietbrock, I., Beeinflussung der Arzneimittelelimination bei Patienten auf einer Beatmungsstation. Anaesthesiologische Informationen *18*, 58 (1977)

[16] Rietbrock, I., Richter, E., Veränderungen der Pharmakokinetik unter der Intensivtherapie. In: P. Lawin, U. Morr-Strathmann (Edit): Aktuelle Probleme der Intensivbehandlung, p. 207. INA, Bd. 12, Thieme, Stuttgart (1978)

[17] Rietbrock, I., Riemenschneider, J., Varianz der Digitoxinkonzentrationen im Plasma.—Eine Analyse der bestimmenden Faktoren bei Intensivpatienten. In: K. Greeff, N. Rietbrock (Edit): Symposium über Digitoxin als Alternative in der Therapie der Herzinsuffizienz. p. 68, Schattauer Verlag (1979)

[18] Rietbrock, I., Lazarus, G., Richter, E., Breimer, D. D., Hexobarbital disposition in intensive care patients. Br. J. Anaesthesiol. (In press).

[19] Rosalki, S. B., Tarlow, D., Rau, D., Plasma gamma-glutamyl-transpeptidase elevation in patients receiving enzyme inducing drugs. Lancet II, 376 (1971)

[20] Schmidt, E., Schmidt, F. W., γ-Glutamyl-Transpeptidase. Dtsch. med. Wschr. *98*, 1572 (1973)

[21] Sotaniemi, E. A., Effects of drug pretreatment on antipyrine levels in blood and tissues: An example of multiple drug interactions. Pharmacology *10*, 306 (1973)

[22] Sotaniemi, E. A., Ylöstalo, P. R., Kauppila, A. J., Factors affecting drug administration in hospital. Europ. J. clin. Pharmacol. *7*, 473 (1974)

[23] Sotaniemi, E. A., Huhti, E. A., Disappearance rate of tolbutamide in patients in medical wards. Ann. Clin. Res.; zit. in Europ. J. clin. Pharmacol. *7*, 473 (1974)

[24] Thiessen, J. J., Sellers, E. M., Denbergh, P., Dolman, I., Plasma protein binding of diazepam and tolbutamide in chronic alcoholics. J. Clin. Pharmacol. *16*, 345 (1976)

[25] Thomson, P. D., Melmon, K. L., Richardson, J. A., Cohn, K., Steinbrunn, W., Cudihee, R., Rowland, M., Lidocaine pharmacokinetics in advanced heart failure, liver disease, and renal failure in humans. Ann. Intern. Med. *78*, 499 (1973)

[26] Whitfield, J. B., Moss, D. W., Neale, G., Orme, M., Breckenridge, A., Changes in plasma

γ-glutamyl transpeptidase activity associated with alterations in drug metabolism in man. Brit. Med. J. I 316 (1973)

[27] Wilkinson, G. R., Shand, D. G., A physiological approach to hepatic drug clearance. Clin. Pharm. Ther. *18*, 377 (1975)

[28] Zilly, W., Arzneimittelelimination (Hexobarbital, Tolbutamid, Digoxin und β-Methyldigoxin) bei Patienten mit akuter Hepatitis und Leberzirrhose. Habil.-Schr., Würzburg (1976)

Chapter 8

Subject (and species) selection in clinical pharmacological studies

The role of patient selection and patient description in clinical pharmacological studies

Roland Gugler and Andrew Somogyi
Department of Medicine, University of Bonn,
Bonn, Federal Republic of Germany

Clinical pharmacological studies have contributed substantially to our understanding of drugs, in particular in the area of clinical pharmacokinetics. We are impressed by the enormous progress in the analytical methodology (GC, HPLC, mass spectroscopy) to an extent, that some simple aspects of clinical studies have been neglected in favor of newer and more sophisticated techniques. Consequently, characterization and selection of patients in published studies is often surprisingly poor and diminishes the quality of otherwise good clinical pharmacological data.

One important factor which determines the disposition of drugs in the body is age. Age dependency of plasma clearance has been shown for a great number of drugs. Figure 1 shows the plasma clearance of cimetidine to be reduced with increasing age [6]. These findings are of clinical significance in the light of an increasing number of reports on mental confusion in elderly patients on cimetidine therapy. The condition seems to be related to high blood and cerebrospinal fluid concentrations of cimetidine [12] whereas previous kinetic reports in young healthy subjects failed to detect this phenomenon.

The disposition of drugs can differ in male and female patients. Elimination of diazepam is reduced in women, and a prolonged plasma half-life as well as a reduced plasma clearance is observed [11].

Drug kinetics in obese patients differ from normal weight subjects even after correction for the weight factor by expressing the kinetic parameters per kg of body weight. In 14 obese subjects, compared with 57 'normal' subjects the plasma elimination half-life of theophylline was prolonged, and plasma clearance per kg of body weight was reduced [4].

The effect of smoking on drug disposition (Figure 2) has been described for theophylline [8], and similar findings have also been obtained with a number of other drugs. Theophylline plasma clearance was still elevated 3 months after cessation of smoking [8].

The concomitant intake of other drugs can profoundly influence pharmacokinetic measurements. In a large study, Levi *et al.* [10] found no difference in plasma half-life of phenylbutazone between healthy subjects and patients with chronic liver disease. However, when the patients who were on other drugs at the time of the study were excluded from statistical analysis, patients with liver disease showed a significantly prolonged phenylbutazone half-life, whilst liver diseased patients on other drugs behaved indentically to the control group.

Table 1 gives a list of clinical parameters essential for adequate subject description in clinical pharmacological studies. This list of information should be available in studies with patients as well as with 'healthy volunteers'. Such data ideally should be presented in every published study in the form of tables listing the data for every patient, so that variations in the study results can eventually be related to peculiarities in these clinical parameters. Clinical pharmacological studies (pharmacokinetic and pharmacodynamic) should be carried out initially in a small group of 4 to 5 healthy subjects in order to obtain the basic data. The major emphasis in subsequent investigations however, should be placed upon studies in patients who will receive the particular drug in the future. At present the role of the healthy volunteer in clinical pharmacological studies is far too great. Reasons for this are that healthy subjects are easy to find, and studies on them can be planned more exactly and also be performed outside the hospital.

Patients in clinical pharmacological studies should cover all age groups. They should be classified according to the severity of their disease state. In general such studies should be performed on pa-

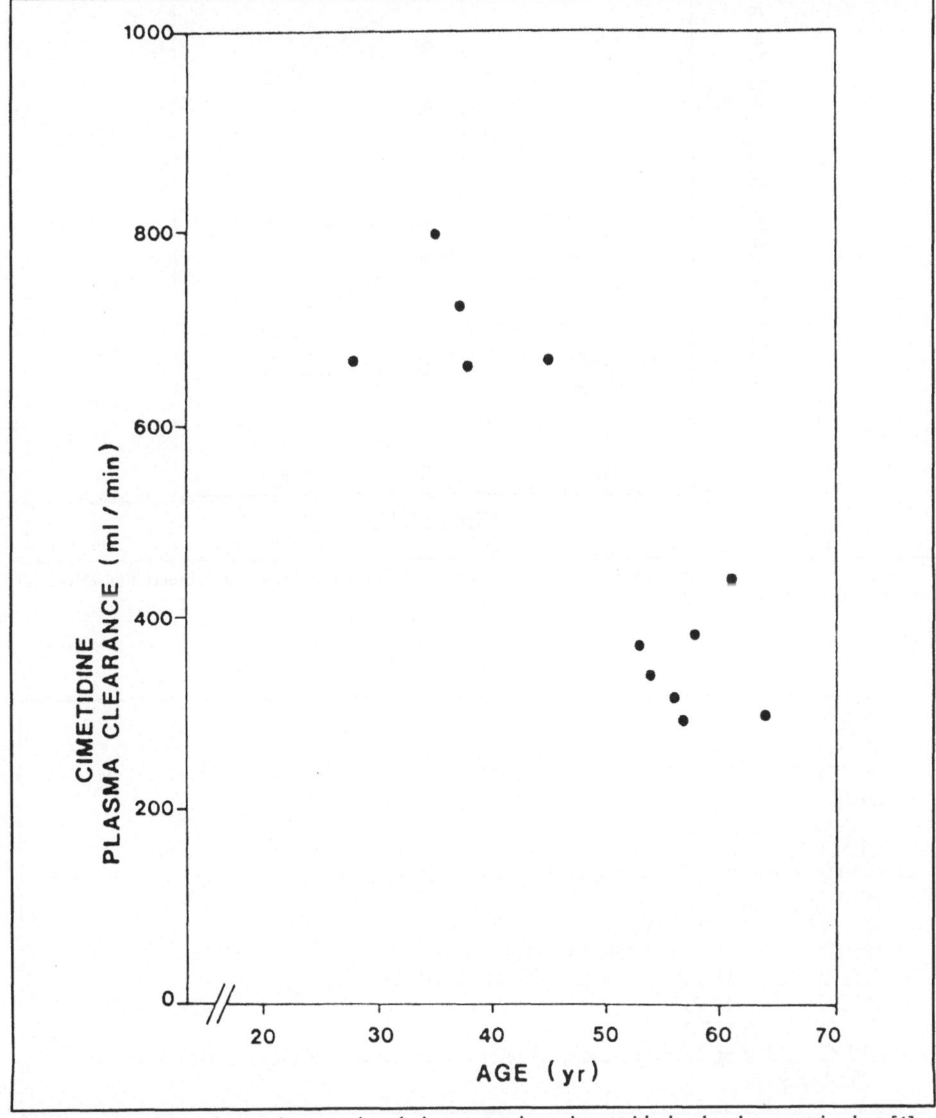

Figure 1: Cimetidine plasma clearance in relation to age in patients with duodenal or gastric ulcer [6].

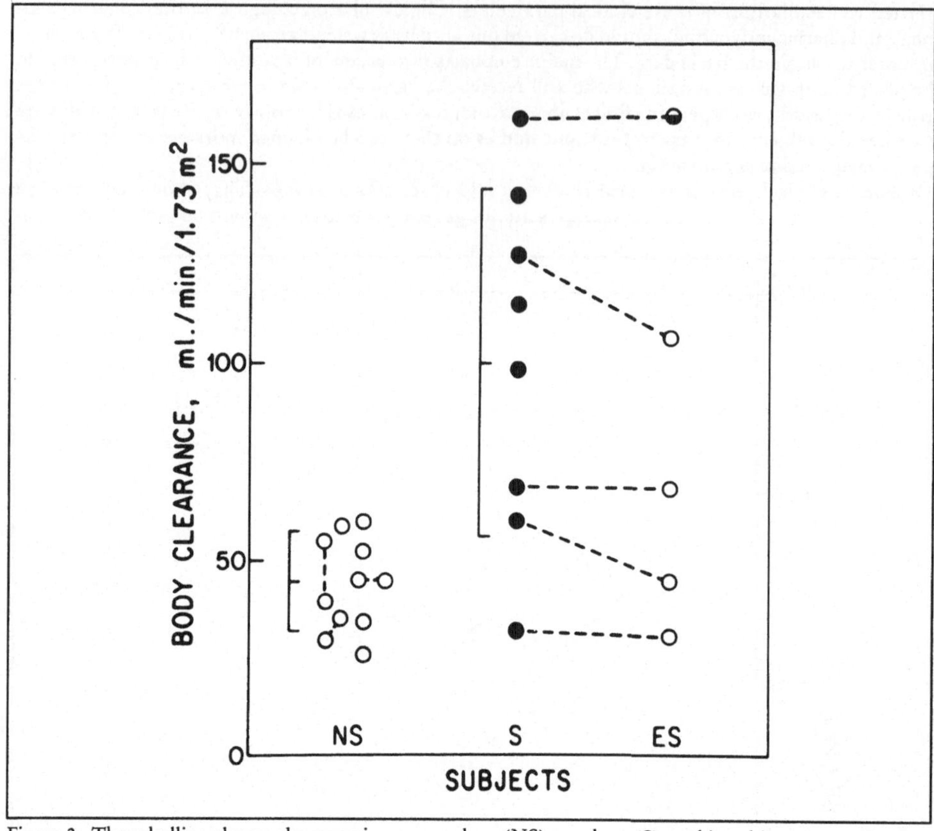

Figure 2: Theophylline plasma clearance in non-smokers (NS), smokers (S), and in subjects 3 months after cessation of smoking (ES) [8].

- AGE
- SEX
- WEIGHT
- HEIGHT
- HEMOGLOBIN
- HEMATOCRIT
- SERUM CREATININE (CREATININE CLEARANCE)
- SERUM BILIRUBIN
- SERUM TRANSAMINASES
- SERUM ALKALINE PHOSPHATASE
- TOTAL PLASMA PROTEIN & ELECTROPHORESIS
- SMOKING HABITS
- DRINKING HABITS
- DRUGS including laxatives, tranquillizers, oral contraceptives, aspirin etc.
- DISEASES

Table 1: List of essential clinical data for adequate patient description in clinical pharmacological studies.

tients who are not on any other drugs. Multiple drug therapy is common practice however and patients may need to be included in the trials who receive additional drug therapy. This is the case in the treatment of hypertensive disease, and also in tuberculostatic treatment which at present is commonly practised using a triple drug combination therapy with rifampicin, a drug with a strong capability of inducing the metabolism of other compounds.

On reviewing the effect of liver disease on the disposition of drugs, it becomes obvious that conflicting results on some drugs are reported by different authors (Table 2), [16]. In some cases these differences can be explained by two major deficiencies: 1. imprecise diagnosis; 2. inaccurate definition of severity of the disease. Branch and coworkers studied the plasma elimination of antipyrine in a large group of patients with liver disease [1]. Impaired elimination was detected when the total group of liver patients were compared to a group of healthy subjects, but only when subdividing the patients according to the exact histological diagnosis was it revealed that antipyrine disposition was affected differently in the different groups: half-life was markedly prolonged in cirrhotic patients, less in patients with chronic active hepatitis, and was only slightly altered in patients with acute hepatitis and with biliary obstruction (Figure 3). Since the disposition of highly protein bound drugs may be altered when binding is decreased as a result of reduced serum albumin concentration [5], information on the protein concentration pattern is essential. This is often unchanged in acute hepatitis, steatosis, and chronic persistant hepatitis, but is reduced in most patients with chronic active hepatitis and liver cirrhosis [13].

Zilly and coworkers have shown that the pharmacokinetics of hexobarbital are significantly altered in all patients with liver cirrhosis [17]. However, while changes were only minor in patients with compensated liver cirrhosis, dramatic changes were observed in decompensated cirrhotics, and significant differences in all kinetic parameters tested were also present between the two groups of cirrhotic patients. These results demonstrate that classifying patients as being cirrhotics alone is insufficient in allowing definite conclusions on the changes to be expected in a particular patient. Klotz and coworkers observed in patients with viral hepatitis a small increase in the plasma elimination half-

Difference reported	no difference reported
Acetaminophen	Aminopyrine
Acetanilide	* Antipyrine
Amylobarbital	p-Aminosalicylic Acid
* Antipyrine	Barbiturates
Carbenicillin	* Chloramphenicol
* Chloramphenicol	Chlorpromazine
Clindamycin	Dicoumarol
Clofibrate	Pentobarbital
Diazepam	* Phenylbutazone
Hexobarbital	Phenytoin
Isoniazid	Salicylic Acid
Lidocaine	* Tolbutamide
Meperidine	* Valproic Acid
Meprobamate	
Pentobarbital	
Phenobarbital	
* Phenylbutazone	
Prednisone	
Rifampicin	
Theophylline	
* Tolbutamide	
* Valproic Acid	

Table 2: Effect of liver disease on the elimination of drugs.
*) Results of different studies controversial

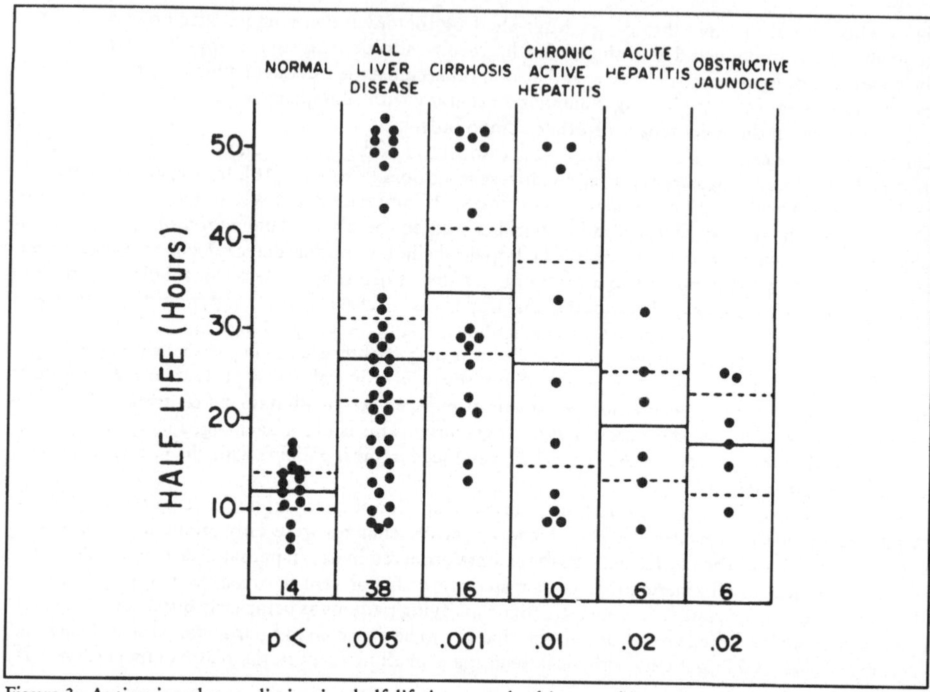

Figure 3: Antipyrine plasma elimination half-life in normal subjects and in patients with liver disease. Liver disease patients are presented as a total group and according to the specific diagnosis [1].

life, but no significant change in the plasma clearance of valproic acid [9], while we detected a significant prolongation of half-life and reduction of plasma clearance in an apparently identical group of patients [7]. The patient groups were, however, not comparable as to the stage of their disease; while in the first study patients were in the recovery phase after acute hepatitis and showed relatively low values of serum transaminases, patients of the latter study were investigated during the first week of hospital admission when they were in the acute phase of hepatitis.

The severity of a disease can also change from day to day as shown by Vozeh and coworkers using theophylline clearance as an indicator (Figure 4 [15]). Plasma concentration of theophylline varied considerably in relation to the patient's condition. In some patients who improved during the time course of observation, plasma concentration decreased as the plasma clearance increased; in others plasma levels increased due to a reduced plasma clearance as their condition deteriorated.

A list of factors considered necessary for adequate judgment on the actual clinical condition of any patient with liver disease is shown on Table 3. In addition to the exact histological diagnosis (not in acute viral hepatitis) clinical data on ascites and portal hypertension is required, as both can affect drug disposition. Specific laboratory tests include enzymes, bilirubin, serum proteins and clotting factors. Indocyanine green clearance or galactose elimination rate will give some general information on the drug elimination capacity by the liver. When Branch and coworkers studied the relationship between several biochemical parameters and antipyrine elimination in patients with liver disease, they found a close correlation with prothrombin time and serum albumin concentration, but no correlation with serum bilirubin, alkaline phosphatase and serum transaminases [1]. Indocyanine green clearance is closely correlated to the plasma elimination of various drugs. Although antipyrine clearance is determined primarily by the metabolic capacity through the liver, and propranolol clearance is dependant on liver blood flow and active transport through the liver cell, the clearance of both drugs can be accurately predicted by the indocyanine green test [2, 3].

Because of the importance of clinical patient description, clinical pharmacological studies in patients

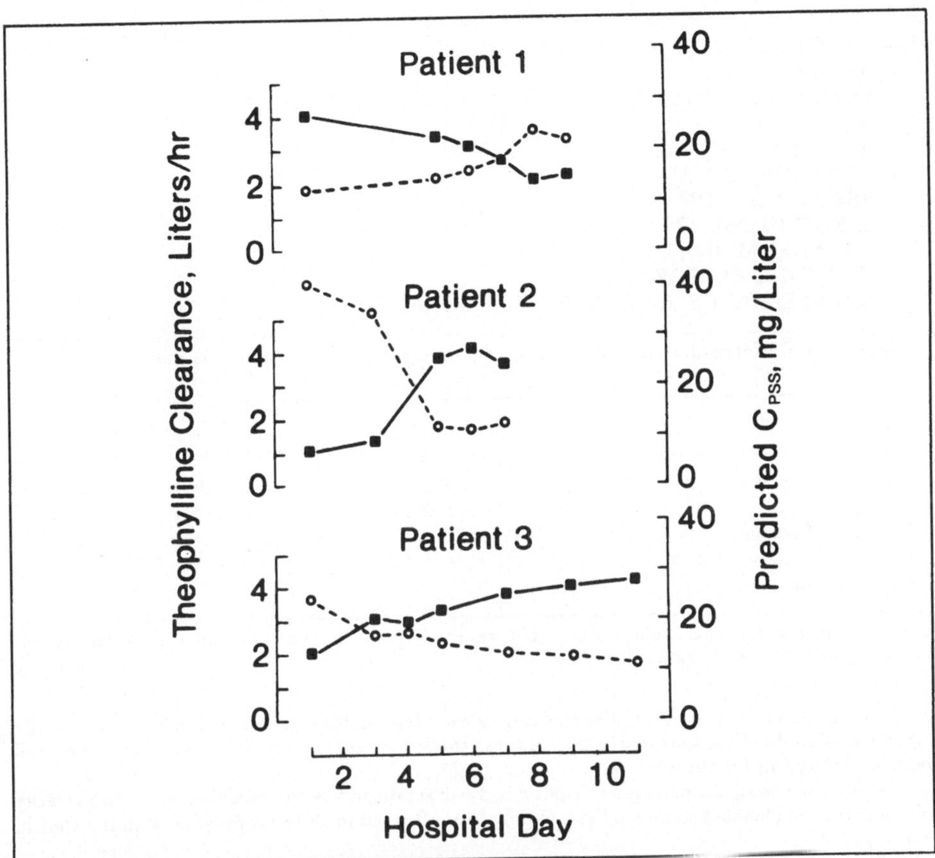

Figure 4: Measured theophylline clearance (solid lines) and predicted steady state theophylline plasma concentration (broken lines) per hospital day in 3 patients [15].

can only be carried out in close cooperation between the clinical pharmacologist and the clinical specialist, since the clinical pharmacologist has in most cases insufficient insight into all aspects of a specific disease and the most appropriate tests to define the severity of the disease. One possibility for overcoming several of these problems involves clinical pharmacological studies performed as an intrapatient comparison, i. e. to study the patient during the acute phase of the disease and again after recovery.

Whenever possible, pharmacokinetic parameters in disease states should be determined in combination with pharmacodynamic tests. Only after proving that the patient reacts to a given drug plasma concentration with a response identical to the healthy organism, can we apply our pharmacokinetic data to the sick patient. Pancuronium plasma clearance is reduced in patients with biliary obstruction by about 50 percent compared to a control group, and the plasma half-life is doubled [14]. A very important piece of information is, however, the fact that the minimum plasma concentration at which an effect from pancuronium can be recorded is identical in both groups (Table 4).

Conclusion

1. A large list of clinical data is essential for meaningful clinical pharmacological studies. Data should be listed individually for each patient in the form of tables.

- EXACT HISTOLOGICAL DIAGNOSIS
- ASCITES?
- PORTAL HYPERTENSION?
- BILIRUBIN
- ALKALINE PHOSPHATASE
- TRANSAMINASES
- SERUM ALBUMIN
- SERUM GLOBULIN
- PROTHROMBIN TIME
- CLOTTING FACTORS
- ICG CLEARANCE or GALACTOSE ELIMINATION

Table 3: Clinical information required for clinical pharmacological studies in patients with liver disease.

Parameter		Control group	Biliary obstruction
Plasma clearance	(ml/min)	105 ± 34	59 ± 21
Half-life	(min)	125 ± 26	241 ± 89
Duration of action	(min)	71 ± 37	114 ± 46
Minimum effective Plasma concentration	(μg/ml)	0.24 ± 0.08	0.25 ± 0.14

Table 4: Pharmacokinetic and pharmacodynamic results on pancuronium in patients with biliary obstruction compared to 'normal' surgical patients [14].

2. Pharmacokinetic studies should be performed on a few healthy volunteers to obtain some basic information on the drug; the target group of these studies should however be those patients who will receive the drug in the future.
3. The basis for adequate patient description is the exact diagnosis and reliable data on the severity of the disease. Valuable patient studies can only be performed in close cooperation with the clinical specialist.

References

[1] Branch, R. A., Herbert, C. M., Read, A. E.: Determinants of serum antipyrine half-lives in patients with liver disease. Gut 14, 569—573 (1973).

[2] Branch, R. A., James, J., Read, A. E.: A study of factors influencing drug disposition in chronic liver disease using the model drug (+)-propranolol. Brit. J. Clin. Pharmacol. 3, 243—249 (1976).

[3] Branch, R. A., James, J. A., Read, A. E.: The clearance of antipyrine and indocyanine green in normal subjects and in patients with chronic liver disease. Clin. Pharmacol. Ther. 20, 81—89 (1976).

[4] Gal, P., Jusko, W. J., Yurchak, A. M., Franklin, B. A.: Theophylline disposition in obesity. Clin. Pharmacol. Ther. 23, 438—444 (1978).

[5] Gugler, R., Azarnoff, D. C.: Drug protein binding and the nephrotic syndrome. Clin. Pharmacokin. 1, 25—35 (1976).

[6] Gugler, R., Somogyi, A.: Reduced cimetidine clearance with age. New Engl. J. Med., *301,* 435 (1979).

[7] Gugler, R., Hartlapp, J.: Unpublished results.

[8] Hunt, S. N., Jusko, W. J., Yurchak, A. M.: Effect of smoking on theophylline disposition. Clin. Pharmacol. Ther. 19, 546—551 (1976).

[9] Klotz, U., Rapp, T., Müller, W. A.: Disposition of valproic acid in patients with liver disease. Europ. J. Clin. Pharmacol. 13, 55—60 (1978).

[10] Levi, A. J., Sherlock, S., Walker, D.: Phenylbutazone and isoniazid metabolism in patients with liver disease in relation to previous drug therapy. Lancet 1, 1275—1278 (1968).

[11] MacLeod, S. M., Giles, H. G., Bengert, B., Liu, F. F., Sellers, E. M.: Age- and gender-related differences in diazepam pharmacokinetics. J. Clin. Pharmacol. 19, 15—19 (1979).

[12] Schentag, J. J., Cerra, F. B., Calleri, G., De Glopper, E., Rose, J. Q., Bernhard, H.: Pharmacokinetic and clinical studies in patients with cimetidine-associated mental confusion. Lancet 1, 177—181 (1979).

[13] Skrede, S., Blomhoff, J. P., Elgjo, K., Gione, E.: Serum proteins in diseases of the liver. Scand. J. Clin. Lab. Invest. 35, 399—406 (1975).

[14] Somogyi, A. A., Shanks, C. A., Triggs, E. J.: Disposition kinetics of pancuronium bromide in patients with total biliary obstruction. Brit. J. Anaesth. 49, 1103—1108 (1977).

[15] Vozeh, S., Powell, J. R., Riegelman, S., Costello, J. F., Sheiner, L. B., Hopewell, P. C.: Changes in theophylline clearance during acute illness. J. A. M. A. 240, 1882—1884 (1978).

[16] Wilkinson, G. S., Schenker, S.: Drug disposition and liver disease. In: F. Di Carlo: Drug Metab. Rev. IV (Marcel Dekker, New York and Basel), 139—175 (1976).

[17] Zilly, W., Breimer, D. D., Richter, E.: Hexobarbital disposition in compensated and decompensated cirrhosis of the liver. Clin. Pharmacol. Ther. 23, 525—534 (1978).

Role of volunteer selection in human pharmacology studies

Leopold, G., Pabst, J., and Ungethüm, W.
Medical Research (Head H. P. Wolf),
Human Pharmacology Center, E. Merck,
Box 4119, D-6100 Darmstadt, W. Germany

Before the first administration of a new drug to patients many pharmacokinetic and—if possible—pharmacodynamic questions and problems, concerning the new substance, are studied in healthy volunteers. Usually a relatively small number of volunteers participate in these studies. These subjects must be carefully selected to avoid undesired and misleading distortion of the results.
The criteria for the selection of volunteers can basically be divided into three groups: somatic characteristics, psychic characteristics, and habits and conditions of living (Figure 1). Each individual aspect within these groups can influence one or more factors of the biopharmaceutical LADME-system (*l*iberation, *a*bsorption, *d*istribution, *m*etabolism and *e*limination) and thus modify results of the pharmacologic objectives of a study. This relates to pharmacokinetics—basic kinetics and bioavailability—as well as to pharmacodynamics—efficacy and tolerance.
The *somatic characteristics* of volunteers are listed in Table 1. They comprise firstly the usual *anthropometric data* of the volunteers, i. e. specification of race, sex, age, weight, height, and/or ponderal index etc.

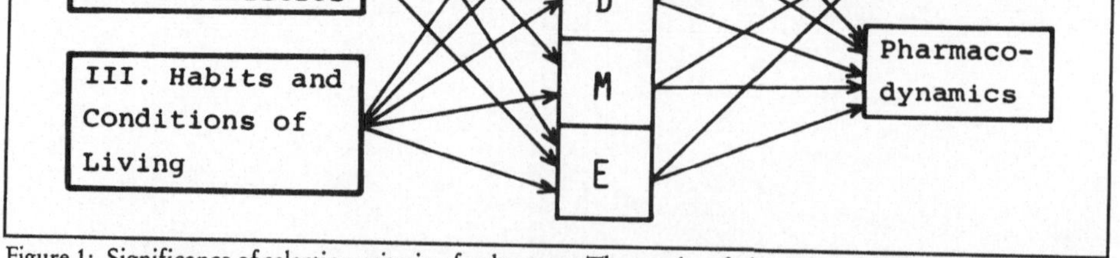

Figure 1: Significance of selection criteria of volunteers: The results of pharmacological studies may be distorted via influence on factors of the biopharmaceutical LADME-system.

1. Anthropometric Data Race, Sex, Age, Weight, Height, Ponderal-Index 2. Physical State Physical Examination, Laboratory Data: Clinical Chemistry, Hematology, Hemostaseology, Urinalysis 3. Special Physiologic Functions Liver, Kidney, Stomach, Thyroid

Table 1: Somatic characteristics

The *clinical examination* ensures that the volunteers are actually healthy. Sometimes volunteers who want to participate in pharmacologic trials tend to conceal or diminish former or present limitations of their physical condition. This leads to the obligation to search very carefully by anamnesis, medical examination, and laboratory analyses for past diseases, disposition for allergies and present limitations of the physical state.

Special attention must also be paid to several *physiologic functions*. Even moderate disorders of the physiologic functions of the gastrointestinal tract, the thyroid, the liver and the kidneys may result in clinically relevant distortion of the results of pharmacologic studies.

It may also be favourable to know in advance *genetic differences in the activity of drug metabolizing enzyme systems* of the volunteers or to exclude volunteers with known enzymatic deficiencies. For example, when it can be expected from preclinical investigations that acetylation of a drug will be an important metabolic step in man, the study should involve a group of volunteers with a defined or ethnically balanced number of slow and rapid acetylators.

Figure 2 shows the well-known influence of the acetylation polymorphism on the serum-concentration-time curve of acetyl-sulfadimidine after oral administration of sulfadimidine. With this substance the assessment of the individual acetylator phenotype of volunteers is easily possible [26].

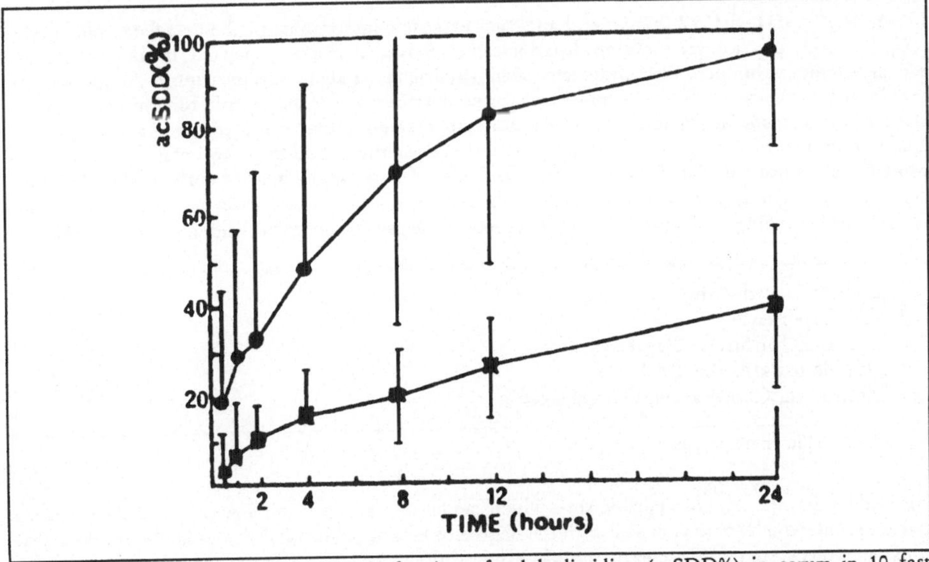

Figure 2: Time course of the acetylated fraction of sulphadimidine (acSDD%) in serum in 10 fast (●——— ●) and 11 slow (■———■) acetylator volunteers. Oral administration of SDD 160 mg/kg metabolic active mass (mean dose 3.33 g). Mean acSDD% was significantly ($p < 0.001$) higher in the fast acetylators at every observation point. Thin vertical bars indicate ± 3 SD (limited at 100%).

(Talseth and Landmark, 1977)

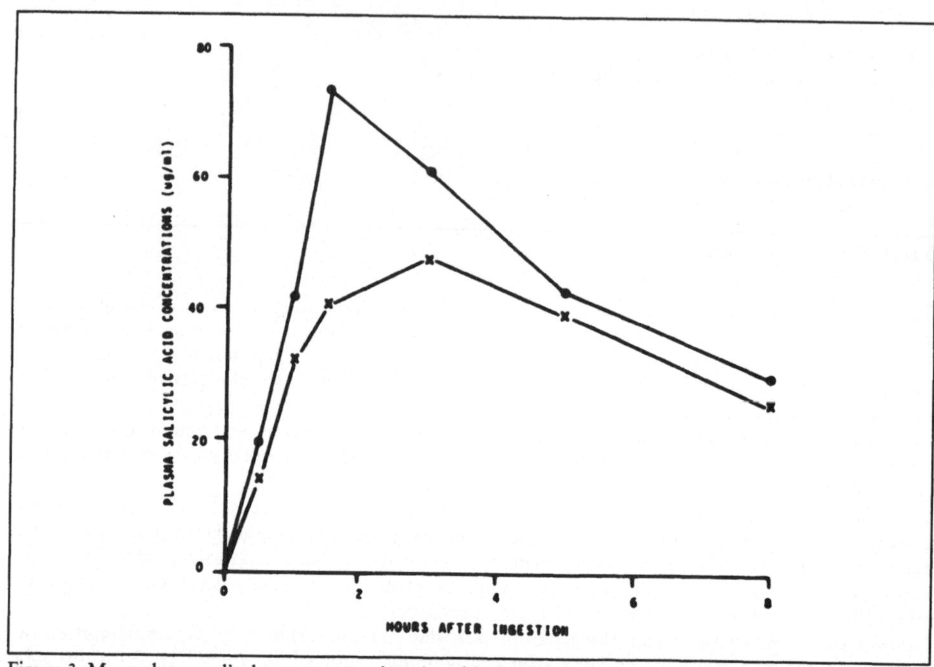

Figure 3: Mean plasma salicylate concentrations in achlorhydric and control patients following an oral dose of 900 mg of acetylsalicylic acid. ●———● Achlorhydric (n = 6); x———x controls (*n* = 6) (Prescott, 1974)

Lunde *et al.* reviewed 1977 the general and very extensive importance of the acetylator phenotype [16]. The other physiologic functions listed in table 1 may also be easily checked. It can definitely be prevented, that volunteers with undetected achlorhydria take part in a study. Figure 3 demonstrates that in such a case normal kinetics may be distorted. Disturbance of the thyroid function may lead to changes of characteristic parameters of drug metabolism and elimination (Figure 4).
The importance of somatic characteristics as criteria for the selection of volunteers is widely accepted. This is not true for the *psychic characteristics* which generally are not sufficiently taken into consideration. The systematic investigation of their significance as criteria for the selection of volunteers is just beginning. The most important aspects of the psychic characteristics are listed in table 2.

1. Level of Neuroticism
2. Trial Experience
Tolerance for Stress; Degree of Stress
3. Attitude towards the Trial
Motivation, Cooperation, Compliance

Table 2: Psychic characteristics

It is evident that the level of neuroticism—which can be assessed in a simple way by special questionnaires [4] and which correlates well with the degree of emotional instability and lability in the autonomic nervous system [30]—clearly modifies the results of pharmacodynamic studies. But even the results of pharmacokinetic studies can be influenced. Nakano *et al.* recently demonstrated that rate and extent or the absorption of diazepam was significantly greater in volunteers exhibiting a high level of neuroticism as compared to volunteers with a low level of neuroticism (Figure 5). This was probably due to enhanced gastric motility and faster gastric emptying in the volunteers with a high

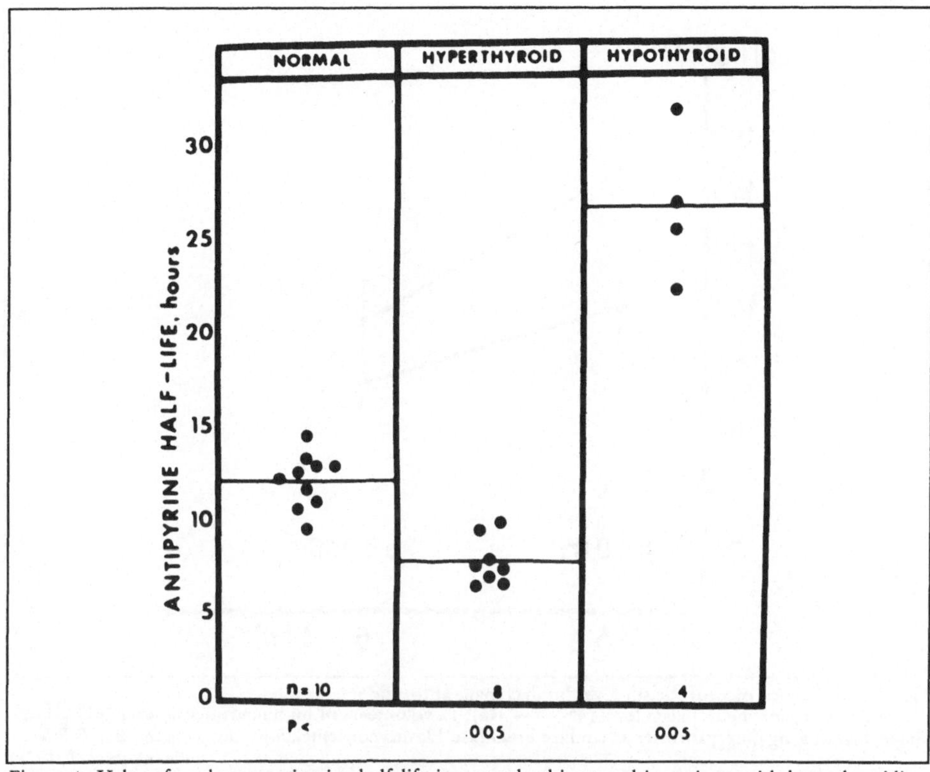

Figure 4: Values for plasma antipyrine half-life in normal subjects and in patients with hyperthyroidism and hypothyroidism. Each closed circle represents the value for a single individual.

(Vesell *et al.*, 1975)

level of neuroticism [18]. Besides the level of neuroticism the degree of test-experience of the volunteers is important for the objective tolerance for stress and for their subjective degree of being stressed.

Our group could demonstrate by studies utilising experimental stress situations* that during a period of psychic stress the enteral absorption of sulfaperine and indomethacin is delayed in comparison to the control situation [14, 15].

Figure 6 shows clearly that after cessation of the stress the absorption deficit is compensated. This fact is not only important for adequate planning of human pharmacology studies but is also clinically relevant in therapy and diagnosis [1, 29]. For practical reasons the *individual attitude of volunteers towards a trial* may be very important. The lack of motivation, cooperation and compliance—especially in the case of very complex protocols—can reduce the quality of the results. Also the third group of selection criteria, the *habits and conditions of living* (table 3), are now becoming more important.

This group does not comprise the *external* conditions *during* a study, but all individual habits and conditions of living and environment which have *persistently* affected the *internal* milieu of a volunteer *before* a study.

One major point is the *individual eating habits.* Kappas *et al.* demonstrated (Figure 7) that a change from normal food to a high protein/low carbohydrate diet was accompanied by a significant reduc-

* part of a research program, supported by the German Federal Government Department for Research and Technology (BMFT)

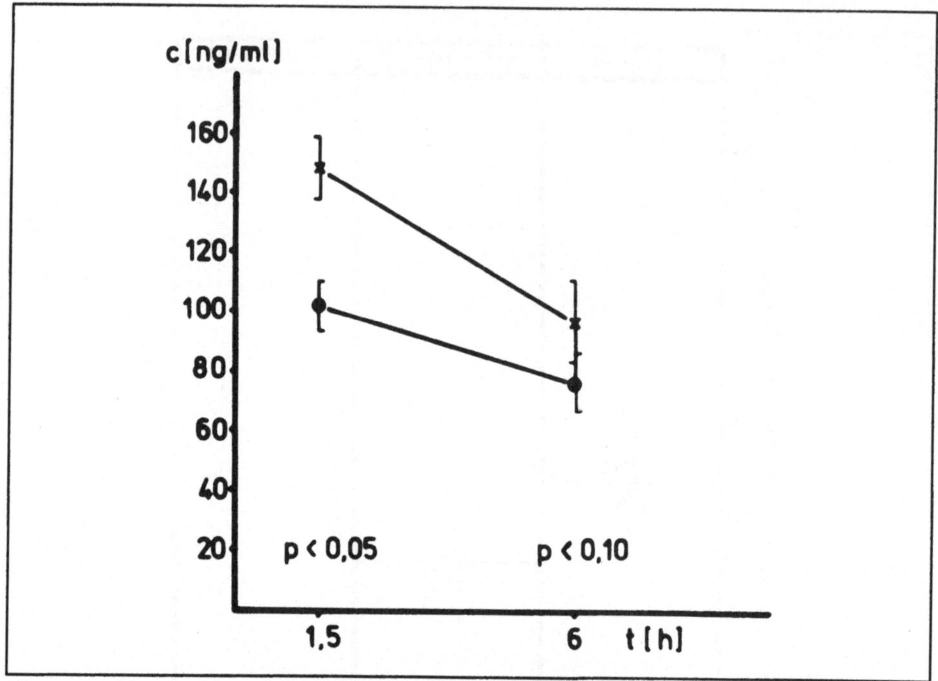

Figure 5: Influence of neuroticism level on diazepam absorption.
12 volunteers of low neuroticism level (●———●); 12 volunteers of high neuroticism level (x———x); single dose of 5 mg diazepam after a standard breakfast. Plasma concentrations of diazepam, $\bar{x} \pm$ S.E.M.
(NAKANO *et al.*, 1979)

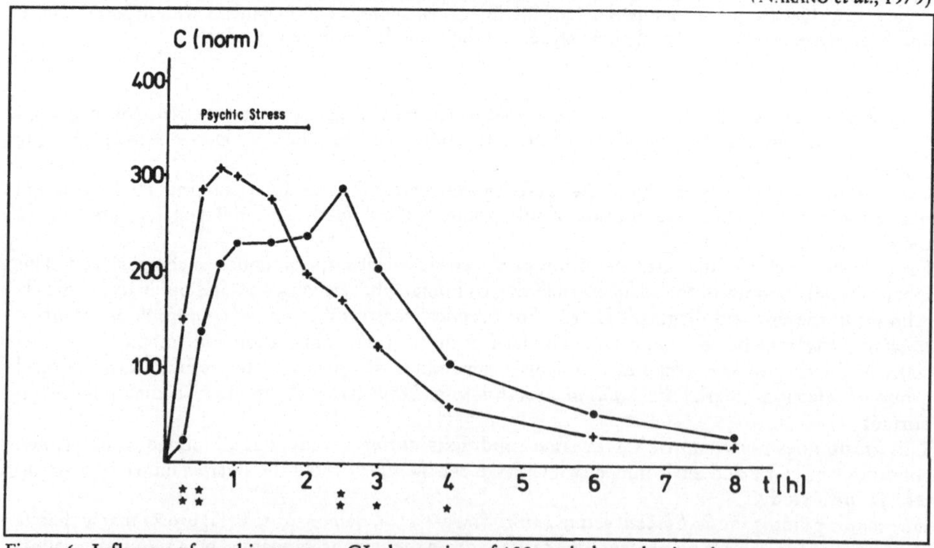

Figure 6: Influence of psychic stress on GI-absorption of 100 mg indomethacin; plasma concentration time curves after oral administration of 2 × 50 mg Amuno®capsules under and without psychic stress.
Psychic stress: acoustical vigilance test of 2 h duration (identifying discrete signals under white noise of 90 dB). $\bar{x}$, $n = 16$ (8 emotionally labile and 8 emotionally stable volunteers), 2-way cross-over, *)$p \leq 0.1$; **)$p \leq 0.05$. +———+ control; ●———● under psychic stress. (LEOPOLD *et al.*, 1979)

1. Eating Habits Meal times; Quantity and Composition of Food; Fluid Intake, Type and Volume. 2. Social Drugs (Type and Quantity) Alcohol, Tobacco, Coffee/Tea. 3. Drugs (Contraceptive Pill, Hypnotics, Laxatives, Vitamins, Antacids, Analgesics, Sedatives) 4. Micturition (Deliberate Control) 5. Defecation (Normal Frequency) 6. Physical Activity 7. Employment

Table 3: Habits and conditions of living

tion of the elimination half-life of theophylline, whilst a change back to a low protein/high carbohydrate diet lead, within two weeks, to a restoration of the original half-life. The same is true for antipyrine [2, 9]. This is consistent with results of FRASER *et al.* who observed generally a longer elimination half-life for antipyrine in vegetarians than in non-vegetarians [6]. The mechanism which

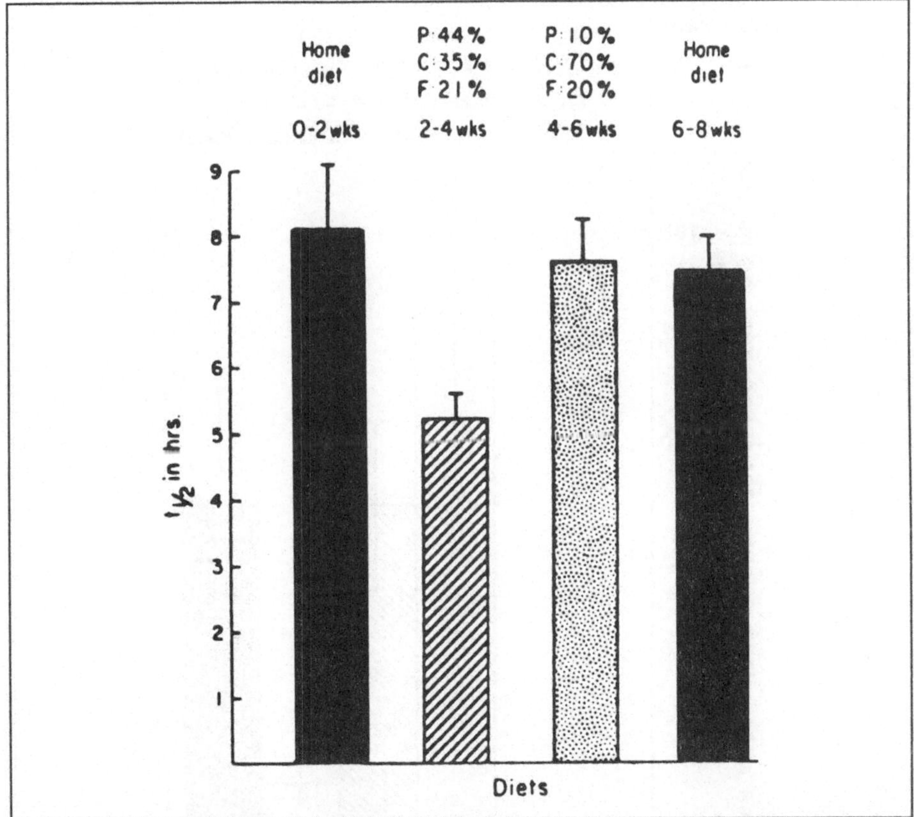

Figure 7: Theophylline half-lives in 6 normal subjects maintained on their usual home diets and on two test diet periods.
Each bar represents mean ± SE for the 6 subjects. The abbreviations are: P, protein; C, carbohydrate; and F, fat. After 2 wk on their usual home diets (diet 1), subjects were maintained on the low C—high P diets (diet 2) for 2 wk, followed by 2 wk on the high C—low P diets (diet 3), followed by 2 wk on their usual home diets (diet 4). The values for diets 1, 3, and 4 are not significantly different from each other. The value for diet 2 is significantly different from that of diet 1 ($p < 0.05$) and diet 3 ($p < 0.01$). (KAPPAS *et al.*, 1976)

is responsible for the change of microsomal enzyme activities caused by differences in the protein-carbohydrate-relationship of the food is at this time not quite clear.
In the meantime it has been explained why food rich in charcoal broiled beef or rich in cabbage induces drug metabolizing enzyme. Figure 8 demonstrates that a diet rich in charcoal broiled beef, already after 4 days results in a significant reduction of the area under the plasma-concentration-time curve of phenacetin [2]. The situation is quite similar for antipyrine and theophylline [2, 10]. The factors responsible for the induction of drug metabolizing enzymes are polycyclic hydrocarbons which are present in the smoke of the charcoal fire. PANTUCK *et al.* described an enzyme inducing effect of a diet containing cabbage and Brussels sprouts on the metabolism of antipyrine and phenacetin [3, 20]. Figure 9 shows the relative change of antipyrine-half-life and of area under plasma-concentration-time-curve of phenacetin. Compounds with indol-structure which are common in cabbage and Brussels sprouts are responsible for the enzyme induction.
Healthy volunteers *fasting* for weight reduction should not take part in pharmacologic studies.

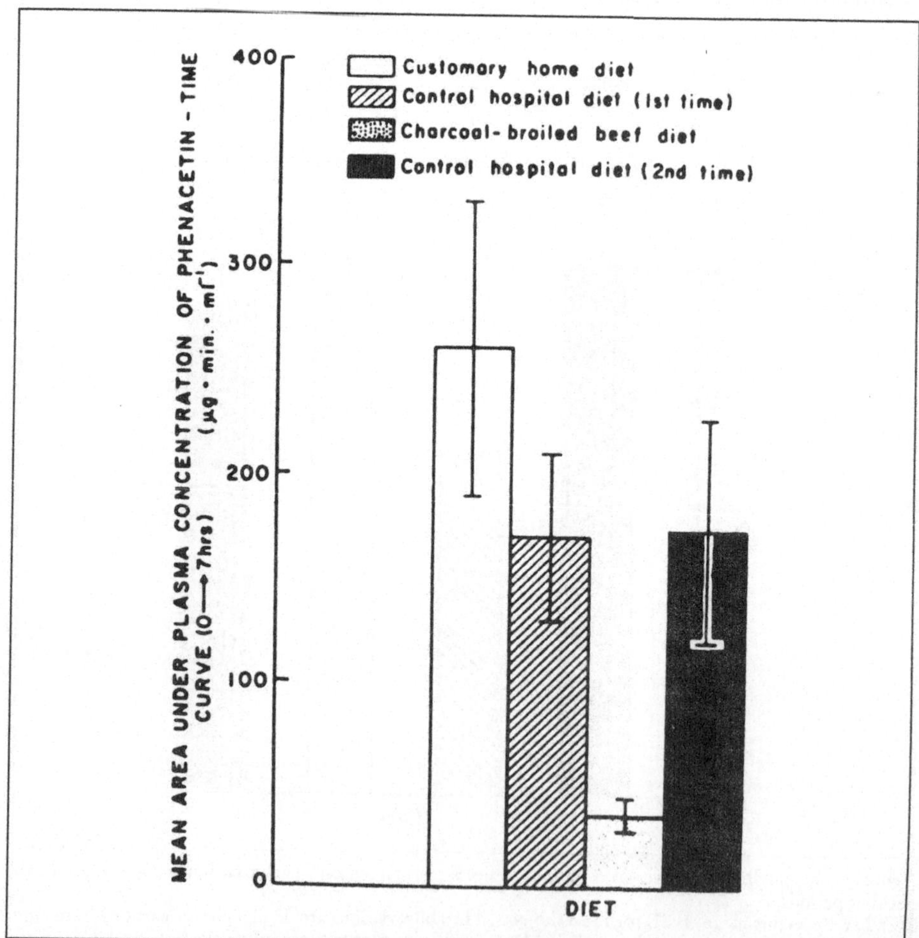

Figure 8: Effect of a diet containing charcoal-broiled beef on the area under the phenacetin plasma concentration-time curve (0→7 hr) in humans. Phenacetin (900 mg) was administered orally to 9 subjects after each dietary regimen. Each value represents the mean ± SE. (CONNEY *et al.*, 1977)

Reidenberg reviewed the changes of the elimination half-lives of some drugs before and during fasting [23]. Another major point in this third group of selection criteria is the habitual and regular consumption of so called *social drugs*. Since the classical publication of Pantuck *et al.* (1972) demonstrating for the first time lower plasma concentrations of phenacetin in cigarette smokers [19], many similar and related papers appeared and have recently been reviewed [8]. Figure 10 might serve as an example for the influence of *cigarette smoking* on the elimination half-life of drugs [7]. It demonstrates that the elimination half-life of theophylline in smokers is significantly smaller than in non-smokers. It could also be shown that the enhancement of the clearance rate is directly proportional to the daily cigarette consumption [8]. If smoking is stopped, it takes 3 months and longer until the elimination characteristics for theophylline in ex-smokers become similar to those in non-smokers. Polycyclic hydrocarbons present in the tobacco smoke are responsible for the induction of primarily hepatic microsomal enzymes. Today it is regarded as "malpractice" to study the bioavailability of theophylline products in a panel of volunteers including smokers. Recently Murdock of the FDA demanded that in all reports on clinical pharmacokinetic studies the individual smoking habits of the volunteers should be stated [17].

The next and very important social drug is *ethanol.* The drinking habits of the volunteers should be carefully explored and documented and the liver function should be checked. The influence of chronic ingestion of alcohol on pharmacokinetics has recently been reviewed [24]. Figure 11 shows that tolbutamide is significantly faster eliminated from the blood of alcoholic subjects as compared to non-drinking adults. During abstinence this difference disappears [13]. It is evident that the influence of the factor alcohol depends very much on type, concentration, daily volume and duration of regular alcohol consumption.

Methylxanthine containing beverages, primarily coffee and tea, play a major role as mild stimulants. Type and amount of the daily consumption should be recorded as a characteristic feature of each volunteer. This is very important as there is probably a tendency to a more intensive consumption of more than one "social drug". So heavy smokers tend to drink more coffee. It has been presumed that heavy smoking causes a higher clearance rate for caffeine which in turn is compensated by a higher consumption of coffee [21].

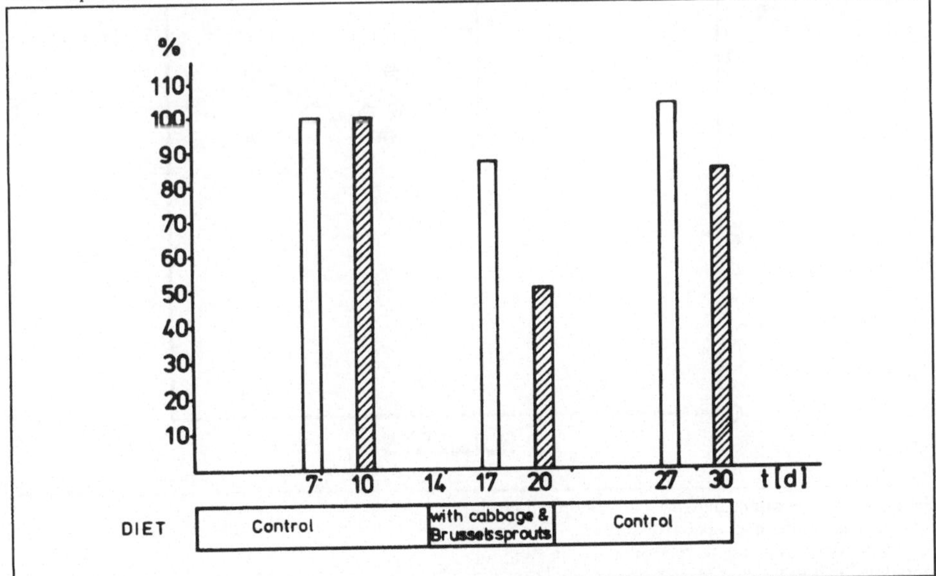

Figure 9: Effect of a cabbage and Brussels sprouts containing diet on antipyrine and phenacetin metabolism in man; 10 volunteers. Antipyrine: 1.8 mg/kg p.o. on day 7, 17 and 27. Phenacetin: 900 mg p.o. on day 10, 20 and 30. Results as relative changes of: antipyrine half-life; open columns; phenacetin $AUC_{(0-7h)}$; hatched columns (Pantuck *et al.*, 1978, Conney *et al.*, 1979)

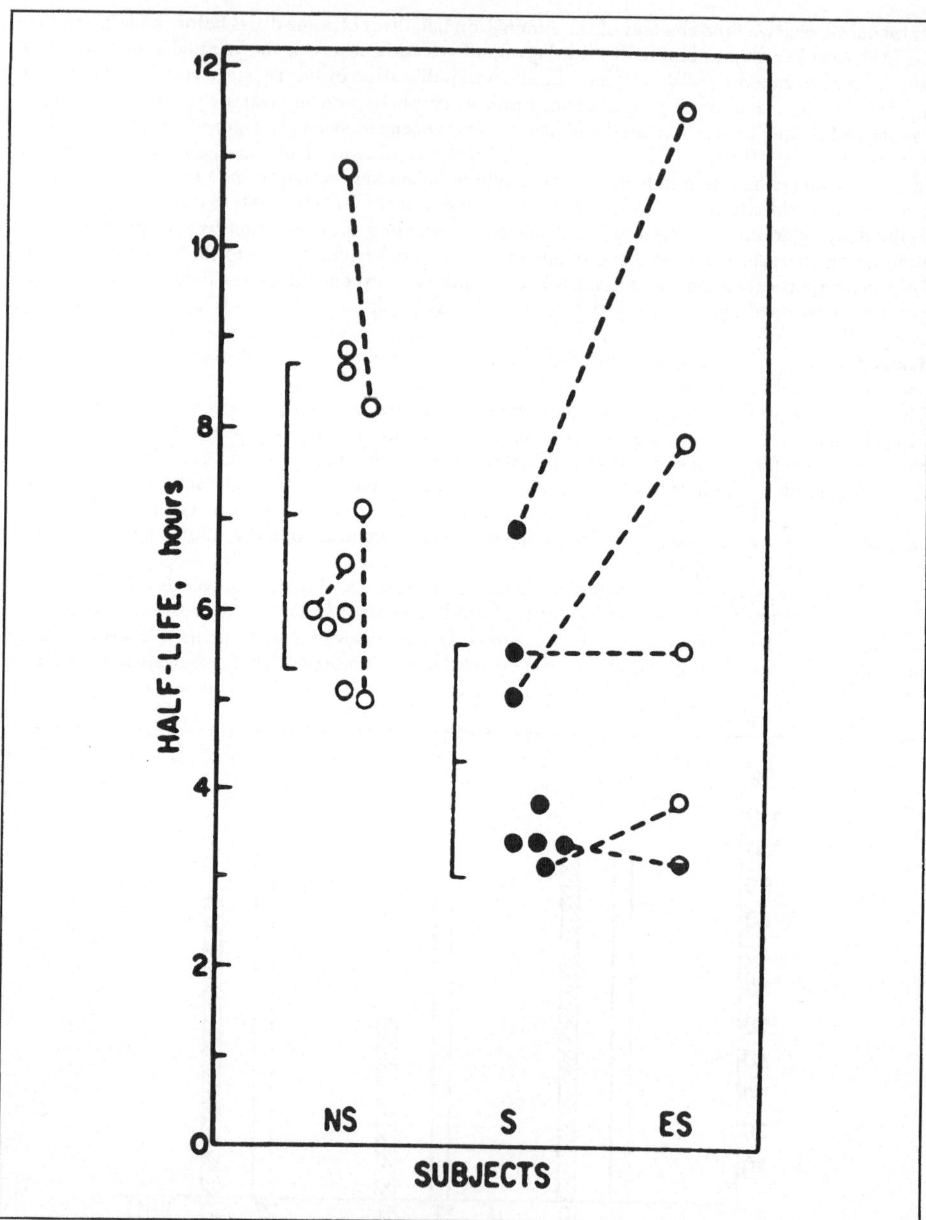

Figure 10: Elimination half-life of theophylline in non-smokers (NS) and cigarette-smokers (S). Some of the smoking subjects were studied after stopping smoking for 3 months (ES), but one of the latter did not fully quit smoking (ha'ed circle). Broken lines connect data from repeated studies in individual subjects. The vertical lines depict the mean ± 1 standard deviation of the data sets. (HUNT *et al.*, 1976)

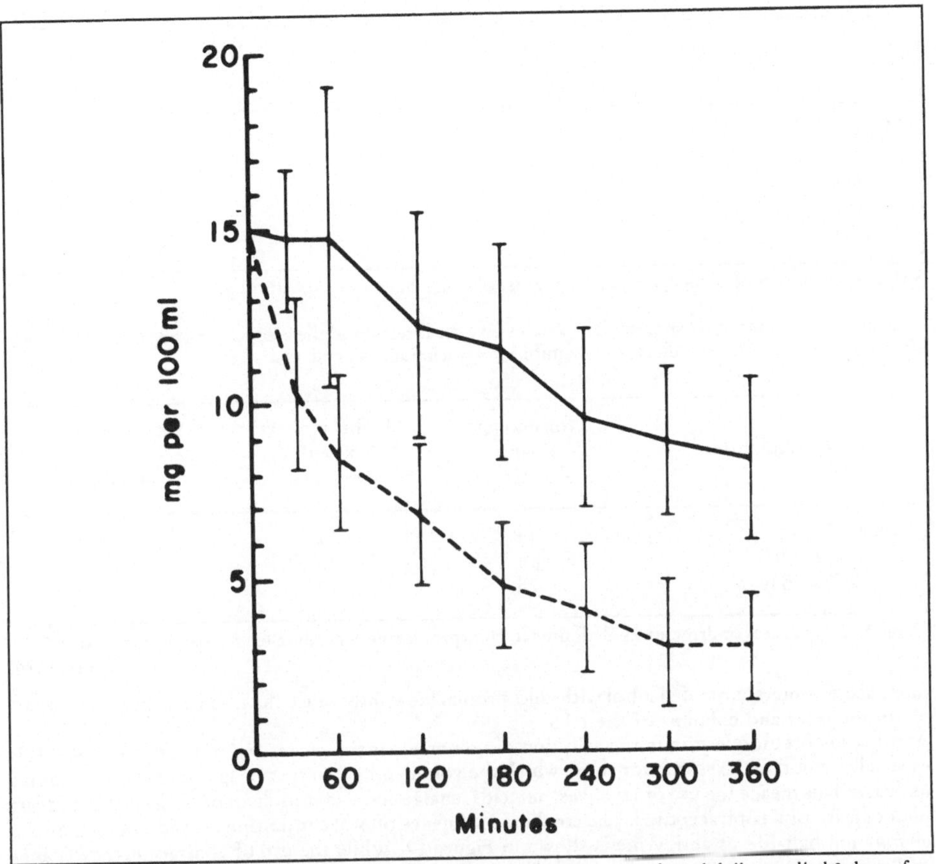

Figure 11: Ten alcoholic subjects (– – –) drinking more than 200 gm ethanol daily, studied 3 days after cessation of alcohol, and 6 non-drinking adults (———), all male and all with no history of any drug intake, were given 1 gm tolbutamide intravenously at zero time and subsequent blood levels of tolbutamide were measured. All values (mean and SD) after 3 hr are significantly different at the $p<0.05$ level, which indicates that such alcoholic subjects remove tolbutamide from the blood faster than normal subjects. (KATER *et al.*, 1969).

The *simultaneous influence of several factors* on the metabolism of antipyrine was investigated by VESTAL *et al.* [28]. Table 4 summarizes the associations which have been observed between metabolic clearance rate, age and habits by multiple analysis of variance. The metabolic clearance of antipyrine is reduced with rising age and goes up under smoking and coffee-drinking. Under alcohol (only consumption of moderate amounts in this study!) no change could be observed. This table also shows that smoking is associated with a higher consumption of coffee.

The simultaneous influence of several social drugs is not only important for pharmacokinetic studies, but also for pharmacodynamic investigations. Table 5 is taken from a paper of SWETT who investigated the frequency of the side effect *drowsiness* under chlorpromazine in a large group of patients [25].

He subdivided the patients according to their smoking and drinking habits into non-smokers, light smokers and heavy smokers and no drink at all, up to 5 drinks per day and more than 5 drinks per day. It can be easily read from Table 5 that with rising cigarette consumption the frequency of drowsiness declines, while with rising alcohol consumption drowsiness becomes more frequent. These findings can be plausibly interpreted: The enzyme inducing effect of smoking and the—in this case

	MCR	Age	Smoking	Caffeine	Alco-hol
MCR	—				
Age	↓	—			
Smoking	↑	↓	—		
Caffeine	↑	↓	↑	—	
Alcohol	0	↓	↑	↑	—

Table 4: Summary of associations among metabolic clearance rate, age and habits[1)]

1) Simple associations by χ^2 analysis. The arrows give the direction of the association and all are statistically significant at $p < 0.025$; 0 indicates no significant association. (Vestal *et al.*, 1975)

Alcohol consumption	Nonsmokers % with drowsiness	Light smokers % with drowsiness	Heavy smokers % with drowsiness
None	14	11	0
≤ 5 Drinks/day	18	10	2
> 5 Drinks/day	25	17	8

Table 5: Frequencies of drowsiness attributed to chlorpromazine according to alcohol consumption. (Swett, 1974)

more acute—interaction of alcohol with chlorpromazine jointly cause the trend that becomes apparent in the rows and columns of the table.

Another important question in the selection of volunteers is the recent *ingestion of other drugs.* It is especially important to search for those which the volunteers often do not spontaneously recognize as drugs. This means the use of laxatives, antacids, analgesics, vitamins, hypnotics, sedatives and last but not least, oral contraceptives. The combined influence of oral contraceptives and smoking on the elimination half-life of antipyrine is shown in Figure 12. While the use of contraceptive pills generally causes a prolongation of the elimination half-life, smoking reduces it. Both effects are clearly independent.

For the practical performance of pharmacokinetic studies it may be important to select volunteers whose normal *frequency of defecation* and ability for optimal *control of micturition* meet the requirements of the protocol.

Another characteristic of volunteers which should be listed is the *employment* or profession and the *usual physical activity.* From this the physical condition can be estimated which may be important in pharmacodynamic studies. There is yet another reason for finding out the conditions of employment of the volunteers. It might give a first indication for the possibility of hepatic enzyme induction by relevant environmental exposure. The last example (Figure 13) demonstrates this situation impressively. The upper panel shows the frequency distribution of antipyrine half-lives of workers who have been exposed to insecticides in comparison to those of unexposed workers in the lower panel [12].

In summary, to avoid distorted results in human pharmacological studies one has to select carefully the volunteers whilst giving attention to a number of important aspects. The criteria for selection can be divided into 3 groups; somatic characteristics, psychic characteristics and habits and conditions of living. The importance of each individual aspect within these groups varies with regard to type and objective of the study. It is impossible and even unnecessary to control all criteria in one study. But as Figure 14 points out schematically, when writing up a protocol, the investigator must check each selection criterion considering the objectives of the trial, the biopharmaceutic principles and the relevant preclinical data, in order to find out which of these criteria are critical in a given situation.

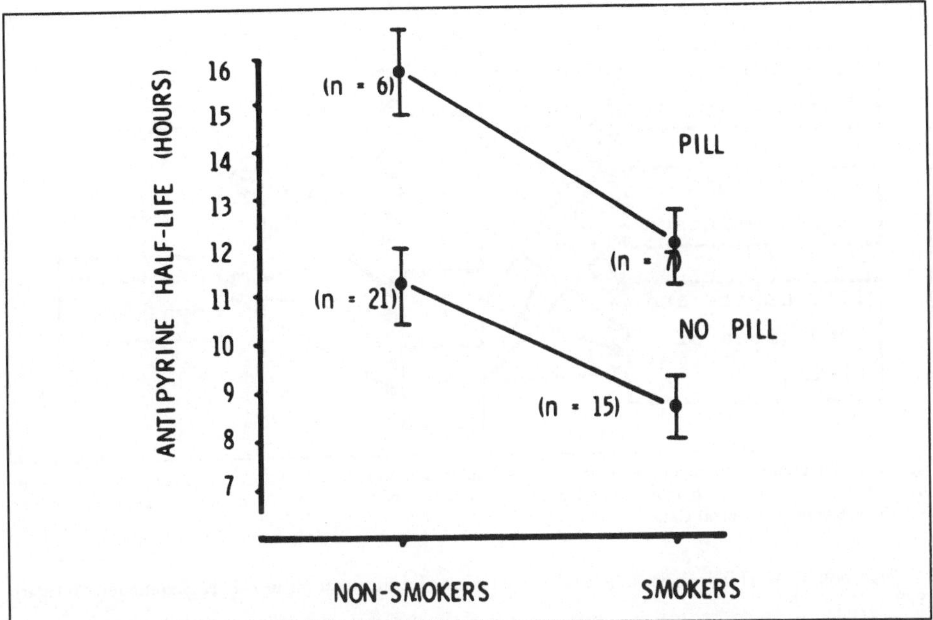

Figure 12: Antipyrine half-life in non-vegetarian women in relation to smoking habits and use of the contraceptive pill (mean ± SEM). (FRASER *et al.*, 1977)

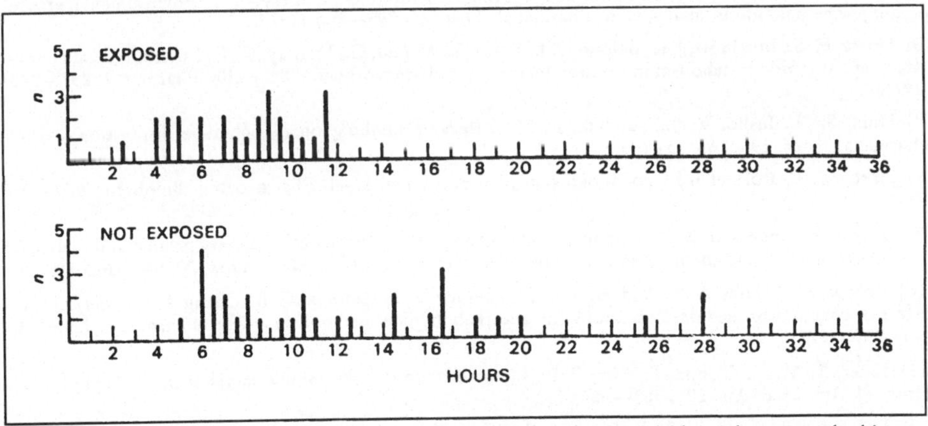

Figure 13: Distribution of antipyrine half-lives in workers exposed to insecticides and unexposed subjects. (KOLMODIN *et al.*, 1969)

References

[1] Carstairs, L. S.: Headache and gastric emptying time.—Proc. Roy. Soc. Med. 51, 790—791 (1958).

[2] Conney, A. H., Pantuck, E. J., Kuntzman, R., Kappas, A., Anderson, K. E., Alvares, A. P.: Nutrition and chemical biotransformations in man.—Clin. Pharmacol. Ther. 22, 707—719 (1977).

[3] Conney, A. H., Pantuck, E. J., Pantuck, C. B., Buening, M., Jerina, D. M., Fortner, J. G., Alvares, A. P., Anderson, K. E., Kappas, A: Role of environment and diet in the regulation of human drug metabolism.—

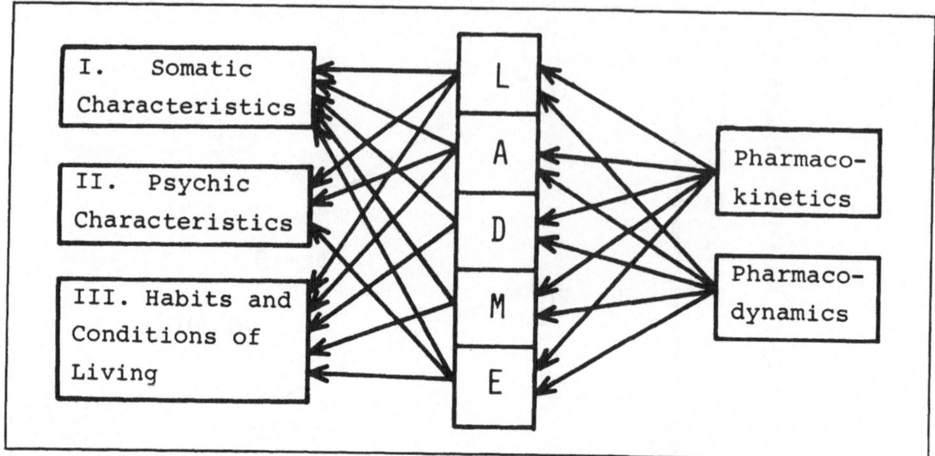

Figure 14: Assessment of the importance of individual selection criteria of volunteers: each criterion within the three groups must be checked considering the objectives of the study, the biopharmaceutic principles and the relevant preclinical data.

In: Estabrook, R. W., Lindenlaub, E. (ed.): The induction of drug metabolism.—F. K. Schattauer, Stuttgart 1979.

[4] Eysenck, H. J., Eysenck, S. B. G.: Manual for the Eysenck Personality Inventory.—University Press, London 1964.

[5] Fraser, H. S., Mucklow, J. C., Bulpitt, C. J., Kahn, C., Mould, G., Dollery, C. T.: Environmental effects on antipyrine half-life in man.—Clin. Pharmacol. Ther. 22, 799—805 (1977).

[6] Fraser, H. S., Mucklow, J. C, Bulpitt, C. J., Kahn, C., Mould, G., Dollery, C. T.: Environmental factors affecting antipyrine metabolism in London factory and office workers.—Br. J. clin. Pharmac. 7, 237—243 (1979).

[7] Hunt, S. N., Jusko, W. J., Yurchak, A. M.: Effect of smoking on theophylline disposition.—Clin. Pharmacol. Ther. 19, 546—551 (1976).

[8] Jusko, W. J.: Role of tobacco smoking in pharmacokinetics.—J. Pharmacokin. Biopharm. 6, 7—39 (1978).

[9] Kappas, A., Anderson, K. E., Conney, A. H., Alvares, A. P.: Influence of dietary protein and carbohydrate on antipyrine and theophylline metabolism in man.—Clin. Pharmacol. Ther. 20, 643—653 (1976).

[10] Kappas, A., Alvares, A. P., Anderson, K. E., Pantuck, E. J., Pantuck, C. B., Chang, R., Conney, A. H.: Effect of charcoal-broiled beef on antipyrine and theophylline metabolism.—Clin. Pharmacol. Ther. 23, 445—450 (1978).

[11] Kater, R. M. H., Tobon, F., Iber, F. L.: Increased rate of tolbutamide metabolism in alcoholic patients.—J. Am. Med. Ass. 207, 363—365 (1969).

[12] Kolmodin, B., Azarnoff, D. L., Sjöquist, F.: Effect of environmental factors on drug metabolism: Decreased half-life of antipyrine in workers exposed to chlorinated hydrocarbon insecticides.—Clin. Pharmacol. Ther. 10, 638—642 (1969).

[13] Kostelnik, M. E., Iber, F. L.: Correlation of alcohol and tolbutamide blood clearance rates with microsomal alcohol-metabolizing enzyme activity.—Am. J. Clin. Nutr. 26, 161—164 (1973).

[14] Leopold, G., Pabst, J., Nowak, H.: Einfluß äußerer Faktoren auf die Bioverfügbarkeit enteral verabreichter Pharmaka.—In: Rietbrock, N., Schnieders, B. (ed.): Bioverfügbarkeit von Arzneimitteln.—G. Fischer, Stuttgart 1979.

[15] Leopold, G., Burow, H. M., Breitstadt, A., Nowak, H.: Modification of the bioavailability of drugs by external factors.—In: Gladtke, E., Heimann, G. (ed.): 25 years of pharmacokinetics.—G. Fischer, Stuttgart 1980.

[16] Lunde, P. K. M., Frislid, K., Hansten, V.: Disease and acetylation polymorphism.—Clin. Pharmacokin. 2, 182—197 (1977).

[17] Murdock, Jr. H. R., Robillard, N. F.: Use of smokers in bioavailability studies.—Clin. Pharmacol. Ther. 25, 238 (1979).

[18] Nakano, S., Ogawa, N., Kawazu, Y.: Influence of neuroticism level on diazepam absorption.—Clin. Pharmacol. Ther. 25, 239 (1979).

[19] Pantuck, E. J., Kuntzman, R., Conney, A. H.: Decreased concentration of phenacetin in plasma of cigarette smokers.—Science 175, 1248—1250 (1972).

[20] Pantuck, C. B., Pantuck, E. J., Garland, W. A., Min, B., Wattenberg, L. W., Anderson, K. E., Kappas, A., Conney, A. H.: Effect of a cabbage and Brussels sprouts containing diet on antipyrine and phenacetin metabolism in man.—Pharmacologist 20, 170 (1978).

[21] Parsons, W. D., Neims, A. H.: Effect of smoking on caffeine clearance.—Clin. Pharmacol. Ther. 24, 40—46 (1978).

[22] Prescott, L. F.: Gastrointestinal absorption of drugs.—Med. Clin. North Am. 58, 907—916 (1974).

[23] Reidenberg, M. M.: Obesity and fasting-effects on drug metabolism and drug action in man.—Clin. Pharmacol. Ther. 22, 729—734 (1977).

[24] Sellers, E. M., Holloway, M. R.: Drug kinetics and alcohol ingestion.—Clin. Pharmacokin. 3, 440—452 (1978).

[25] Swett, C., Jr.: Drowsiness due to chlorpomazine in relation to cigarette smoking.—Arch. Gen. Psychiatry 31, 211—213 (1974).

[26] Talseth, T., Landmark, K. H.: Polymorphic acetylation of sulphadimidine in normal and uraemic man.—Eur. J. clin. Pharmacol. 11, 33—36 (1977).

[27] Vesell, E. S., Shapiro, J. R., Passanati, G. T., Jorgensen, H., Shively, C. A.: Altered plasma half-lifes of antipyrine, propylthiouracil, and methimazole in thyroid dysfunction.—Clin. Parmacol. Ther. 17, 48—56 (1975).

[28] Vestal, R. E., Norris, A. H., Tobin, J. D., Cohen, B. H., Shock, N. W., Andres, R.: Antipyrine metabolism in man: influence of age, alcohol, caffeine, and smoking.—Clin. Pharmacol. Ther. 18, 425—432 (1975).

[29] Volans, G. N.: Migraine and drug absorption.—Clin. Pharmacokin. 3, 313—318 (1978).

[30] Wilson, G. D.: Personality.—In: Eysenck, H. J., Wilson G. D. (ed.): Human Psychology.—MTP Press Ltd., Lancaster 1976.

Comparative pharmacokinetics of furosemide in animals and man

F. Sörgel**, *, E. Mutschler***, M. Hropot**, R. Muschaweck**, and M. Schäfer***

* Institut für Gerontologie der Universität Erlangen-Nürnberg (Present address)
** HOECHST AG, Frankfurt/Main
*** Pharmakologisches Institut für Naturwissenschaftler, Frankfurt/Main

Introduction

Species differences in pharmacokinetics and metabolism are well known for many drugs. When drug metabolism in the test species leads to the compound emerging as biologically inactive, this may mislead and prevent the compound from being further developed since it could have biological activity in man. Similarly, in toxicity studies, species differences may be of great importance for the evaluation of a new compound. These problems became very important during development in the case of several diuretics.

Aims of the investigations

The fate of furosemide in the body was investigated in rhesus monkeys, beagles, rats and compared to literature data for man, in order to determine the presence of possible species differences. These investigations should help to elucidate whether pharmacokinetic and metabolic studies in monkeys, dogs and rats have significance for man.

Methods

Electrolytes were measured by standard procedures.
Furosemide and its metabolites were measured by quantitative thin layer chromatography using HPTLC-plates.

- Plasma TLC — Addition of methanol (with internal standard), centrifugation and spotting plates with supernatant.
- Urine TLC — directly spotted onto the plate.
- Bile TLC — addition of methanol (with internal standard), centrifugation and spotting the plates with specific amounts of supernatant.

Results

The diuretic action of furosemide is similar in beagles and rhesus monkeys. A rapid onset of action was seen, the maximum effect being observed during the first ten minutes after administration. In man the maximum effect of furosemide was observed 30—40 minutes after i. v. administration. Urinary excretion of furosemide in beagles and rhesus monkeys was also very rapid, the maximum excretion rate being observed during the first ten minutes after administration. There are no comparable literature data available from investigations in man.

Species	% ur. excr.	Method	Ref.
rhesus monkeys	55—65	Quantitative TLC (Fluo)	[2]
beagles	55	Quantitative TLC (Fluo)	[3]
man	90	Total ^{14}C-activity	[4]
man	87	Total ^{35}S-activity	[5]
man	63	TLC, elution, Fluo	[6]

Table 1: Urinary excretion of furosemide after i. v. administration was as follows:

Species	Comp. model	$t_{1/2}$ α (min.)	$t_{1/2}$ β (min.)	Vol. distr.	Vol. distr. % of b.w.	(Ref.)
rhesus monkeys	II	15.6	96	0.128 l/kg	13%	[2]
beagles	II	5.0	133	0.2 l/kg	~ 20%	[3]
man	II	10.9	51	0.110 l/kg	~ 11%	[7]

Table 2: The elimination of furosemide from plasma:

Significant metabolism of furosemide was observed; the major part of metabolism seems to be conjugation to a glucuronide of furosemide. In rats there were only very small amounts of furosemide conjugate present in urine.

Discussion

In our investigations, done mainly in animals, some differences emerged in comparison with man. The rapid excretion of furosemide in rhesus monkeys and beagles is responsible for the very rapid and marked onset of diuretic action in these species. In man, however, the maximum diuretic effect of furosemide was seen 30—40 minutes after administration. It remains to be shown whether this is a result of different distribution or different tubular secretion of furosemide in man. The urinary excretion of furosemide also revealed species differences. It is, however, still unclear whether this is really due to different metabolism and excretion or only a question of different methods of measurement of furosemide. We have established that glucuronide fomation of furosemide did occur in all species, although it was very low in the rat. As glucuronidation is a very important factor in furosemide metabolism, our findings might be of interest for toxicological studies. MITCHELL's [8] in vitro studies, showing cytochrome P_{450} metabolism of furosemide, did not consider the fact that glucuronidation might be a major elimination pathway of furosemide.

Literature:

[1] Schäfer, M., Dissertation, Frankfurt/M. 1978

[2] Sörgel, F., Muschaweck, R., Mutschler, E., Hropot, M., Naunyn-Schmiedeberg's Arch. Pharmacol. Suppl. to Vol. 302, R 169 (1978)

[3] Sörgel, F., Muschaweck, R., Hropot, M., Naunyn-Schmiedeberg's Arch. Pharmacol. Suppl. to Vol. 303, E 189 (1979)

[4] Rupp, W., Zapf, R. M., Arzneim.-Forsch. (Drug Res.) *23*, 1665—1668 (1973)

[5] Honari, J., Blair, A. D., Cutler, R. E., Clin. Pharmacol. Ther. *22*, 395—401 (1977)

[6] Andreasen, F., Hansen, H. E., Mikkelsen, E., Europ. J. clin. Pharmacol. *13*, 41—48 (1978)

[7] Andreasen, F., Mikkelsen, E., Europ. J. clin. Pharmacol. *12*, 15—17 (1977)

[8] Mitchell, J. R., Potter, W. Z., Hinson, J. A., Jollow, D. J. Nature, *251*, 508 (1974)

Chapter 9

Protein binding

Methods for the measurement of drug binding to plasma proteins

W. Edward Lindup
Department of Pharmacology and Therapeutics, University of Liverpool, Liverpool

Introduction

Binding to plasma proteins can have a marked effect on the distribution, pharmacological activity and rate of elimination of a drug. In general it is considered that the unbound fraction of drug is pharmacologically active [23] and that the bound fraction is not immediately available for distribution through body water or for certain routes of elimination. Gillette [16] and others [33] have indicated how binding to plasma proteins may either hasten or retard elimination, depending on the mechanism involved. Since plasma protein binding affects the intensity and duration of pharmacological activity, the influence of disease and/or drug-induced changes in binding can be important clinically. Klotz [20] summarised more than 30 *in vitro* methods which are available for measurement of drug binding. However this brief review will concentrate on those methods likely to give the most physiological results.

Qualitative and quantitative aspects

Any experimental investigation of drug binding to plasma proteins usually seeks to answer one or more of the questions posed by Scatchard [29]: *How many* (molecules bound)? *How tightly? Where?* (which protein) and *Why?* To these may be added *"What of it?"* a pertinent question for clinical pharmacologists.

Separation of plasma proteins by various forms of electrophoresis and column chromatography can provide qualitative information on the identity or nature of the binding protein(s) for a particular drug [25].

These separation methods often use unphysiological experimental conditions which means that the results will not yield precise quantitative information on the extent of binding. Nevertheless there is increasing evidence that albumin is neither the sole nor the major binding protein for weak organic bases in plasma [13].

Disease or drug-induced changes in either the binding properties or the pattern of plasma protein may occur. Renal failure in man [27] and animals [6, 7] for example increases the unbound concentration of many acidic drugs. However the binding of weak organic bases tends to be unaffected. Changes in the pattern of plasma proteins can occur, e. g. in rheumatoid arthritis, and if the binding proteins for a particular drug have been identified it should become possible to anticipate the direction of changes in binding and make any necessary adjustments to the dosage. The methods for quantitation of the unbound fraction can be broadly divided into two categories: (i) direct methods for measurement of unbound drug, such as equilibrium dialysis (ii) indirect methods which include the determination of drug in saliva.

Direct methods

The four methods which have predominated are: equilibrium dialysis, ultrafiltration, ultracentrifugation and gel filtration [24] and their relative merits are summarized in Table 1. The method of plasma or serum collection itself may produce errors: difficulties have occurred with a plasticizer leached from "Vacutainers" [2] and from the use of an indwelling heparinized cannula [34].

Equilibrium Dialysis

This has been the most used method but the conventional bag and beaker technique is slow and cumbersome and until the advent of the new dialysis cells, ultrafiltration and gel filtration were becoming more commonly used.
The main factors which influence the rate at which a dialysis system approaches equilibrium are the concentration gradient of drug for diffusion, the rate of mixing, the surface area of the membrane and its particular characteristics such as its molecular weight cut-off. The low (membrane surface area)/(volume) ratio is the main reason for the slow (up to 48 hours) approach to equilibrium with the conventional system.
Scholtan [30] devised a closed dialysis cell in which narrow protein and buffer compartments of equal volume were separated by the membrane. This design has been developed further [32] and cells, manufactured from "Teflon", are now commercially available in 200 μl to 5000 μl half-cell sizes (Diachema, Switzerland; MSE-Fisons, U.K.). The surface area to volume ratio of a conven-

METHOD	ADVANTAGES	DISADVANTAGES
Equilibrium dialysis	Accurate quantitive data. Most used method, so comparison easy. Simple apparatus and good temperature control. Relatively rapid with dialysis cells.	Membrane binding, osmosis and Donnan inequalities. Non physiological: original equilibrium disturbed by dilution effect of buffer compartment
Ultrafiltration	Accurate quantitative data. No dilution. Simple apparatus. Rapid and approximates physiological situation.	Membrane binding, sieve effect and Donnan equilibrium. Protein concentrated—equilibrium disturbed. Temperature and pH control needed.
Ultracentrifugation	No membrane-related effects or change in total drug concentration.	Sedimentation of drug molecules—control samples? Protein concentrated. Floating lipid layer. Expensive apparatus and time consuming. Temperature and pH Control needed.
Gel filtration	No membrane effects. Separation of several binding proteins possible. Can use high molecular weight drugs.	Binding to gel. Larger amounts of drug and plasma needed. Time consuming unsuitable for multiple samples.

Table 1: Some methods for the measurement of drug binding to plasma proteins

tional dialysis experiment where lml of plasma is dialysed against 10 ml of buffer is about 0.9 whereas this ratio for the l ml cell is at least 4.5 and may be higher, depending on the particular design. Temperature control and mixing is straightforward since banks of 20 cells can be immersed and rotated in a water bath. The relatively short equilibration times needed (Table 2) may decrease further if recent improvements in membranes (e. g. Spectrapor®, Spectrum Medical Industries Inc., Los Angeles, U.S.A.) continue.

Ligand	Molecular Weight	Equilibration Time (hr)
Bromocresol green	720	5
HABA	242	3
Methyl orange	327	3
Methyl red	269	2
Phenytoin	252	4
Salicylic Acid	138	3
L-Tryptophan	204	4
Warfarin	308	4

Table 2: Typical equilibration times used for various ligands
Data from Bowmer & Lindup [4, 6, 7]

Donnan problems can be avoided by either prior dilution of whole plasma or the use of a buffer of sufficient ionic strength. Binding to the dialysis membrane and, less commonly, to the cell material may occur. Control binding experiments with various concentrations of drug in the absence of protein will indicate the maximum extent of such non-specific adsorption. However correction for such losses can also be made by measurement of drug concentration in both protein and buffer compartments and calculation of the percentage recovery.
Volume changes due to osmosis could be relatively easily assessd with the conventional bag and beaker system but this is not so easy with small cell systems, especially those of 200 μl capacity. One possibility is to measure total protein concentration before and after dialysis. Another method is to include an inert non-dialysable polymer such as dextran or a polyethylene glycol derivative in the buffer compartment to prevent osmosis. Polyethylene glycol 6000 ($0.5\%\frac{w}{v}$) in the buffer compartment will abolish the osmotic effect of whole plasma. In practice this may be unnecessary because the binding of salicylic acid, a drug with binding characteristics relatively sensitive to protein concentration, was unaffected by osmosis (Bowmer & Lindup, unpublished results).

Ultrafiltration

This technique is in principle similar to equilibrium dialysis. A single solution of drug in plasma or serum is filtered through a semi-permeable membrane to separate a small volume of protein-free phase in which the concentration of unbound drug can be measured. Ultrafiltration frequently employs the same type of membrane as dialysis but must be supported to withstand the filtration pressure which is provided either by centrifugal force in a centrifuge ($\sim$ 1000 g) or by gas pressure. The volume of ultrafiltrate should not generally exceed 10% of the total sample volume to prevent an undue increase in concentration of the protein and hence any change in binding. Care must therefore be taken to avoid errors from dilution of the ultrafiltrate by residual moisture left from preparation of the membrane. This may mean discarding the first portion of ultrafiltrate which will also help to minimise errors from membrane binding. The possible sieve effect [22] has been investigated little so far but could be a serious source of error which leads to an overestimate of the binding of drugs of high molecular weight. The sensitivity of the analytical method may be a severe limitation to this technique with a highly bound drug.

Loss of dissolved carbon dioxide increases the pH of plasma but Toribara *et al* [31] devised a closed system for use in a centrifuge. It is difficult to carry out ultrafiltration at 37° by centrifugation unless a good centrifuge is available. Campion and Olsen [8] have described an ultrafilitration device using gas pressure and various commercial devices are available (Amicon Corporation; Millipore Corp.). If pH and temperature are adequately controlled then ultrafiltration offers a relatively fast and simple way to measure binding under physiological conditions. The hydrostatic pressures employed are usually comparable to renal filtration pressure [12].

Ultracentrifugation

This method involves application of a high centrifugal force (100000 g or more) to a drug-protein solution for a prolonged period, say 15 hours. The binding of fenoprofen has been studied by this method for example [28]. The protein sediments to the bottom of the tube, no membrane is required and the unbound drug concentration in the protein-free supernatant is measured. Problems connected with the use of a membrane are avoided and there is no change in concentration of either total drug or total protein.
However despite the superficial attractiveness of this method there are a number of drawbacks (Table 1) which have yet to be thoroughly investigated. The plasma protein(s) are concentrated at the bottom of the tube but the inherent assumption that binding constants are independent of protein concentration is not warranted for all drugs [5]. A lipid rich layer may be present on top of a plasma sample after centrifugation and this can cause sampling difficulties. Drug molecules will be sedimented to various extents, depending or their shape and size, by the high g-force used [22]. Ultracentrifugation will therefore tend to overestimate binding unless the results are corrected for sedimentation of drug in a control sample. However it is difficult to constitute such a control solution which must contain inert macromolecules of a similiar shape and size to plasma proteins and also have a similar viscosity to plasma.

Gel Filtration

The original approach, sometimes called the "zonal" method, involved separation of the drug-protein mixture into two zones, one containing unbound drug, the other containing protein and protein-bound drug [17]. This method tends to underestimate binding because bound drug dissociates from the drug-protein complex during migration through the column. The method of Hummel & Dreyer [19] and the 'frontal analysis' method [9] are two ways of circumventing this problem. Gel filtration avoids membrane-related problems and so may be particularly useful for the investigation of drugs of higher molecular weight. It can also be used to assess the relative contribution of various plasma proteins to the overall extent of drug binding. Dextran gels have also been used in a batch method [26] and this avoids the need to prepare columns.

Indirect methods

Ideally it would be useful to estimate the unbound fraction without having to use a separation technique. This could have application for the routine monitoring of patients, particularly where the fluid to be analysed can be obtained non-invasively.

Salivary drug concentration

A number of drugs appear in saliva at a concentration corresponding to that of the unbound unionized concentration in plasma. Therefore measurement of salivary drug concentration should provide, after correction for any ionisation, an estimate of the unbound fraction *in vivo*. The saliva/plasma ratio of aminopyrine, antipyrine, carbamazepine, digoxin, phenacetin, phenytoin, primidone

and theophylline are reasonably similar to their respective unbound fractions in plasma [10, 18]. Thus the salivary concentrations of these drugs provide an estimate of the unbound fraction in plasma.
Attempts to correlate salivary drug concentration with total and unbound drug concentrations in plasma have shown considerable variation and this may be caused by the method used to collect saliva, the nature and volume of the fraction studied and also the method used to measure plasma protein binding. Parotid saliva has been suggested as the best predictor of the concentration of phenytoin in serum ultrafiltrate [1] and more detailed investigations of this sort are required to validate the technique.

Blood: plasma ratio

The uptake of several drugs such as diazepam, pentobarbital and phenytoin into erythroytes is a function of the unbound drug concentration [3, 14, 21]. Therefore measurement of either the (blood)/(plasma) or (erythrocyte)/(plasma) drug concentration ratios may offer a rapid and simple method to estimate the unbound drug concentration in a blood sample. Only phenytoin has been studied in any detail but the results look promising [21].

Miscellaneous

Some drugs may be present in various body fluids, such as cerebrospinal fluid, semen, synovial fluid and tears at approximately the unbound concentration in plasma. This feature may be exploitable in certain circumstances.

Graphical analysis of results

Graphical procedures are commonly used for analyses of binding data to obtain the apparent association constant (*k*) and the number of binding sites (*n*). The conventional procedures (see [11]) such as the double-reciprocal and Scatchard plots have several disadvantages including the amount of calculation required. The direct linear plot [15] was developed for use in enzyme kinetics but can be applied to steroid [35] or drug [7] binding data which are linear. The method is directly analogous to that of Eisenthal & Cornish-Bowden [15] except that concentrations of bound and unbound drug are plotted as ordinate and abscissa respectively. This plot offers a non-parametric approach to the calculation of binding constants and has several advantages over other methods: it is simple to draw, no calculations are involved and the binding constants are read directly off the graph. However in many cases the Scatchard plot may be a better way to display results for publication.

Summary

Equilibrium dialysis with the multiple cell system is a relatively rapid way of simultaneously measuring the plasma protein binding of up to 20 samples. However this is still not satisfactory on a routine basis and the measurement of either salivary drug concentration or the blood/plasma ratio are possibly more convenient ways to assess binding *in vivo*. The direct linear plot is recommended as a simple graphical procedure for the calculation of binding constants from linear data.

References

[1] Anavekar, S. N., Saunders, R. H., Wardell, W. M., Shoulson, I., Emmings, F. G., Cook, C. E., Gringeri, A. J.: Parotid and whole saliva in the prediction of serum total and free phenytoin concentrations.—Clin. Pharmacol. Ther. 24, 629—637 (1978).

[2] Borgå, O., Piafsky, K. M., Nilsen, O. G.: Plasma protein binding of basic drugs. 1. Selective displacement from α_1-acid glycoprotein by tris (2-butoxyethyl) phosphate.—Clin. Pharmacol.-Ther. 22, 539—544 (1977).

[3] Borondy, P., Dill, W. A., Chang, T., Buchanan, R. A., Glazko, A. J.: Effect of protein binding on the distribution of 5,5'-diphenylhydantoin between plasma and red cells.—Ann. N. Y. Acad. Sci. 226, 82—87 (1973).

[4] Bowmer, C. J., Lindup, W. E.: Binding of phenytoin, L-tryptophan and o-methyl red to albumin. Unexpected effect of albumin concentration on the binding of phenytoin and L-tryptophan.—Biochem. Pharmacol. 27, 937—942 (1978a).

[5] Bowmer, C. J., Lindup, W. E.: Scatchard plots with a positive slope and role of albumin concentration.—J. Pharm. Sci. 67, 1193—1195 (1978b).

[6] Bowmer, C. J., Lindup, W. E.: Decreased binding of drugs to plasma proteins from rats with acute renal failure: effects of ureter ligation and intramuscular injection of glycerol.—Brit. J. Pharmacol. 66, 275—281 (1979a).

[7] Bowmer, C. J., Lindup, W. E.: Investigation of the drug binding defect in plasma from rats with glycerol-induced acute renal failure.—J. Pharmacol Exp. Ther. (1979b) in press.

[8] Campion, D. S., Olsen, R.: Measurement of drug displacement by continuous ultrafiltration.—J. Pharm. Sci. 63, 249—252 (1974).

[9] Cooper, P. F., Wood, G. C.: Protein-binding of small molecules: new gell filtration method.—J. Pharm. Pharmac. 20, 150S—156S (1968).

[10] Danhof, M., Breimer, D. D.: Therapeutic drug monitoring in saliva.—Clin. Pharmacokin. 3, 39—57 (1978).

[11] Davison, C.: Protein binding *in* Fundamentals of Drug Metabolism and Drug Disposition (Eds: B.N. La Du, H. G. Mandel, E. L. Way), 63—75 (1971), Williams & Wilkins, Baltimore.

[12] Dixon, P. F., Booth, M., Butler, J.: *in* Hormones in Blood (Eds: C. H. Gray, A. L. Bacharach) 2, 305—389 (1967), Academic Press, London.

[13] Editorial: Drug binding to α_1 acid glycoprotein—clinically important? Lancet, 1, 368 (1979).

[14] Ehrnebo, M., Odar-Cederlöf, 1.: Binding of amobarbital, pentobarbital and diphenylhydantoin to blood cells and plasma protein in healthy volunteers and uraemic patients—Europ. J. Clin. Pharmacol. 8, 445—453 (1975).

[15] Eisenthal, R., Cornish-Bowden, A.: The direct linear plot. A new graphical procedure for estimating enzyme kinetic parameters.—Biochem. J. 139, 715—720 (1974).

[16] Gillette, J. R.: Overview of drug-protein binding.—Ann. N. Y. Acad. Sci. 226, 6—17 (1973).

[17] Hardy, T. L., Mansford, K. R. L.: Gel filtration as a method of studying drug protein binding.—Biochem. J. 83, 34P (1962).

[18] Horning, M. G., Brown, L., Nowlin, J., Lertratanangkoon, K., Kellaway, P., Zion, T. E.: Use of saliva in therapeutic drug monitoring.—Clin. Chem. 23, 157—164 (1977).

[19] Hummel, J. P., Dreyer, W. J.: Measurement of protein-binding phenomena by gel filtration.—Biochim. Biophys. Acta 63, 530—532 (1962).

[20] Klotz, I. M.: Physicochemical aspects of drug-protein interactions: a general perspective.—Ann. N. Y. Acad. Sci. 226, 18—35 (1973).

[21] Kurata, D., Wilkinson, G. R.: Erythrocyte uptake and plasma binding of diphenylhydantoin.—Clin. Pharmacol. Ther. 16, 355—362 (1974).

[22] Kurz, H., Trunk, H., Weitz, B.: Evaluation of methods to determine protein-binding of drugs. Equilibrium dialysis, ultrafiltration, ultracentrifugation, gel filtration.—Arzneim.-Forsch. 27, 1373—1380 (1977).

[23] Levy, G.: Effect of plasma protein binding of drugs on duration and intensity of pharmacological activity.—J. Pharm. Sci. 65, 1264—1265 (1976).

[24] Lindup, W. E.: Drug-albumin binding.—Biochem. Soc. Trans. 3, 635—640 (1975).

[25] Parke, D. V., Lindup, W. E.: Quantitative and qualitative aspects of the plasma protein binding of carbenoxolone, an ulcer-healing drug.—Ann. N. Y. Acad. Sci. 226, 200—213 (1973).

[26] Pearlman, W. H., Crépy, O.: Steroid-protein interaction with particular reference to testosterone binding by human serum.—J. Biol. Chem. 242, 182—189 (1967).

[27] Reidenberg, M. M.: The binding of drugs to plasma proteins and interpretation of measurements of plasma concentrations of drugs in patients with poor renal function.—Amer. J. Med. 62, 466—470 (1977).

[28] Rubin, A., Warrick, P., Wolen, R. L., Chernish, S. M., Ridolfo, A. S., Gruber, C. M.: Physiological disposition of fenoprofen in man. III. Metabolism and protein binding of fenoprofen.—J. Pharmacol. Exp. Ther. 183, 449—457 (1972).

[29] Scatchard, G.: The attractions of proteins for small molecules and ions.—Ann. N. Y. Acad. Sci. 51, 660—672 (1949).

[30] Scholtan, W.: Über die Bindung der Langzeitsulfonamide an die Serumeiweißkörper.—Makromol. Chem. 54, 24—59 (1962).

[31] Toribara, T. Y., Terepka, A. R., Dewey, P. A.: The ultrafiltrable calcium of human serum. I. Ultrafiltration methods and normal values.—J. Clin. Invest. 36, 738—748 (1957).

[32] Weder, H. J., Bickel, M. H.: Interactions of drugs with proteins II: Experimental methods, treatment of experimental data, and thermodynamics of binding reactions of thymoleptic drugs and model dyes.—J. Pharm. Sci. 59, 1563—1569 (1970).

[33] Wilkinson, G. R., Shand, D. G.: A physiological approach to hepatic drug clearance.—Clin. Pharmacol. Ther. 18, 377—390 (1975).

[34] Wood, M., Shand, D. G., Wood, A. J. J.: Altered drug binding due to these use of indwelling heparinized cannulas (heparin lock) for sampling.—Clin. Pharmacol. Ther. 25, 103—107 (1979).

[35] Woosley, J. T., Muldoon, T. G.: Comparison of the accuracy of the Scatchard, Lineweaver-Burk and direct linear plots for the analysis of steroid-protein interactions.—J. Steroid Biochem. 8, 625—629 (1977).

Chapter 10

New analytical and diagnostic methods

Analytical reliability of methods to determine theophylline in serum or plasma

K. Borner[1], A. H. Staib[2], D. Schuppan[2], K. H. Molz[2], R. Lissner[2], and J. Lichey[3]
1 Institut für Klinische Chemie und Klinische Biochemie der Freien Universität Berlin
2 Klinikum der Universität Frankfurt, Zentrum der Pharmakologie,
Abteilung Klinische Pharmakologie, Frankfurt/Main
3 Medizinische Klinik und Poliklinik, Klinikum Steglitz der Freien Universität Berlin

Introduction

Theophylline is frequently used in patients with acute or chronic reversible airway disease. Its analysis in serum or plasma is required both for pharmacological studies and the individual control of drug therapy. Therapeutic drug monitoring is necessary because of wide individual variation of the liver capacity to metabolize the drug under various physiologic or pathologic circumstances. Five basic methods are recommended for the analysis of theophylline in serum or plasma, most of them in many variants:

1. Extraction and UV-spectrophotometry (UV) [6, 18, 19]
2. Radioimmunoassay (RIA) [2, 11)
3. High pressure liquid chromatography (HPLC) [3, 10, 13, 14, 22, 23, 24]
4. Homogeneous enzymeimmunoassay (EIA, EMIT®) [4, 5, 8, 12]
5. Gaschromatography (GC) [7, 9, 15, 16, 20, 21]

We evaluated the methods 1—4 with regard to analytical reliability, reagent cost and practicability.

Materials and Methods

Materials: Analytical grade chemicals were obtained from E. Merck (Darmstadt, Germany), anhydrous theophylline from Sigma (München, Germany).

Methods and Instruments

1. Extraction and UV-Spectroscopy according to Schwerdtner [19] using a Zeiss DMR 21 recording spectrophotometer.
2. High pressure liquid chromatography [14] using a Hewlett-Packard LC model 1082 A with a Lichrosorb RP 8 column and a fixed wavelength detector.
3. Radioimmunoassay using the Gamma Dab [125]theophylline kit of Clinical Assays (Cambridge,

Ma.). Counting was performed with a Packard model 5130 gamma counter.
4. The homogeneous enzyme immunoassay (EMIT®) was performed with kits obtained from Syva/Palo Alto through Merck/Darmstadt. A line spectrophotometer (Eppendorf M 1001) with an attached recorder was used for the measurements.
Clinical specimens were obtained from adult patients with chronic respiratory disease of the Medical Department of the Klinikum Steglitz, Berlin, and from children treated for acute bronchial asthma at the Pediatric Department of the Frankfurt University Clinic.
Common statistical procedures were performed according to a standard text book [17] and bivariate regression analysis according to a previous publication [1].

Results

Detection limits: All methods can measure theophylline concentrations down to 2—2.5 mg/l without modification. But whereas HPLC, RIA and EIA require sample volumes of 10—25 µl per measurement the UV-method needs at least 500 µl of sample. Thus it is much less sensitive and is unsuitable for pediatric specimens. Since for pharmacokinetic studies even lower concentrations must be measurable, enrichment of the analyte by extraction and concentration was performed thereby gaining a tenfold increase in sensitivity of the RIA and HPLC.

Accuracy and precision: The recovery of theophylline added in concentrations from 5 to 40 mg/l to bovine serum and charcoal treated human serum was 94.3—102.6% (HPLC), 95.0—103.6% (RIA) and 91.2—105.6% (EMIT). Table 1 shows results obtained with control sera. Deviations from the stated value ranged maximally from −6.8% to +15.3%. Between-batch precision is about 6% (CV)

Material	Number of Samples	Concentration assigned mg/l	Concentration found mg/l	bias %	CV day-to-day %
UV-Method					
Pooled sera + theophylline	12	15	15.4	+ 2.5	3.9
Control serum (Syva)	10	15	17.3	+ 15.3	5.5
HPLC					
Control serum (Syva)	3	15	14.9	− 1.0	–
RIA					
Control serum (Clin. Assays)	12	15	14.8	− 1.2	5.9
Control serum (Clin. Assays)	8	35	32.6	− 6.8	6.0
EIA (EMIT®)					
Control serum (Syva)1)	32	15	16.5	+ 10.0	11.4
Control serum (Syva)2)	15	15	16.7	+ 11.0	9.1

Table 1: Precision and Accuracy Studies

1) lot G 03; 2) lot H 03

for UV, HPLC and RIA at c = 15 mg/l whereas for the EMIT-method precision appears to be somewhat less i. e. with coefficients of variation between 9% and 11%.

Interferences: The UV-method is severely impaired by concomitant drug therapy. In 47 out of 98 samples from in-patients UV-spectra indicated an interfering substance, thus making an analysis of theophylline impossible. Attempts to identify interfering substances by the patients drug history and by running spectra of implicated substances led to the identification of sulfamethoxazole, noraminopyrinemethanesulfonate, S-carboxymethylcysteine and phenylbutazone in a few cases, the remainder being unexplained. We have no evidence for similar interferences in enzyme immunoassays, but in HPLC an occasional interference in the following chromatogram may occur, if injections are made too closely.

Methods comparison: Comparing analytical data obtained from the same clinical specimens by different methods yielded the following results:
HPLC and EMIT yield the best correlation (Figure 1).
The RIA in contrast shows a constant error compared with the enzyme immunoassay and—in addition—a small but definitive number of outliers [5 out 91] (Figure 2). Furthermore, in pharmacokinetic studies, RIA-values were grossly different from results obtained using HPLC and EMIT.

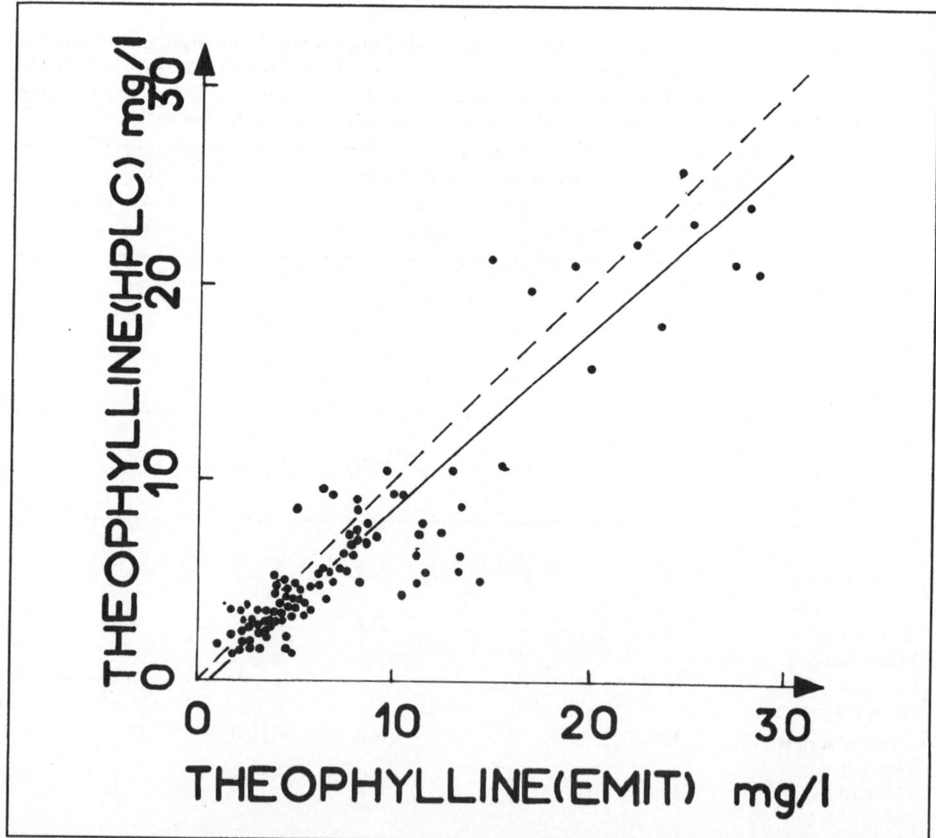

Figure 1: Comparison of results of 106 samples assayed by enzyme immunoassay (EMIT) and high pressure liquid chromatography (dashed line $y = x$; $\bar{x} = 7.74$ mg/l; $\bar{y} = 6.52$ mg/l; $\check{C}_{HPLC} = 0.907 \times C_{EMIT} - 0.50$ mg/l; $r = 0.951$; $p < 0.01$)

Practicability and cost: Each of the methods studied requires skilful personnel. Only the immunological methods (RIA, EIA) are suitable for handling large batches of samples either in manual or partly mechanized procedures. The homogeneous enzyme immunoassay only, can be totally automated [14]. The obvious advantage of the EIA is the avoidance of handling radioactive materials.
The cost for suitable measuring instruments is substantial for each of the 4 methods tested. Prices of reagents per test (!) are estimated to be below 1 DM for the UV-method and HPLC and around 8 DM for the immune assays. Since each series of measurements comprises a fixed number of standards and controls, the price per analysis strongly depends upon the batch size.

Conclusions

1. The classical spectrophotometric UV-method is outdated for therapeutic drug monitoring for several reasons (sample size, interferences, practicability).
2. Enzyme immunoassay and radioimmunoassay are equally suited for therapeutic drug monitoring. The choice of test depends largely upon available equipment and experience of personnel. The cost of reagents and equipment is substantial. The particular radioimmunoassay that we tested appears to be less reliable with regard to specificity than the enzyme immunoassay.
3. High pressure liquid chromatography appears to be the most promising candidate for a reference

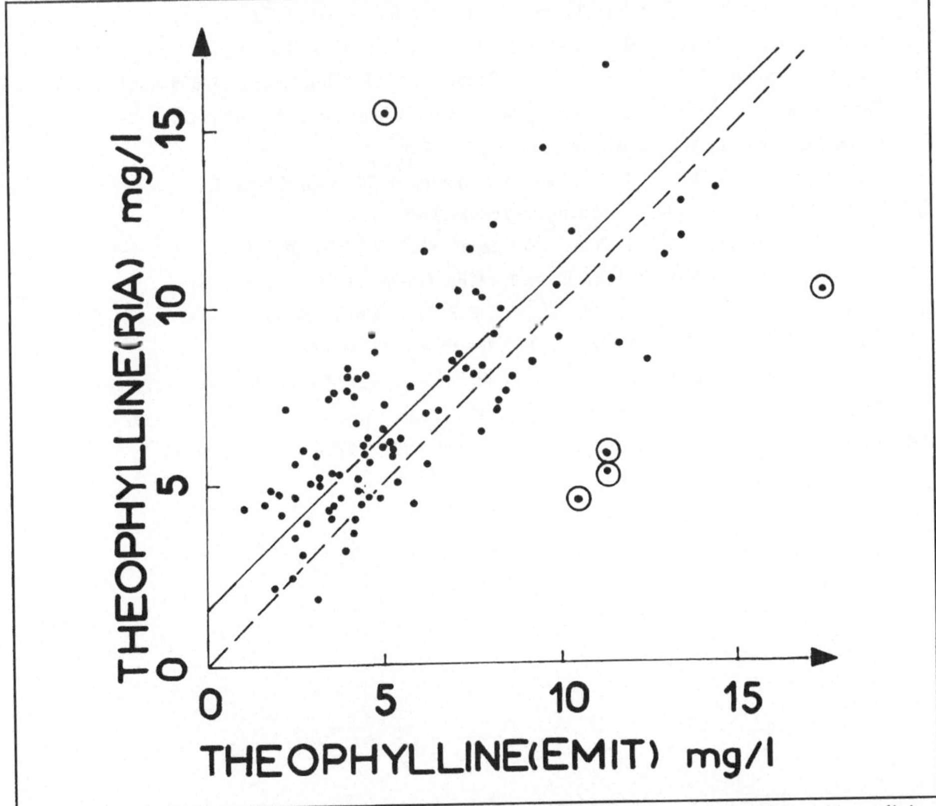

Figure 2: Comparison of results of 86 samples assayed by enzyme immunoassay (EMIT) and by radioimmunoassay. The encircled 5 outliers are excluded from calculations. ($\bar{x}$ = 5.74 mg/l; $\bar{y}$ = 7.02 mg/l; $\tilde{C}_{RIA} = 0.951 \times C_{EMIT} + 1.57$ mg/l; $r = 0.788$; $p < 0.01$)

method. It is less suited to process large batches of samples, and it is occasionally susceptible to interferences by concomitant drug therapy.

References

[1] Averdunk, R., Borner, K.: Z. Kin. Chem. Klin. Biochem. *8*, 263—268 (1970)

[2] Cook, C. E., Twine, M. E., Myers, M., Amerson, E., Kepler, J. A., Tegler, G. F.: Res. Comm. Chem. Path. Pharm. *13*, 497—505 (1976)

[3] Evenson, M. A., Warren, B. L.: Clin. Chem. *22*, 851—855 (1976)

[4] Gushaw, J. B., HU, M. W., Singh, P., Miller, J. G., Schneider, R. S.: Clin. Chem. *23*, 1144 (1977)

[5] Ishizaki, T., Watanabe, M., Morishita, N.: Br. J. Clin. Pharmac. *7*, 333—341 (1979)

[6] Jatlow, P.: Clin. Chem. *21*, 1518—1520 (1975)

[7] Johnson, G. F., Dechtiaruk, W. A., Solomon, H. M.: Clin. Chem. *21*, 144—147 (1975)

[8] Koup, J. R., Brodsky, B.: Amer. Rev. Resp. Dis. *117*, 1135—1138 (1978)

[9] Least, C. J., Johnson, G. F., Solomon, H. M.: Clin. Chem. *22*, 765—768 (1976)

[10] Manion, C. V., Shoeman, D. W., Azarnoff, D. L.: J. Chromatogr. *101*, 169—174 (1974)

[11] Neese, A. L., Soyka, L. F.: Clin. Pharmacol. Ther. *21*, 631—641 (1977)

[12] Oellerich, M., Sybrecht, G. W., Haeckel, R.: J. Clin. Chem. Clin. Biochem. *17*, 299—302 (1979)

[13] Orcut, J. J., Kozak, P. P., Gillman, Sh. A., Cummins, L. H.: Clin. Chem. *23*, 599—601 (1977)

[14] Peng, G. W., Gadallah, M. A. F., Chiou, W. T.: Clin. Chem. *24*, 357—360 (1978)

[15] Perrier, D., Lear, E.: Clin. Chem. *22*, 898—900 (1976)

[16] Reid, R., Fareed, J., Bermes, E. W., Ivery, D., Messmore, H.: Clin. Chem. *22*, 1166 (1976)

[17] Sachs, L.: Angewandte Statistik. Springer-Verlag, Berlin, 1974

[18] Schack, J. A., Waxler, S. H.: J. Pharmacol. Exper. Ther. *97*, 283—291 (1949)

[19] Schwerdtner, H. A., Wallace, J. E., Blum, K.: Clin. Chem. *24*, 360—361 (1978)

[20] Schwerdtner, H. A., Ludden, T. M., Wallace, J. E.: Clin. Chem. *22*, 1167 (1976)

[21] Sheehan, M., Hertel, R. H., Kelly, Ch. T.: Clin. Chem. *23*, 64—68 (1977)

[22] Sitar, D. S., Piafsky, K. M., Ragno, R. E., Ogilvie, R. I.: Clin. Chem. *21*, 1774—1776 (1975)

[23] Thompson, J. D., Nagasawa, H. T., Jenne, J. W.: J. Lab. Clin. Med. *84*, 584—593 (1974)

[24] Weinberger, M., Chidsey, Ch.: Clin. Chem. *21*, 834—837 (1975)

Evaluation of clonidine plasma levels in man using a highly sensitive radioimmunoassay

D. Arndts, H. Stähle, C. J. Struck
C. H. Boehringer Sohn, P.O.B. 200, D-6507 Ingelheim am Rhein, FRG

Introduction

Within the past few years the need for safe, sensitive, and specific drug determination methods has become increasingly necessary.
Strict safety regulations in many countries have made the use of radioisotopes in clinical pharmacological studies almost impossible. Therefore GC, GC/MS, HPLC, and RIA became more important as techniques for the evaluation of pharmacokinetic properties of various drugs.
For the determination of clonidine, a highly active antihypertensive drug [1, 2], therapeutically applied in doses of 75—300 µg (yielding plasma-levels of approx 0.6—2.5 ng/ml), several sensitive and specific, yet very time-consuming, gas-chromatographic or GC/MS techniques have been developed [3, 4]
Like another group [5, 6] we have recently introduced a highly sensitive (0.1 ng/ml) and specific radioimmunoassay for clonidine [7] which enabled us to precisely measure this drug even in large numbers of samples within reasonable time. Since then our assay system has been further improved, mainly by using an iodinized clonidine derivative as tracer ligand.

Materials and Methods

Production of clonidine-antibodies. For antibody production a derivative of clonidine, 4-carboxy-clonidine (code name St 1984) was used as hapten. Synthesis (Figure 1) and analysis of this compound have been described in detail recently [7]. The product of a coupling reaction between St 1984 and serum albumin was injected into rabbits as immunogen for raising antibodies against clonidine. Both the production and characterization of the resulting antiserum has also been extensively described elsewhere [7].

Preparation of iodinized tracer. A tyrosyl-methyl-ester-group (TME) was coupled to St 1984 by means of a carbodiimide-reaction (Figure 1). The coupling-product was then iodinized in a modified Greenwood-Hunter reaction using Chloramine-T as oxidant. (125-I)-labelled St 1984—TME (Figure 2; spec. act. more than 500 Ci/mMol) was subsequently purified using a Sephadex G-25-fine column (0.9 × 60 cm). The complete iodination and purification procedures will be discussed in detail in a further communication [8].

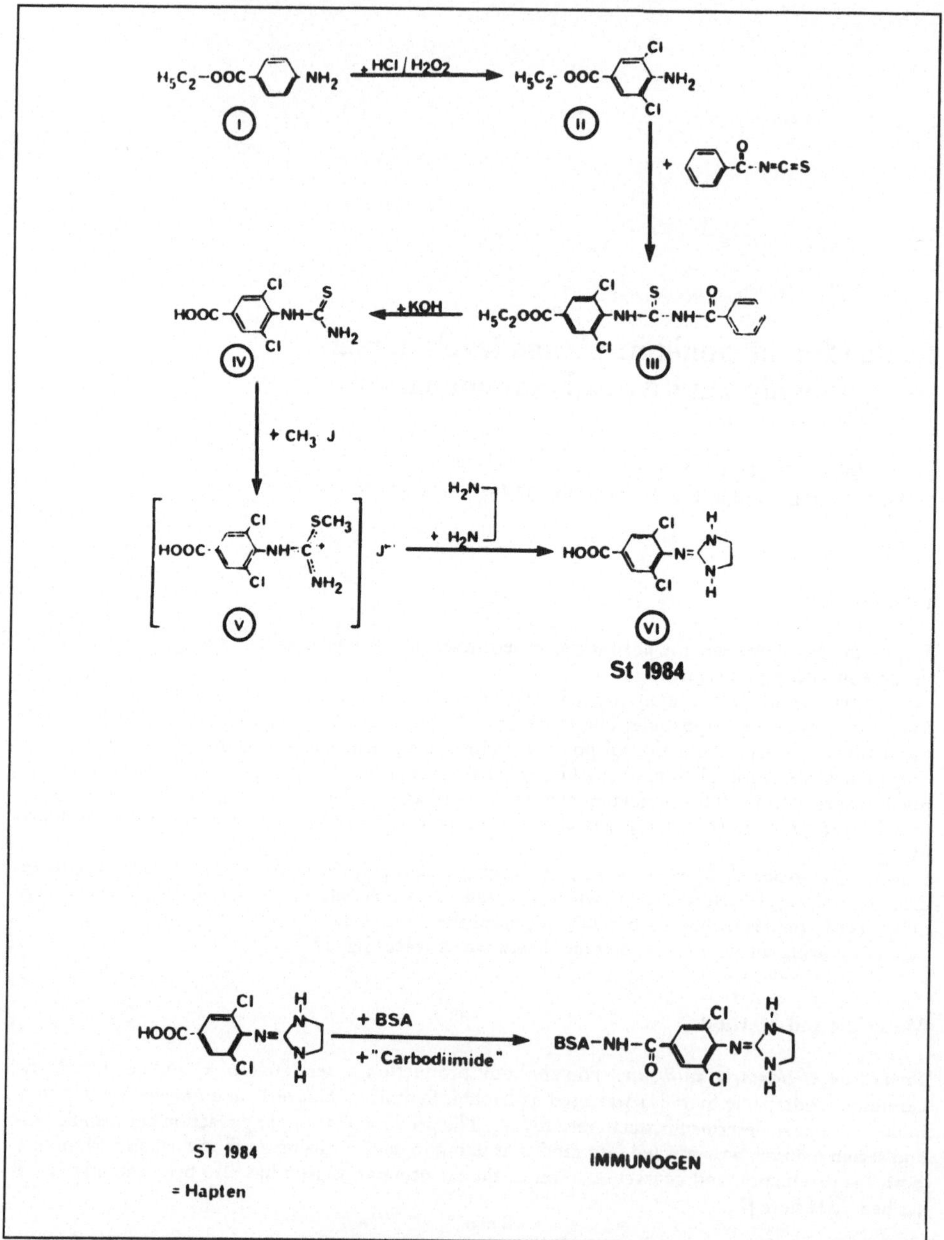

Figure 1: Synthesis of the hapten St 1984, and simplified scheme demonstrating the preparation of the immunogen used for clonidine antibody production.

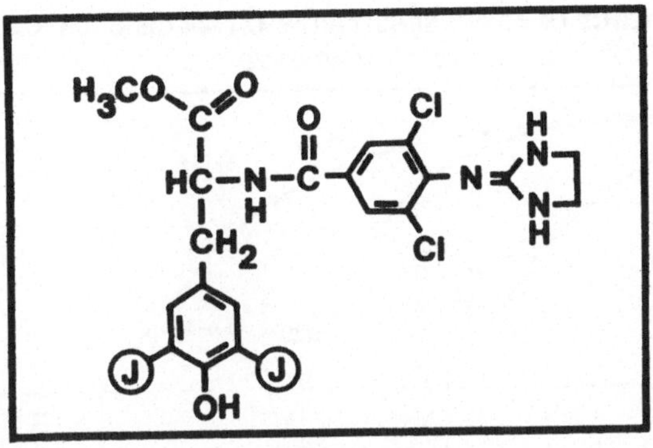

Figure 2: Structure of the radioactive tracer used in the clonidine-RIA. A previously synthesized TME-derivative of St 1984 has been iodinized in a modified Greenwood-Hunter-Reaction. The tracer was purified by chromatography on Sephadex® G-25-fine. The iodination resulted in a labelled product with a specific radioactivity of more than 500 Ci/mMol.

Drug application, blood sampling, and sample handling. In the clinical studies Catapresan®-tablets (clonidine 150 µg) or Catapresan-Perlongetten® (clonidine 250 µg) were given orally with 50 ml water to healthy male volunteers (72—80 kg) kept without food for 10 hours before and 3 hours after drug administration. Blood samples were taken from the cubital vein at different times after application. The blood was centrifuged for 5 min. at 3,000 × g to separate the plasma which was then stored at −20° C until assayed.

Clonidine-RIA. The assay mixture contained (in a total volume of 800 µl): 400 µl sodium phosphate buffer (10 mM, pH 7.4), 200 µl plasma sample (or clonidine standard dilution in normal human plasma), 100 µl (125-I)-St 1984-TME (5,000—10,000 cpm), and 100 µl of an antibody dilution (1:3,000 in normal human plasma). The assay mixture was incubated for a minimum period of 3 h, usually, however, overnight at 4° C. Following incubation the bound and free fractions of radioactivity were separated by addition of a charcoal suspension and subsequent centrifugation after another incubation period of 30 min. Bound radioactivity was measured in a gamma-spectrometer (BF Gammascint 5000).

RIA data processing. Raw data emerging from the gamma-counter (cpm) were processed off-line on a WANG 2200 VP computer using a specially designed program package which we developed to fit our particular requirements. To be processed in this routine, data may be entered either manually via the keyboard or automatically via punched tape. Values for the RIA standard curve are calculated by means of a spline function. A complete set of assay raw data, calculated values, a drawing of the standard curve, and readily identifyable final values for blood plasma clonidine concentrations in the sample are given as a hard-copy printout.

Results

Improvement of clonidine radioimmunoassay. The RIA-system for clonidine [7] using commercially prepared (3-H)-clonidine as tracer ligand (NEN, Dreieich, Germany; spec. act. 26.7 Ci/mMol) already showed obvious improvements in sensitivity (detection limit: 0.1 ng/ml) over a previously established assay using a tracer of lower specific radioactivity (1.6 Ci/mMol; Figure 3) where the detection limit was only 1 ng/ml. However, in clinical trials even higher sensitivity was required.
As shown in Figure 3 this requirement was matched by introducing an iodine-labeled tracer. Due to the increase in specific radioactivity the detection limit was lowered to 0.01 ng/ml. Furthermore, in

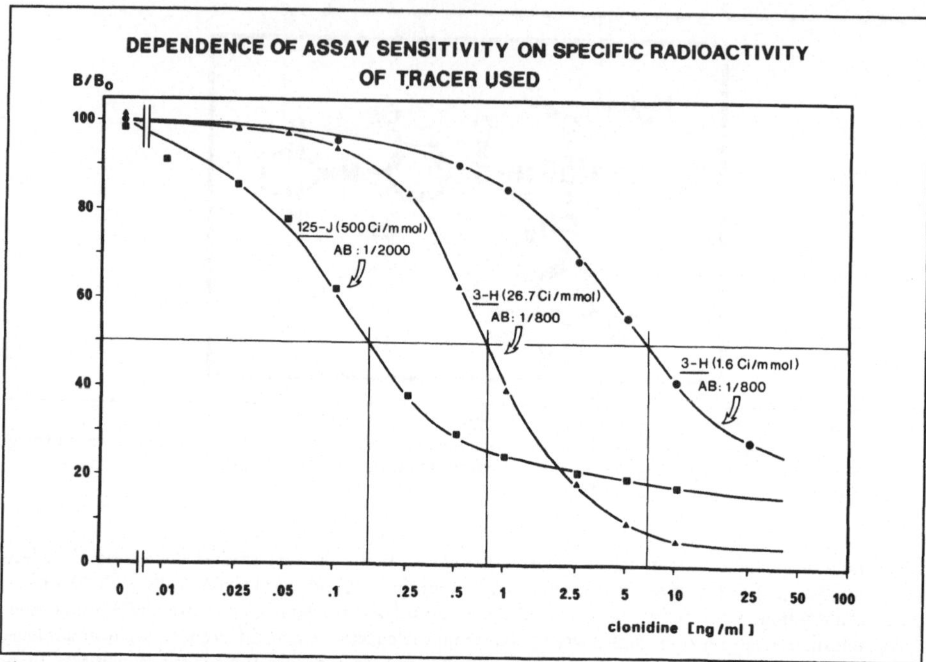

Figure 3: Dependence of RIA-sensitivity on the specific radioactivity of the tracer used. Two different (3-H)-labelled tracers and one (125-I)-labelled clonidine derivative have been used in the RIA system described in the text.

this assay system no other clonidine metabolites or physiologically occurring derivatives interfered significantly with the binding of clonidine to the antibody, except for 4-OH-clonidine (St 666, ref. 9), which showed a cross reactivity of 17% at 50% tracer binding.
The properties, structures, and codes for all substances examined for cross-reactivity are summarized in Figure 4; the corresponding displacement curves evaluated in a RIA-system using (3-H)-clonidine as tracer are given in Figure 5. Using (125-I)-clonidine in a similar experiment (Figure 6) the displacement curves for clonidine and St 666 were found to be clearly separated from each other. This implies that application of an iodine labelled tracer results not only in an increase in assay sensitivity but also in an improvement in the specificity of the clonidine-RIA.

Pharmacokinetic studies in man. In a single-dose experiment, 150 µg clonidine (1 tablet Catapresan®) was given to five healthy volunteers (Figure 7). The peak plasma concentration of 0.6 ng/ml clonidine was recorded 1.5 hours after drug administration. These findings are in good correlation with previous results in our laboratory (not published) and elsewhere [3].
A multiple application trial was performed by giving 250 µg clonidine as a sustained release formulation (1 capsule Catapresan-Perlongetten®/day) to six healthy volunteers over a period of four days (Figure 8). Six hours after application (8.00 a.m.) peak plasma levels for clonidine in 5 subjects were distributed over a range of 0.47 to 1.34 ng/ml. One person exhibited "excessive" 6 hour levels of 2.5 ng/ml during the first two days of the trial. These extraordinarily high blood levels were correlated with marked side effects. Therefore the experiment in that subject was stopped. The reasons for the occurence of such high blood levels is not known.
In the remaining five volunteers the distribution range for peak plasma concentrations narrowed during the course of the experiment whereas basal values measured in samples taken prior to medication each day showed some variability. No significant signs of accumulation phenomena could be observed in this 4 day trial.

No.	Compounds	Structure	Properties	References
1	ST 91	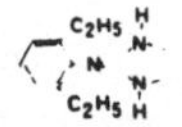	antiarrhythmic	W.HOEFKE et al. 1975 D.ARNDTS et al.1978
2	ST 155 Clonidine	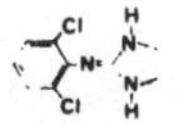	antihypertensive	W. KOBINGER et al. 1978
3	ST 567	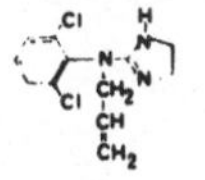	antiarrhythmic	H. STÄHLE et al.1974
4	ST 600	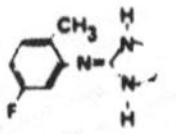	antihypertensive	H.STÄHLE et al. 1974
5	ST666	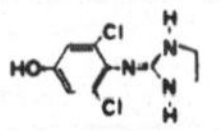	inactive metabolite from St 155	D. REHBINDER et al. 1969 S.DARDA et al. 1978
6	ST 1984	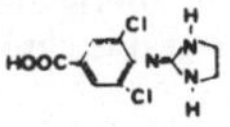	immunogen	unpublished
7	STH 2075	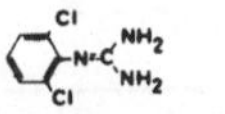	inactive metabolite from St 155	P.HODGES et al. 1976
8	STH 2130	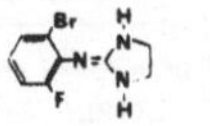	antihypertensive	H.STÄHLE et al.1978
9	STH 2221	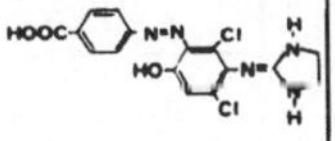	immunogen	B. JARROT et al.1977
10	STH 2236	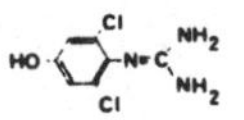	inactive metabolite from St 155	S.DARDA et al. 1978
11	STH 2245	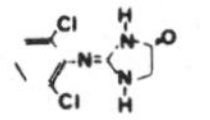	inactive metabolite from St 155	S.DARDA et al. 1978
12	Hoe 440 Tiamenidine	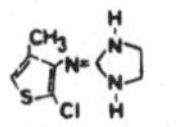	antihypertensive	F.KERSTING et al. 1973
13	STH 2329	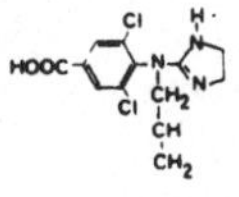	immunogen	unpublished

Figure 4: List of clonidine related compounds tested for cross-reactivity in the clonidine-RIA. The references given may be found in ref. 7.

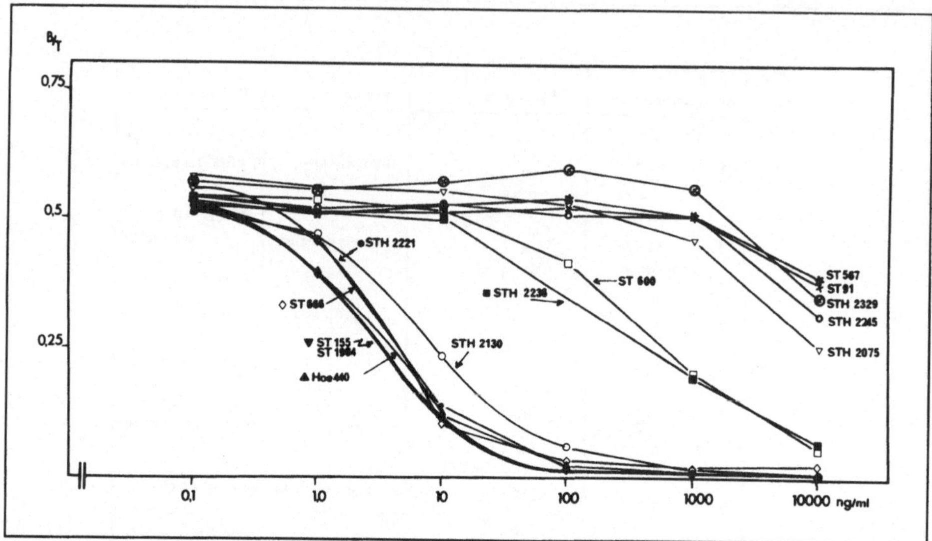

Figure 5: Cross-reactivity of clonidine metabolites and derivatives (listed in Figure 4) in an assay system using (3-H)-labelled tracer ligand. Assay conditions in this case are described in ref. 7.

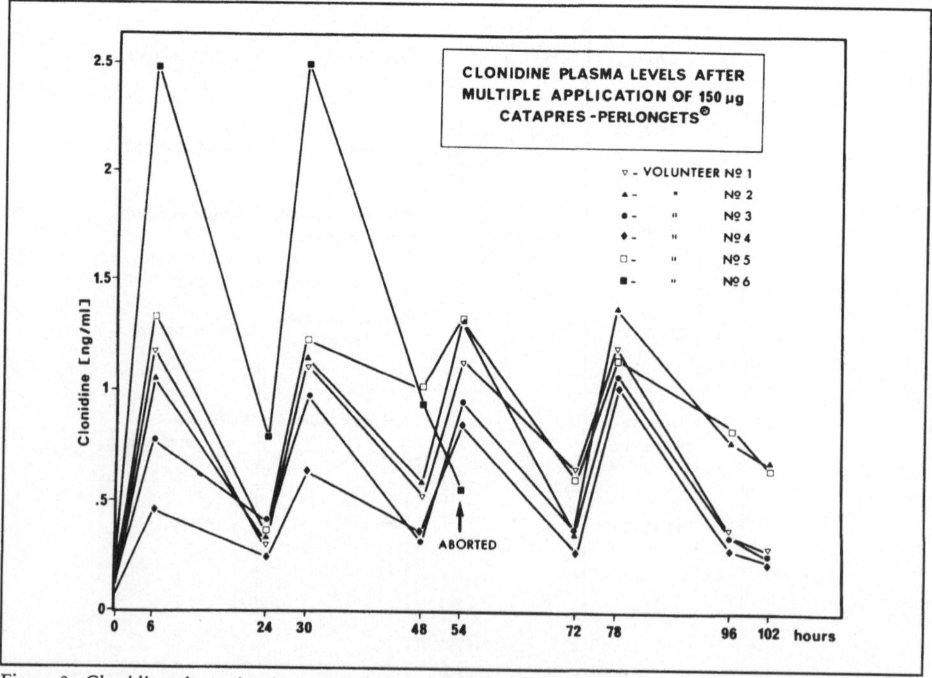

Figure 8: Clonidine plasma levels recorded after multiple application of a slow release formulation of clonidine (1 capsule Catapresan-Perlongetten®, 250 µg clonidine per day).

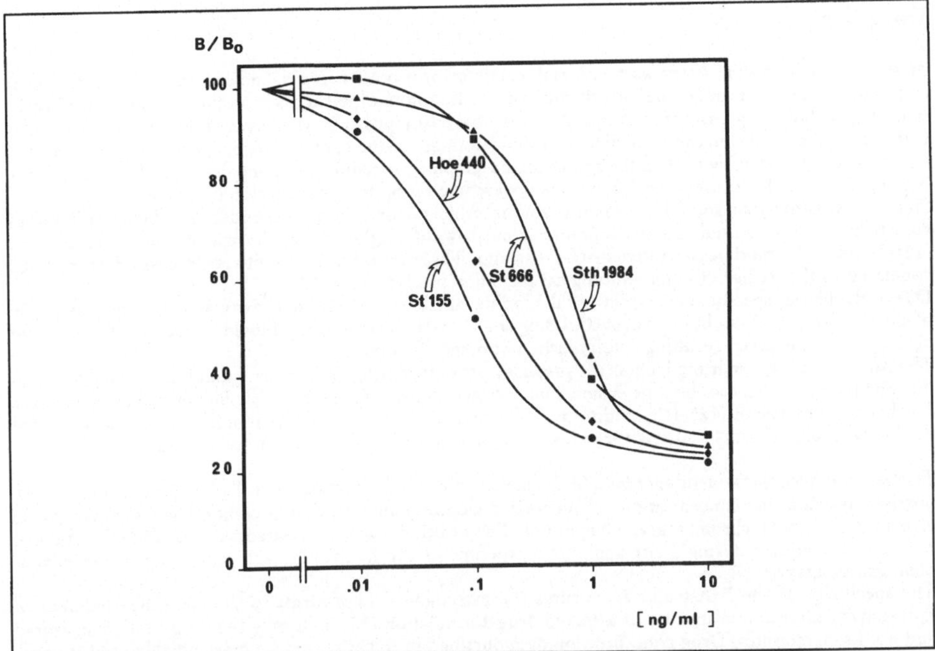

Figure 6: Cross-reactivity of clonidine related compounds evaluated in a RIA-system using (125-I)-labelled tracer.

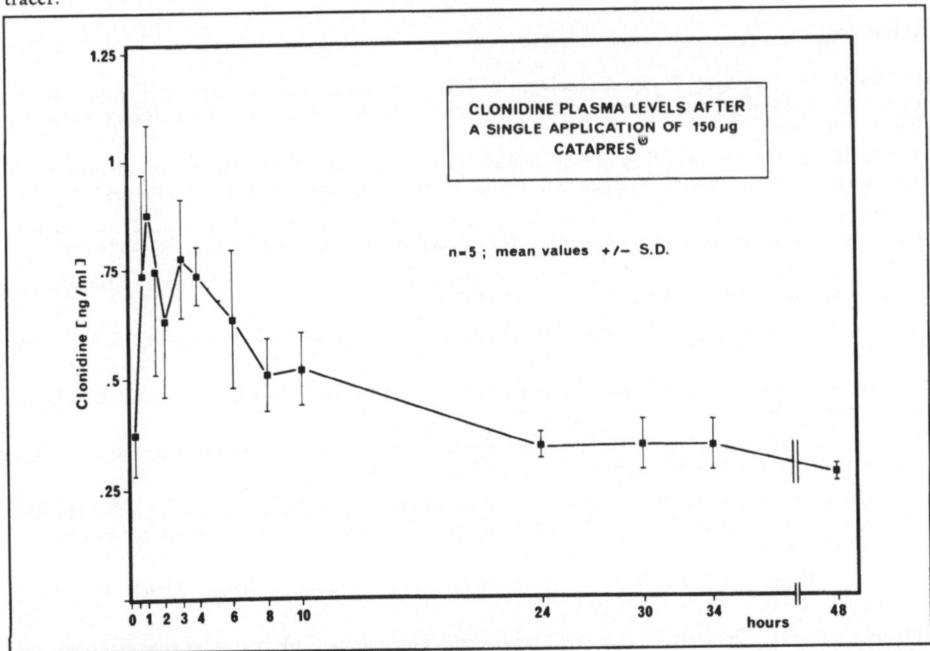

Figure 7: Clonidine plasma levels recorded at different times after single application of 150 µg clonidine (1 Catapresan® tablet).

Discussion

Methodology of clonidine determination. A major step towards precise, rapid, and reproducible measurement of clonidine was achieved by the introduction of a radioimmunological assay method. Thus, instead of 10 samples per day using gas-chromatography, it is now easily possible to analyse several hundred samples with high accuracy within the same time. The disadvantages of the former RIA-methods using tritium label i. e. slightly lower sensitivity than the gas-chromatographic procedures and impaired specificity due to the heterogeneity of the antisera used, have been overcome by optimizing the clonidine RIA.
Since the sensitivity of any RIA system, is among other factors, highly dependent on the specific radioactivity of the tracer used, the main improvement towards higher sensitivity was the introduction of a (125-I)-labelled clonidine derivative as tracer ligand. The increase in sensitivity is close to a factor of 100 compared to the earlier radioimmunological clonidine procedures.
Due to the higher specific radioactivity of the iodine labelled tracer the sensitivity as well as the specificity of the clonidine-RIA could be improved. Using the (125-I)-tracer a more diluted antibody solution could be applied in the assay, resulting in diminished non-specific binding.
The use of a gamma-emitting label made the assay procedure simpler in general and far less time consuming. Sample handling, too, became easier, since extraction procedures may now be omitted in most cases. Furthermore, by use of (125-I)-clonidine as RIA-tracer, (3-H)- und (14-C)-clonidine remain available for double label experiments and recovery-checks in purification and extraction procedures.

Evaluation of pharmacokinetic data by RIA. By means of the radioimmunological assay procedure it is now possible to determine concentrations of unlabelled clonidine in man during clinical trials with much less effort than e. g. with chromatographic methods. The health hazards associated with the administration of radioactive clonidine during pharmacokinetic experiments can be avoided and more samples per experiment can be assayed.
The specificity of the RIA-method reassures the investigator, in contrast to the mere measurement of radioactivity after administration of a spiked drug-formulation [10], that only the drug itself is measured and not its metabolites. Drug concentration data obtained in this way may be more reliably used for subsequent pharmacokinetic computations and simulations.

References

[1] Hoefke, W., Kobinger, W., Pharmakologische Wirkungen des 2-(2,6-Dichlorphenylamino)-2-imidazolidin-hydrochlorids, einer neuen antihypertensiven Substanz. Arzneim. Forsch. (Drug Res.) 16, 1038—1046 (1966)

[2] Schmitt, H., The pharmacology of clonidine and related products. In: Handbuch der experimentellen Pharmakologie. F. Gross, Ed., Springer Verl. Berlin, Heidelberg, New York, Vol 39, 299—396 (1977)

[3] Draffan, G. H., Clare, R. A., Murray, S., Bellward, G. D., Davies, D. S., Dollery, C. T., The determination of clonidine in human plasma. Adv. Mass spectromet. in Biochem. and Med. 2, 389—394 (1976)

[4] Edlund, P.O., Paalzow, L. K., Quantitative gas liquid chromatographic determination of clonidine in plasma. Acta pharmacol. et toxicol. 40, 145—152 (1977)

[5] Jarrot, B., Spector, S., Development of a radioimmunoassay for clonidine, Fed. Proc. 36, 3579 (Abstract) (1977)

[6] Jarrot, B., Spector, S., Disposition of clonidine in rats as determined by RIA, Pharmacol. Exp. Ther. 207, 195—202 (1978)

[7] Arndts, D., Stähle, H., Struck, C. J., A newly developed precise and sensitive radioimmunoassay for clonidine. Arzneim. Forsch. (Drug Res.) 29 (I), 3, 532—538 (1979)

[8] Arndts, D., Stähle, H., Struck, C. J., An improved radioimmunoassay for clonidine using iodine labelled tracer-ligand (Abstract) Int. Theor. and Pract. Course on Radioimmunoassay of Drugs and Hormones, Gardone (Italy) (1979).

[9] Darda, S., Förster, H.-J., Stähle, H., Metabolischer Abbau von Clonidin. Arzneim. Forsch. (Drug Res.) 28, 255—259 (1978)

[10] Rehbinder, D., Deckers, W., Untersuchungen zur Pharmakokinetik und zum Metabolismus des 2-(2,6-Dichlorphenylamino)-2-imidazolidin-hydrochlorid (St 155). Arzneim. Forsch. (Drug Res.) 19, 169—176 (1969)

Simultaneous determination of pyrimidines, purines, azapurines and their metabolites in man by HPLC

Karl Zech, Peter Arnold, Gerhard Ludwig
Byk Gulden Pharmaceuticals, Research Division, D-7750 Konstanz

Introduction:

The analysis of pyrimidine and purine derivatives and their biotransformation products is highly relevant from a clinical point of view.
This applies to:
A) Disorders of purine and pyrimidine metabolism (gout) and subsequent treatment with azapurine [1, 2].
B) Interindividual studies of bioavailability and biotransformation of theophylline [3, 4].

However, purines as well as pyrimidines are polar compounds and HPLC analysis of polar compounds is much more difficult than that of non- or moderately polar compounds. In addition, drug metabolism will normally lead to more hydrophilic compounds in the body. To date, ion exchange chromatography is usually used to analyze polar compounds, including purines and pyrimidines [5], but the unfavourable properties of the ion exchange materials does not permit efficient high-speed separations.
Ion-pair HPLC technique [6] using tetrabutylammonium hydroxide [7] as pairing ion can resolve this problem and will be described in this paper.

Materials and methods

a) Materials

The purines and pyrimidines and their derivatives were obtained from commercial sources (Serva, Heidelberg; Ferak, Berlin, FRG).
Acetonitrile (Lichrosolv®) was obtained from Merck, Darmstadt, FRG; tetrabutylammonium hydroxide from Fluka, Buchs, Switzerland.

b) Apparatus

A Hewlett-Packard (HP) 1084 B liquid chromatograph with HP 79875A UV detector with scanning equipment was employed in this study. Samples (10—30 μl of urine or 40—100 μl of serum) were injected by means of the HP autosampler.

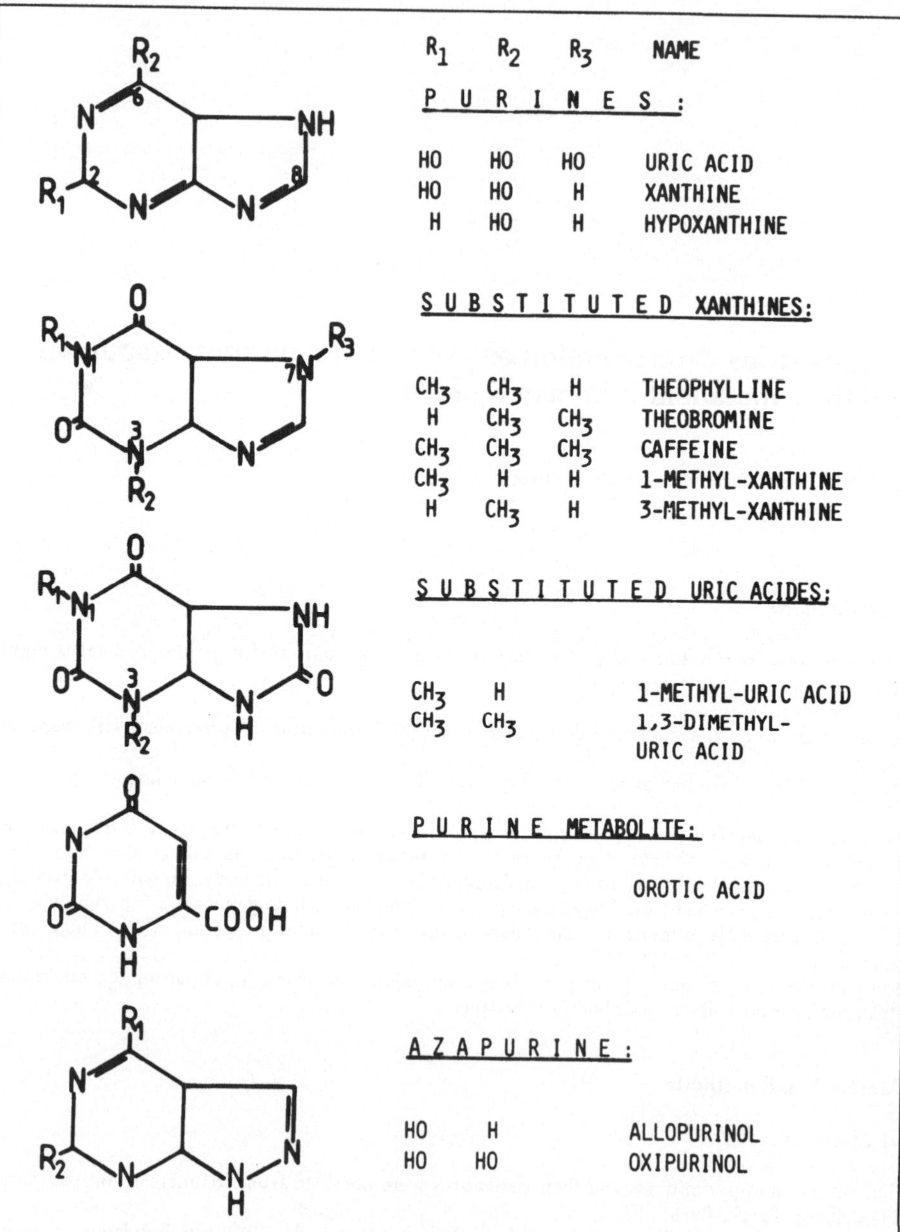

Figure 1: Compounds determined in this study.

A ready-to-use column 4.6 × 250 mm (Knauer, Berlin), filled with RP 18, 10 μ, was used for the chromatographic process.

c) Analytical procedures

Separation of the purines was achieved by means of ion-pair HPLC. Tetrabutylammonium hydroxide 10 mM was used as pairing ion in the mobile phase and the pH was adjusted to 8.0 with phosphoric acid.
All separations were performed in the isocratic mode after addition of 0.2% acetonitrile to the aqueous mobile phase for the determination of substituted xanthines, and 2.5% acetonitrile for the separation of the purines and azapurines.

d) Clean-up of samples for HPLC analysis

Urine:
An aliquot of a urine sample is adjusted to pH 8.0 and diluted with the eluent at a ratio of 1:2. Of this solution, a 10—50 μl aliquot is injected directly into the separation system.

Serum:
0.5 to 1.0 ml of a serum sample in an ultrafiltration tube is centrifuged for 20 min at 4000 rpm and a 40—100 μl aliquot of the obtained ultrafiltrate is injected directly.
The cone-shaped filter inserts used to obtain the ultrafiltrate are from Centriflo (type 2100 CF 50).

Results

Analysis of purines and azapurines

Serum:
Figure 2 shows the analysis of a serum sample after addition of hypoxanthine, xanthine, orotic acid, allopurinol and oxipurinol. The uric acid identified corresponds to endogenous serum uric acid, the only peak found during analysis of a blank sample at this detector setting.

Urine:
Figure 3 shows the analysis of a urine sample (pooled 24-hour urine) of a patient after administration of 300 mg allopurinol. Chromatographic conditions (isocratic mode) have been optimized so as to permit the determination of greater amounts of xanthine than hypoxanthine besides the above compounds. If desired, separation can be improved in the first portion of the chromatogram by slight reduction of the acetonitrile content of the mobile phase.
The investigated substances are normally identified on the basis of retention times by comparison with standards. In addition, the identity of small peaks in the chromatogram was confirmed by peak scanning during the chromatographic process.
Figure 4 shows the UV spectrum of the peak during urine analysis with a retention time of 11.63 min (see Figure 3). Its identification as oxipurinol on the basis of the found retention time is confirmed by the UV spectrum of this peak, as obtained during analysis of the urine sample.

Procedural comparisons of uric acid determination

To examine the clean-up of serum samples, serum uric acid from identical samples is determined separately by two enzymatic methods of analysis, (i. e. the uricase method [8]) with and without deproteinization of the serum samples.

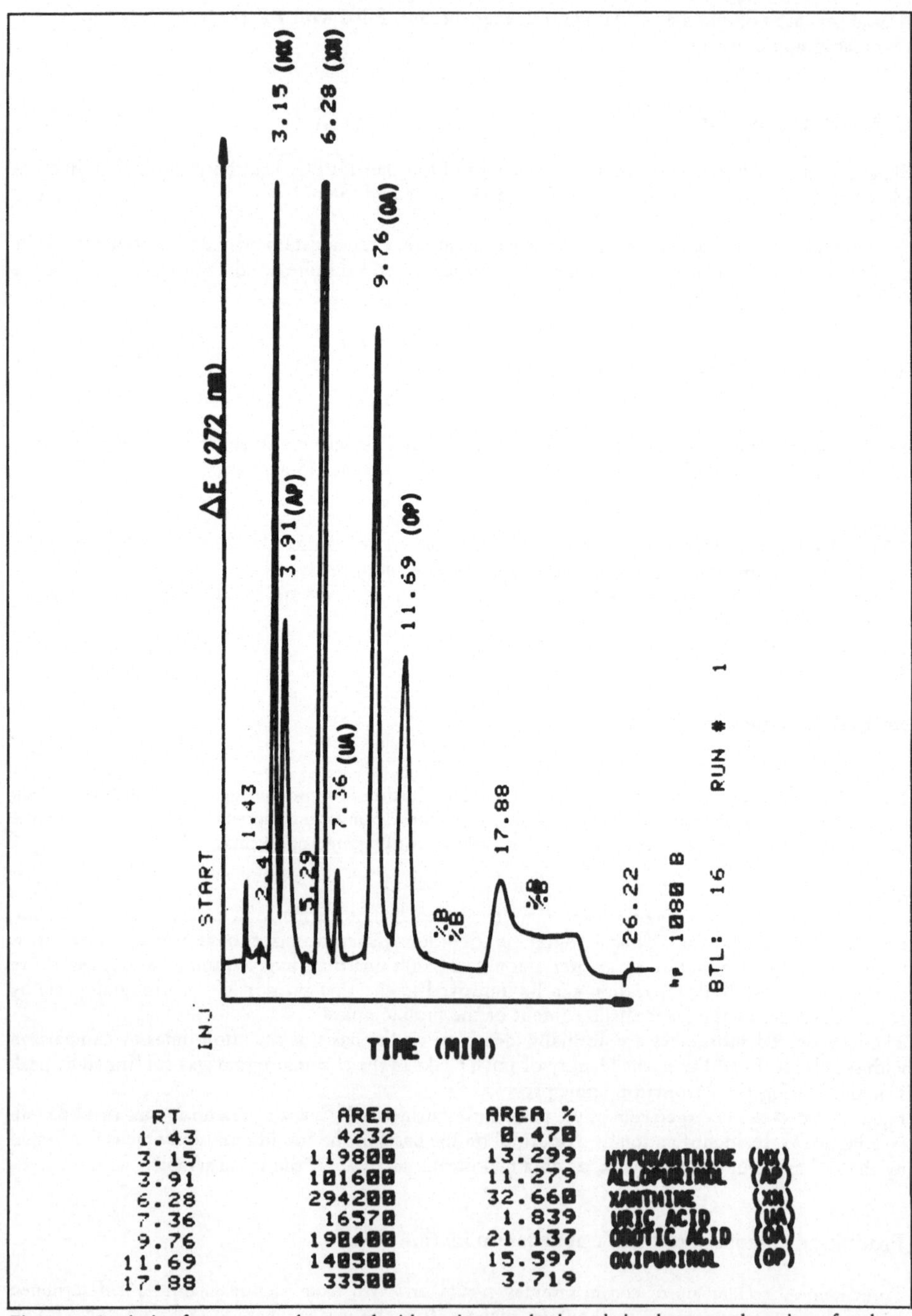

RT	AREA	AREA %	
1.43	4232	0.470	
3.15	119800	13.299	HYPOXANTHINE (HX)
3.91	101600	11.279	ALLOPURINOL (AP)
6.28	294200	32.660	XANTHINE (XN)
7.36	16570	1.839	URIC ACID (UA)
9.76	190400	21.137	OROTIC ACID (OA)
11.69	140500	15.597	OXIPURINOL (OP)
17.88	33500	3.719	

Figure 2: Analysis of serum sample treated with purine standards and simultaneous detection of endogenous serum uric acid; sample size (except uric acid) 400 ng of each compound. Mobile phase: 10 mM tetrabutylammonium hydroxide (pH 8.0) with 0.2% acetonitrile; flow rate 2 ml/min.

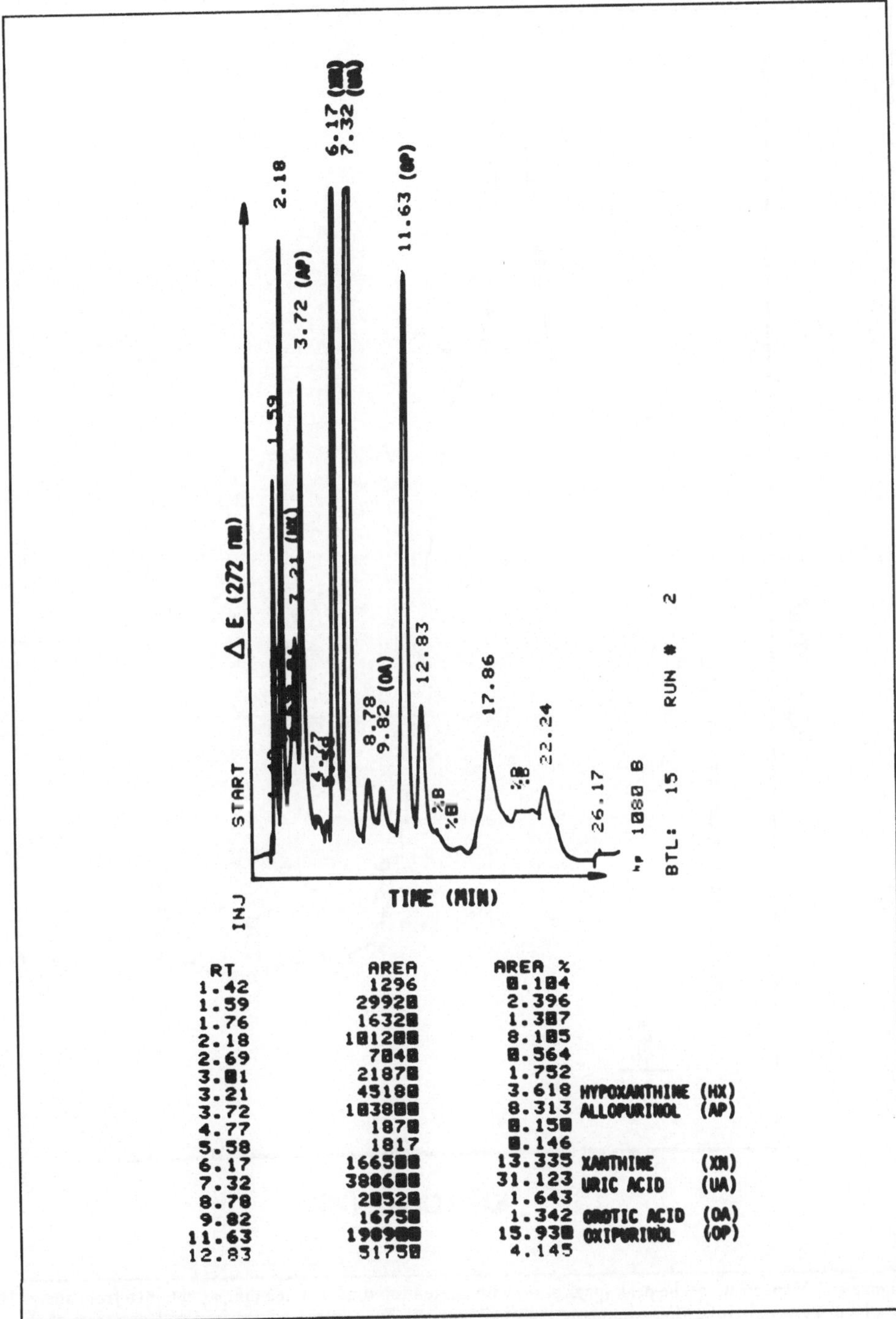

RT	AREA	AREA %	
1.42	1296	0.104	
1.59	29920	2.396	
1.76	16320	1.307	
2.18	101200	8.105	
2.69	7040	0.564	
3.01	21870	1.752	
3.21	45180	3.618	HYPOXANTHINE (HX)
3.72	103800	8.313	ALLOPURINOL (AP)
4.77	1870	0.150	
5.58	1817	0.146	
6.17	166500	13.335	XANTHINE (XN)
7.32	388600	31.123	URIC ACID (UA)
8.78	20520	1.643	
9.82	16750	1.342	OROTIC ACID (OA)
11.63	198900	15.930	OXIPURINOL (OP)
12.83	51750	4.145	

Figure 3: Analysis of urine sample of a patient after treatment with allopurinol.

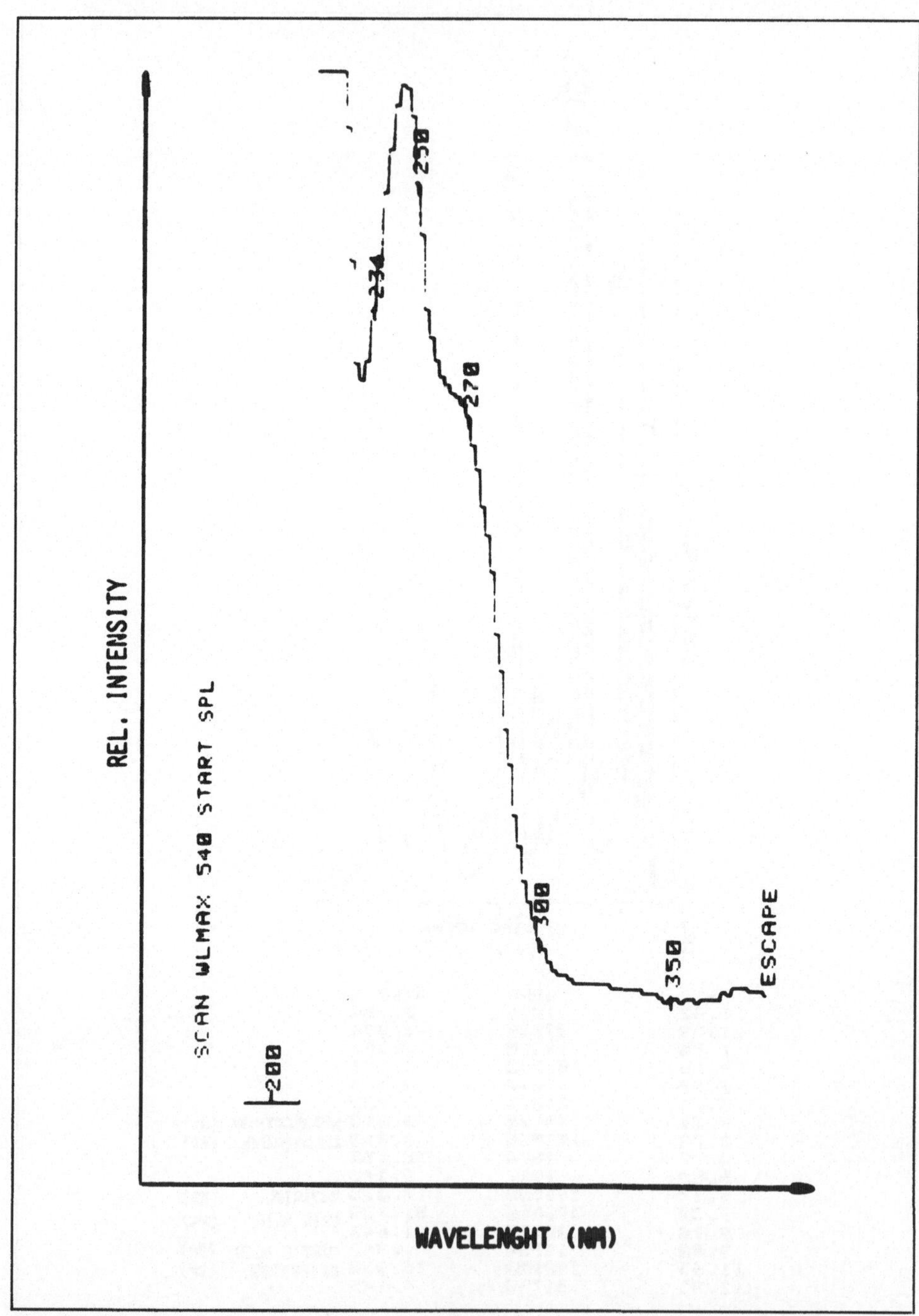

Figure 4: UV spectrum of the peak (peak scan) with a retention time of 11.63 min, as obtained from analysis of a urine sample following administration of allopurinol. For control, comparison with spectrum of an oxipurinol peak, as obtained from HPLC of a standard solution.

Uric acid (μmol/l)		
Uricase method		HPLC
without deprotein	with deprotein	
354.5	321.4	354.7
377.7	348.8	365.3
397.4	367.0	392.4
403.9	368.0	410.2

Table 1: Serum uric acid concentration determined by different methods (repeated tests) before and after allopurinol treatment.

As can be seen from the table, the values obtained during analysis of uric acid in serum by using the uricase method without deproteinization are practically identical to those obtained by HPLC. If the uricase method with deproteinization is used, the values are usually 8—10% lower which may be due to a constant portion of uric acid being lost during protein precipitation.
Analysis of substituted xanthines and uric acids *(theophylline and metabolites)* is shown (Figure 5). Under the chromatographic conditions used the analysis of a blank serum sample shows but one peak, that of uric acid. Consequently, the respective peak in Figure 5 can be assigned to endogenous serum uric acid.

Conclusions

The qualitative and quantitative determination of pyrimidines, purines, substituted purines and azapurines as well as their metabolites by an ion-pair high-performance liquid chromatographic technique, using tetrabutylammonium hydroxide as pairing ion and isocratic chromatographic conditions, is described. The presented method provides a selective and sensitive assay for the substances examined in complex biological fluids. This method requires no pre-extraction step, only ultrafiltration for serum, or dilution of urine samples.

Acknowledgements

We wish to express our thanks to Mrs. M. Näher and Mr. B. Cettier for completing the enzymatic assays. We are also grateful for the valuable assistance of Miss E. Wegmann in preparing the samples.

References

[1] Gröbner, W., Zöllner, N.: Zur Beeinflussung der Purin- und Pyrimidinsynthese durch Allopurinol.—Klin. Wschr. 53, 255 (1975).

[2] Matzkies, F., Berg, G.: Zur Wirkung einer täglichen Einzeldosis von 300 mg Allopurinol auf die Serumharnsäure und Uratausscheidung bei Gichtpatienten.—Dtsch. med. Wschr. 99, 2464 (1974).

[3] Jacob, M. H., Senior, R. M., Kessler, G.: Clinical experience with theophylline relationship between dosage, serum concentration and toxicity. J. Am. Med. Ass. 235, 1983 (1976).

[4] Jenne, J. W., Nagasawa, H. T., Thompson, R. T.: Relationship of urinary metabolites of theophylline to serum theophylline levels.—Clin. Pharmacol. Ther. 19, 375 (1976).

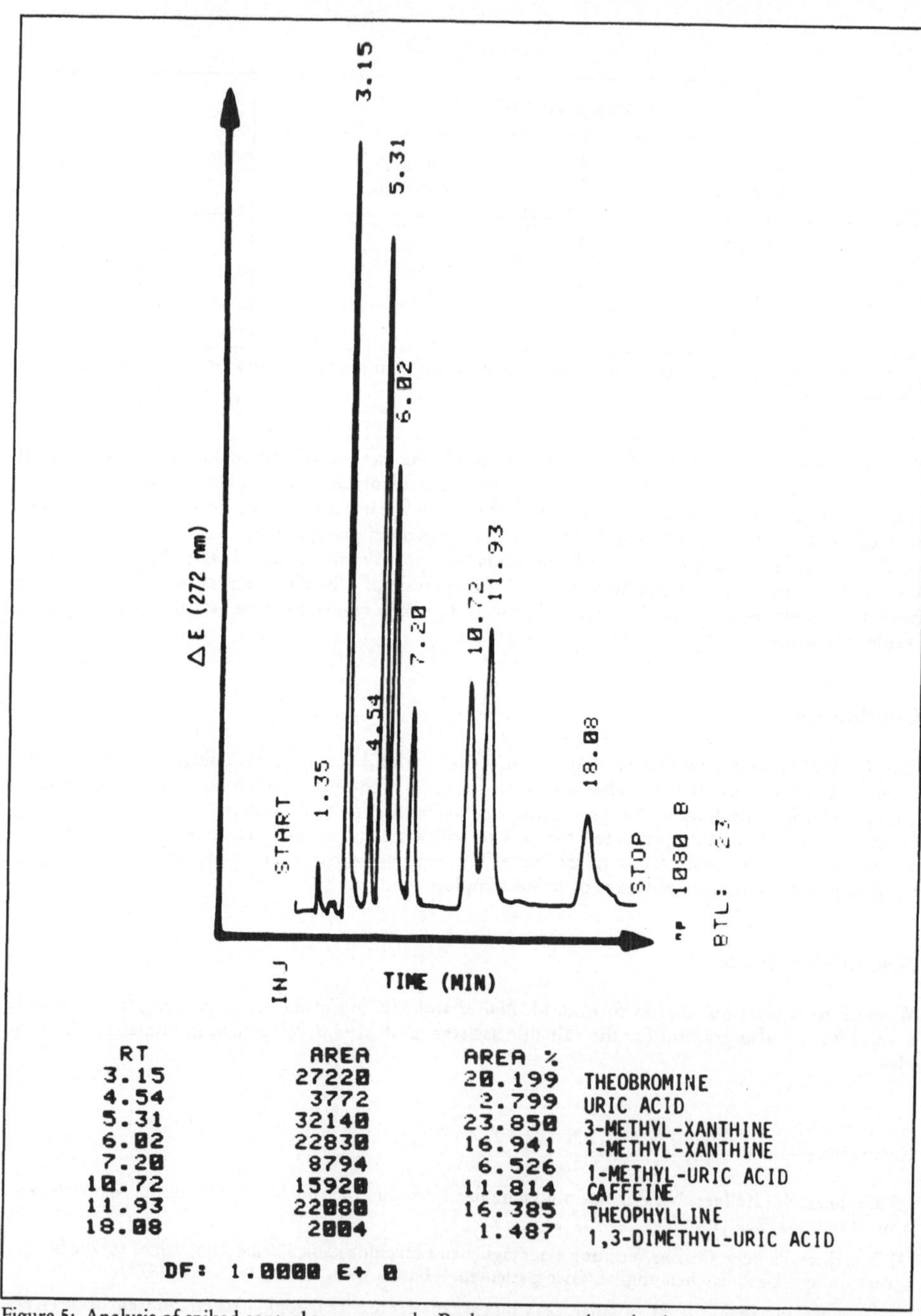

RT	AREA	AREA %	
3.15	27220	20.199	THEOBROMINE
4.54	3772	2.799	URIC ACID
5.31	32140	23.850	3-METHYL-XANTHINE
6.02	22830	16.941	1-METHYL-XANTHINE
7.20	8794	6.526	1-METHYL-URIC ACID
10.72	15920	11.814	CAFFEINE
11.93	22080	16.385	THEOPHYLLINE
18.08	2004	1.487	1,3-DIMETHYL-URIC ACID

DF: 1.0000 E+ 0

Figure 5: Analysis of spiked control serum sample. Peaks correspond to: theobromine 50 ng, 3-methylxanthine 20 ng, 1-methylxanthine 50 ng, 1-methyl-uric acid 100 ng, caffeine 50 ng, theophylline 50 ng, 1.3-dimethyl-uric acid 200 ng. Chromatographic conditions, see Figure 2; instead of 2.5% only 0.2% acetonitrile was used.

[5] Floridi, A., Palmerini, C. A., Fini, C.: Simultaneous analysis of bases, nucleosides and nucleoside mono- and polyphosphates by high-performance liquid chromatography.—J. Chromatogr. 138, 203 (1977).

[6] Tomlinson, E., Jefferies, T. M., Riley, C. H.: Ionpair high-performance liquid chromatography.—J. Chromatogr. 159, 315 (1978).

[7] Wittmer, D. P., Nuessle, N. O., Haney, W. G.: Simultaneous analysis of tartrazine and its intermediates by reversed phase liquid chromatography.—Anal. Chem. 47, 1422 (1975).

[8] Praetorius, E., Poulsen, H.: Enzymatic determination of uric acid.—Scand. J. Clin. Lab. Invest. 5, 273 (1953).

Quantitative thin-layer chromatography of diuretics in clinical pharmacology

M. Schäfer, F. Sörgel, E. Mutschler
Pharmakologisches Institut für Naturwissenschaftler, Universität Frankfurt, Frankfurt/M.

Introduction

In spite of their widespread use there was limited information on the pharmacokinetics of diuretics until recently. This was due to the absence of suitable methods for the quantification of these drugs. There was a lack of sensitivity and specifity in measuring the intrinsic fluorescence in the cuvette (furosemide) and in the derivatisation to coloured products (hydrochlorothiazide, furosemide). During the last few years methods have been developed using GLC and HPLC to separate the drug from plasma constituents. Quantitative thin-layer chromatography has also proved to be successful for measurement of drugs in biological material.
The aim of our investigations was to develop methods using quantitative thin-layer chromatography for the determination of different diuretics in plasma. The methods should be sensitive enough to measure therapeutic doses of the drugs.

Methods

Furosemide

Deproteinisation of plasma by methanol. Development of plates with: Chloroform 70, Ethyl acetate 30, Acetic acid 5.
Enhancement of fluorescence by spraying the plate with a solution of citric acid (10%) followed by quantification (KM 3, Zeiss). It is possible to determine 4-chloro-5-sulfamoylanthranilic acid (CSA), a possible metabolite of furosemide (Figure 1).

Hydrochlorothiazide (HCT)

Extraction from biological material by ethyl acetate. The solvent: ethyl acetate in an unlined tank. Amplification of fluorescence intensity by spraying with a solution of 40% triethanolamine (in methanol) and exposing to U.V.-light (365 nm) prior to measurement (Figure 2, 3).

Bendroflumethiazide (BFT)

Extraction from biological material with ether. The solvent: Chloroform 60, Ethyl acetate 40.

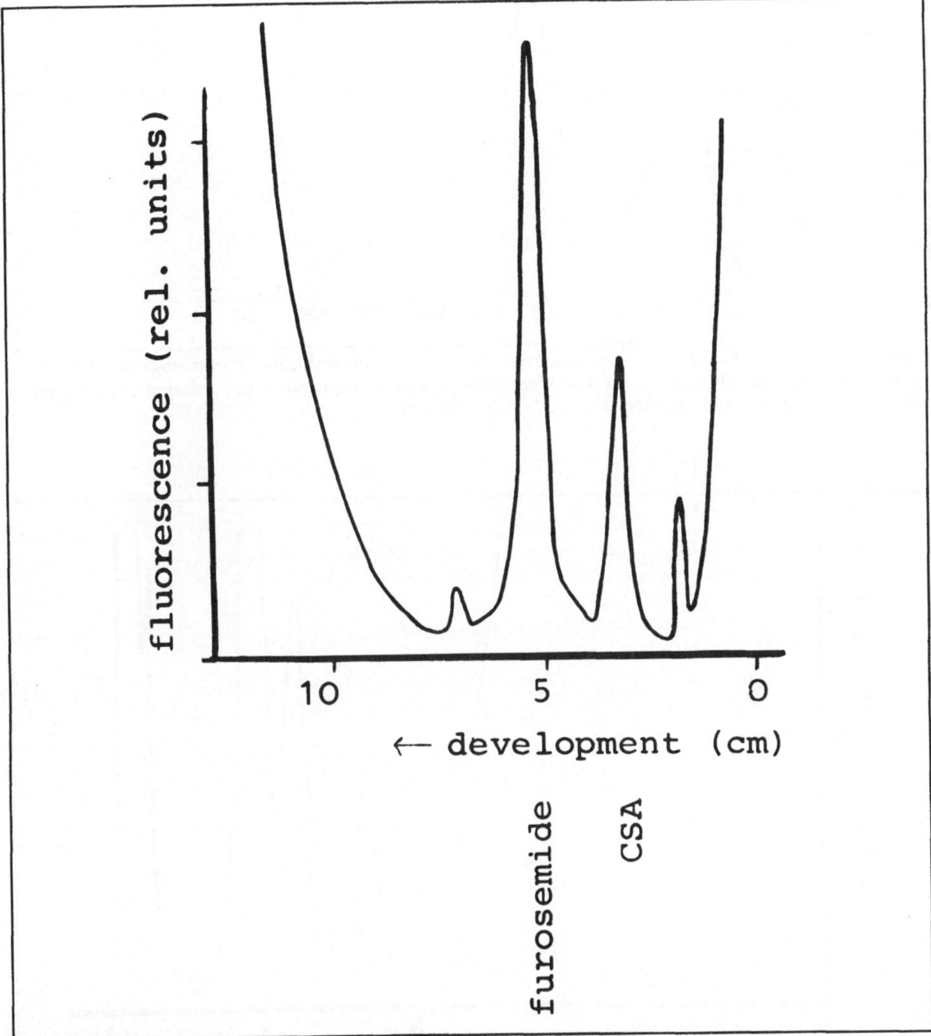

Figure 1: Chromatogram of 1 ml of plasma spiked with 200 ng furosemide and 200 ng 4-chloro-5-sulfamoylanthranilic acid. Deproteinisation with methanol, chromatographed on silica gel 60 plates with the solvent system chloroform—ethylacetate—acetic acid (70:30:5). After drying the plate is sprayed with a solution of 10% citric acid in water—ethyleneglycol (1:1).

%
100
80
60
40
20
240
280
320
360
400
440
480
520
560
nm

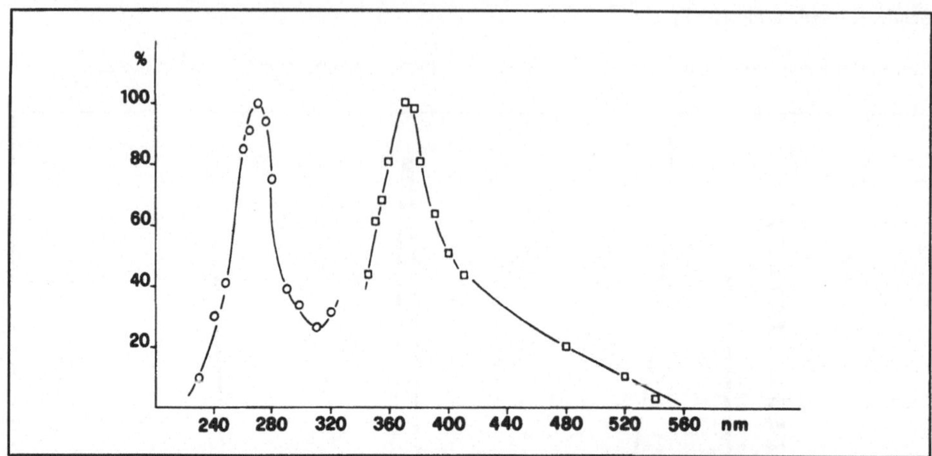

Figure 2: Excitation (O) and emission spectrum (□) of hydrochlorothiazide chromatographed on silica gel 60 plates with the solvent ethyl acetate. After drying the plate is sprayed with a solution of 40% triethanolamine in methanol and radiated with U.V.-light (365 nm).

fluorescence (rel. units)
16
12
8
4
0
← development (cm)
HCT

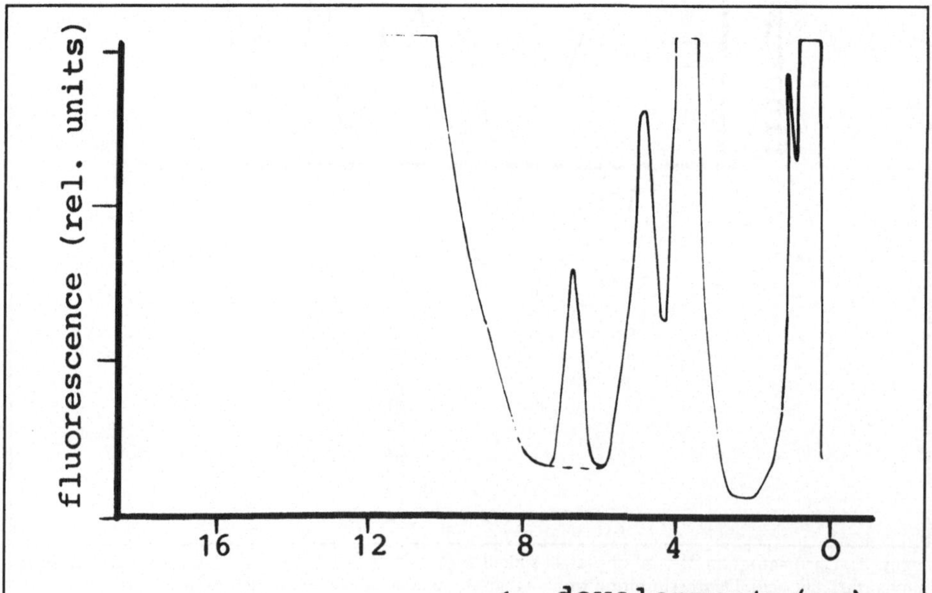

Figure 3: Chromatogram of 50 ng hydrochlorothiazide extracted from 1 ml of plasma by ethyl acetate, chromatographed on silica gel 60 plates with the solvent ethyl acetate. After drying the plate is sprayed with a solution of 40% triethanolamine in methanol and radiated with U.V.-light (365 nm).

Results

		furosemide	HCT	BFT
Linearity	(ng/spot)	0.2—100	5—500	0.3—30
Detection limit	(ng/ml)	20	10	1
Recovery		104%	90%	88%
C.V.		4.7%	8.8%	6.7%
Samples measurable	per day	100	40	40

Pharmacokinetics

In figure 4 the plasma levels after administration of 50 mg hydrochlorothiazide (2 Esidrix®-tablets) to two patients are shown. The curves reveal the influence of renal impairment on the pharmacokinetics of hydrochlorothiazide. In figure 5 plasma levels after a lower dose of HCT (12.5 mg) to a healthy volunteer are shown.

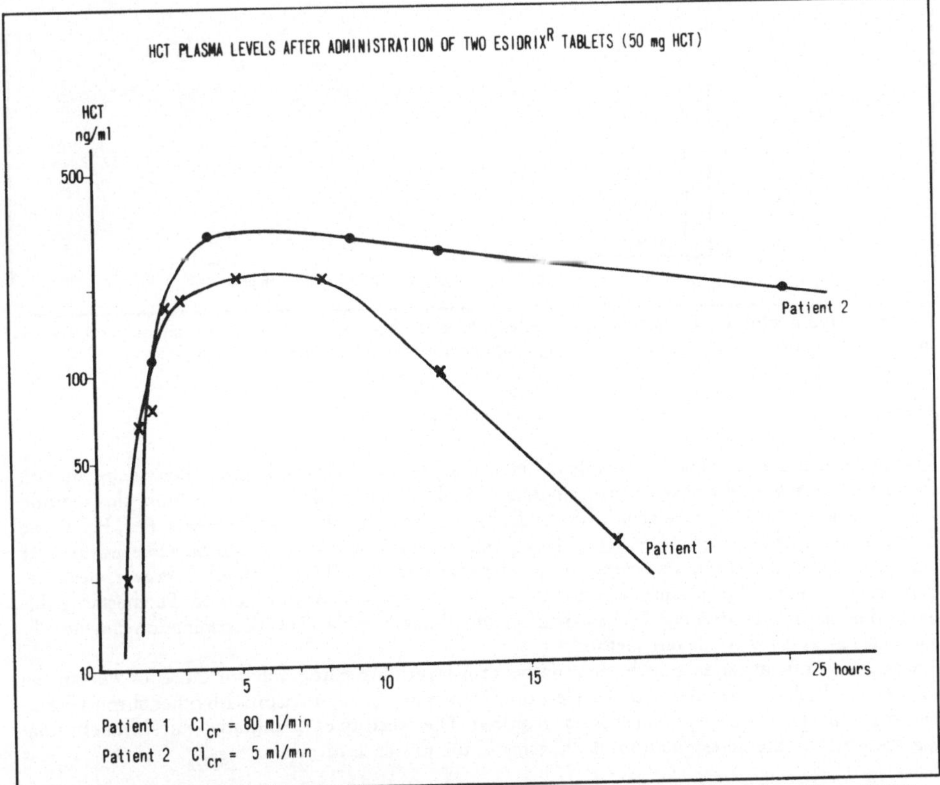

Figure 4: Hydrochlorothizide plasma levels after administration of two Esidrix®-tablets (50 mg HCT) to patients with impaired renal function: patient 1 Cl_{cr} = 80 ml/min, patient 2: Cl_{cr} = 5 ml/min.

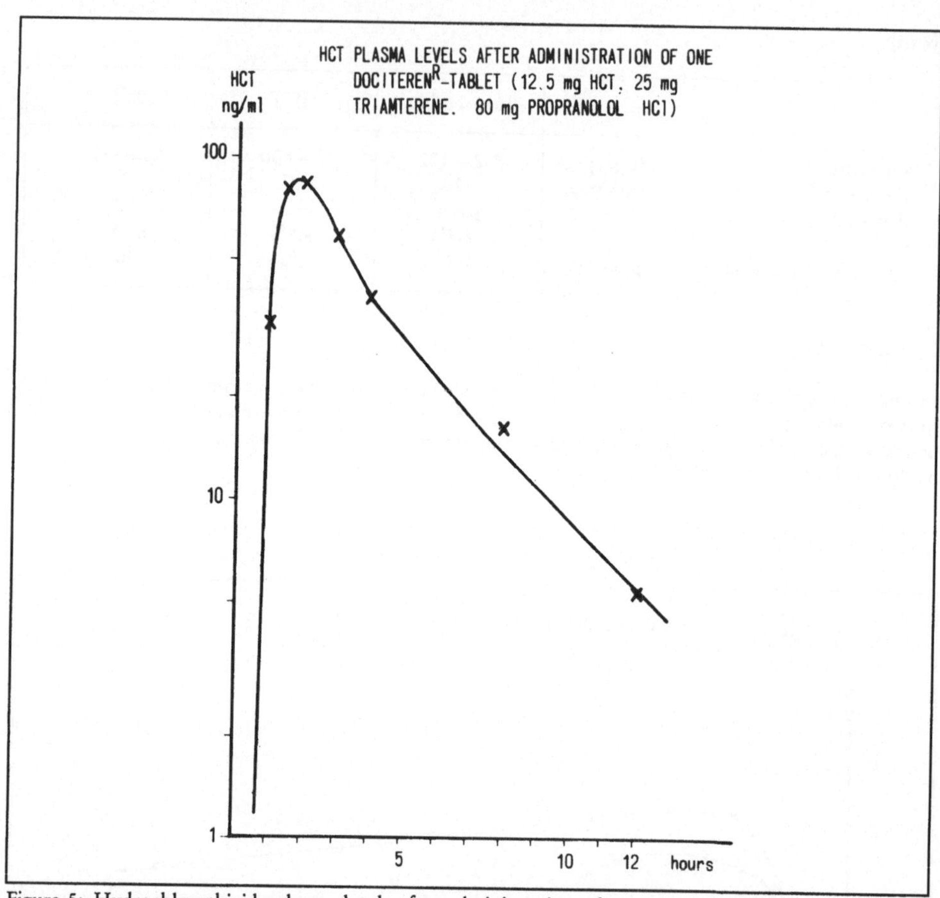

Figure 5: Hydrochlorothizide plasma levels after administration of one Dociteren®-tablet (12.5 mg hydrochlorothiazide, 25 mg triamterene, 80 mg propranolol-hydrochloride) to a volunteer.

Discussion

The methods described make it possible to determine plasma levels of the drug after treatment with therapeutic doses. In the case of furosemide and hydrochlorothiazide determination, this method has been successful for pharmacokinetic studies in healthy volunteers and patients. For, HCT, the detection limit of our method is below 10 ng/ml. A similar sensitivity could be achieved only by high-pressure liquid chromatography or gas-chromatography. These methods, however, often require two or more ml of plasma, whereas 0.5—1 ml is sufficient for our method. Furthermore this method is less time consuming. In the case of bendroflumethiazide, GLC determination may be reliable but not as sensitive as our method.

Summarizing our experience with quantitative thin-layer chromatography of diuretics we can say that our methods are sensitive and often less time consuming in comparison with other chromatographic methods. Expensive equipment is not required. The specifity of quantitative thin-layer chromatography allows the determination of diuretics in the presence of other drugs.

Bibliography

[1] F. Andreasen, P. Jacobsen, Acta Pharmacol. Toxicol. *35*, 49 (1964)

[2] J. E. Baer, H. L. Leidy, A. V. Brooks, K. H. Beyer, J. Pharmacol. Exp. Ther. *125*, 295 (1959)

[3] B. Beermann, M. Groschinsky-Grind, B. Lindström, Eur. J. Clin. Pharmacol. *10*, 295 (1976)

[4] A. D. Blair, A. W. Forrey, T. Meijsen, R. Cutler, J. Pharm. Sci. *64*, 1334 (1975)

[5] K. Carr, A. Rane, J. C. Fröhlich, J. Chromatogr. *145*, 421 (1978)

[6] A. S. Christophersen, K. E. Rasmussen, B. Salvesen, J. Chromatogr. *132*, 91 (1977)

[7] M. J. Cooper, A. R. Sinaiko, M. W. Anders, B. L. Mirkin, Anal. Chem. *48*, 1110 (1976)

[8] P. Hajdu, A. Häussler, Arzneim.-Forsch. *14*, 709 (1964)

[9] B. Lindström, J. Chromatogr. *100*, 189 (1974)

[10] B. Lindström, M. Molander, M. Groschinsky, J. Chromatogr. *114*, 459 (1975)

[11] M. L. MacDougall, D. W. Shoeman, D. L. Azarnoff, Res. Commun. Chem. Pathol. Pharmacol. *10*, 285 (1975)

[12] E. Mikkelsen, F. Andreasen, Acta Pharmacol. Toxicol. *41*, 254 (1977)

[13] W. T. Robinson, L. Cosyns, Clin. Biochem. *11*, 272 (1978)

[14] M. Schäfer, H. E. Geißler, E. Mutschler, J. Chromatogr. *143*, 615 (1977)

[15] M. Schäfer, H. E. Geißler, E. Mutschler, J. Chromatogr. *143*, 636 (1977)

[16] W. J. A. Vandenheuvel, V. F. Gruber, R. W. Walker, E. J. Wolf, J. Pharm. Sci. *64*, 1309 (1975)

Evaluation of positive inotropic and chronotropic activity exhibited by extracts from human kidneys

J. Paraskevova, R. G. Alken, N. Rietbrock
Klinikum der J.-W.-Goethe-Universität, Frankfurt am Main, Abteilung für klinische Pharmakologie

Introduction

There are several methods in use for assaying digoxin concentration in human tissues.
Although GC and HPLC are quite specific, they are not as sensitive as immunological methods and they require prior purification of the sample.
Isolated heart preparations have been used as a digoxin-bioassay for the inotropic action of extracts from human tissues [2].
Another highly sensitive digoxin-bioassay, the inhibition of ^{86}Rb uptake into human erythrocytes has been used but non-specific inhibition and hemolytic effects by the extracts has been observed [1].
In this report forensic studies on ethanolic extracts from human organs were carried out to detect possible presence of digoxin and its cardioactive metabolites.
Immunoassays are commonly used for assaying digoxin in body fluids, but there is a lack of information on cross reactivities in extracts from tissues themselves.
Scholz [4], reported an intrinsic positive inotropic (p. i.) action on the left atria produced by organ extracts from rats and guinea pigs. The different organs showed varying activities (kidneys > heart > liver > plasma). We have confirmed these results and also found that tissue extracts from brain have an exceptionally low activity. This work was done in order to obtain more information about the p. i. activity and was restricted to extracts from human kidneys.

Preparation

Apparently normal kidneys from patients 24 hours post mortem were stored 4° C for 2—60 days. Ethanolic extracts of kidney homogenates were evaporated to near dryness at 40° C, dissoluted in water, and washed with petrolether. The petrol ether phase was pharmacologically inactive. The aqueous phase was centrifuged (18500 rpm for 60 min.). The supernatant was lyophilized, dissoluted in water and stored in aliquots at −20° C.

Pharmacological action

a) Isolated guinea-pig atria

The pharmacological action was tested on an isolated guinea-pig atria preparation (Tyrode pH 7.4, 30° C, preload 1g, right atria spontaneously beating, left atria paced by rectangular impulses 2 Hz, 100 V, 100 msec.). The extract had a p. i. action on the left atria (115 ng/ml), and a slower rate of onset than the p. i. action of adrenaline. On the right atria the extract showed a pronounced positive chronotropic (p. c.) and p. i. action with a fast onset. Both effects were dose dependent and showed no tachyphylaxia. (Figure 1, 2, 3).
Since p. c. action has not been previously reported, the content of adrenaline, noradrenaline and dopamine in our extracts was assayed [3]. The concentrations calculated per bath volume were: adrenaline 0.20 nM, noradrenaline 0.27 nM, dopamine 0.32 nM—resp.: 14, 32, 23 pmol/g tissue. These amines at these concentrations showed no pharmacological action on isolated guinea-pig atria when added as a synthetically prepared mixture.

b) Isolated guinea-pig ileum

On the isolated guinea-pig ileum (Tyrode 34° C, pH 7.4, longitudinal isotonic contractions), the extracts showed a fast sustained spasm, which was fully reversible after wash out. The effect also showed no tachyphylaxia. (Figure 4). Adrenergic substances as well as metadrenalines showed a relaxation under these conditions. Serotonin showed a contraction followed by a spontaneous relaxation. The response of kidney extract was compared to histamine (1×10^{-5}M), carbachol (2×10^{-1} M) and $BaCl_2$ (2×10^{-4} M). Atropine, diphenhydramine and verapamil were added 8 minutes be-

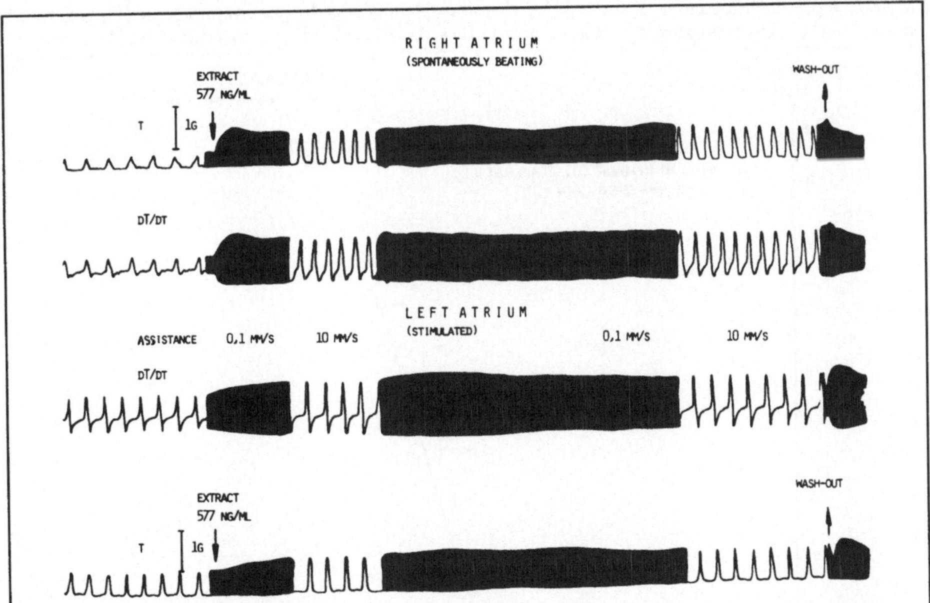

Figure 1: Simultaneously recorded tension (T) and velocity of tension (dT/dt) of the spontaneously beating right atrium (upper graphs) and the stimulated left atrium of one guinea pig at two different recording velocities (0.1 and 10 mm/s). The addition of human kidney extract (final concentration in the bath: 557 ng/ml) exerts a sustained positive chronotropic and inotropic effect on the right atrium and a more slowly developing positive inotropic effect on the left atrium.

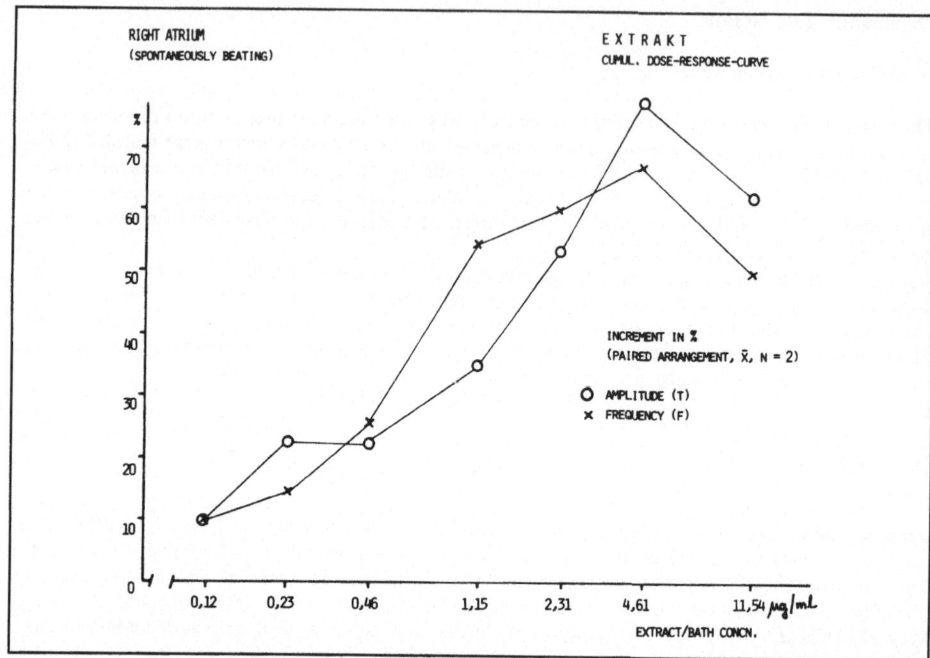

Figure 2: Dose-response curve of the positive chronotropic (X) and the positive inotropic (O) activity of extracts on the right spontaneously beating atrium (n = 2). Abscissa: final concentration of the extract.

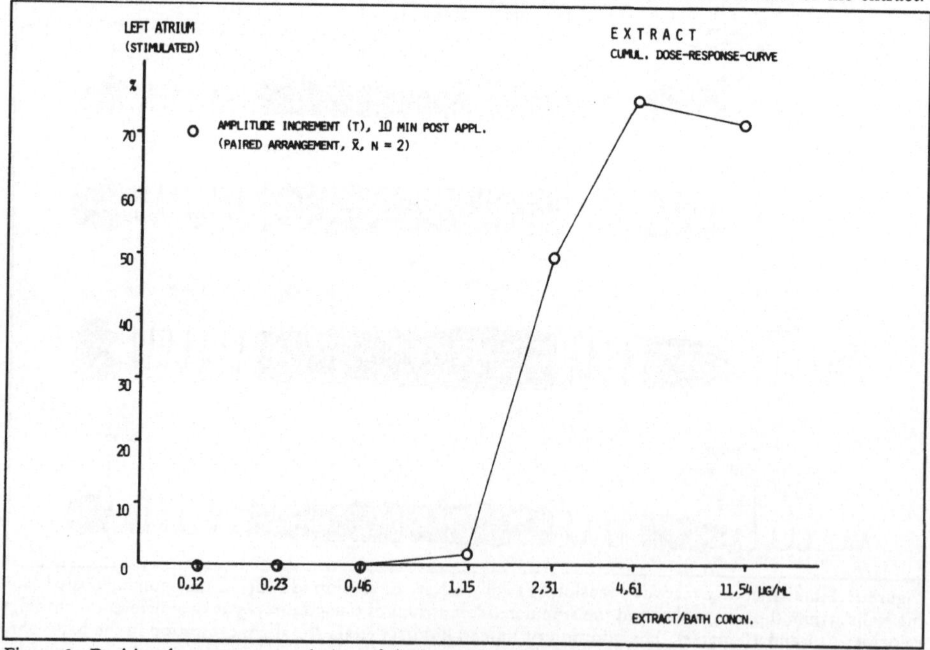

Figure 3: Positive dose-response relation of the inotropic (O) activity of the extracts from human kidneys on paced left guinea pig atria (n = 2). Abscissa: final concentration of the extract.

fore application of each agonist in a cumulated dose-response relationship design. The agonist response was observed for 2 minutes and stopped by wash out. The mean of 3 responses before application of the antagonist was used as a control. The effect of the antagonists are given as a percentage of the control.
Atropine inhibited the carbachol contraction, $ED_{50} = 10^{-8}$ M. $BaCl_2$ contractions and those produced by the kidney extract were little effected, and histamine not at all. (Figure 5)
Diphenhydramine antagonised the contractile response of the kidney extract, $ED_{50} = 5 \times 10^{-8}$ M, and the histamine and carbachol contraction, $ED_{50} = 5 \times 10^{-7}$ M, but antagonised the $BaCl_2$, contraction only weakly, 30% antagonism at 10^{-5} M. (Figure 6)
Verapamil inhibited the guinea-pig ileum contractions during the plateau phase (inhibition of sustained contraction) in the case of all agonists: ED_{50}'s for plateau inhibition were: Extract 5×10^{-8} M; carbachol 2×10^{-7} M; histamine and $BaCl_2$ 10^{-7} M. Initial contractions were strongly inhibited only in the case of the extract and $BaCl_2$, ED = 2×10^{-7} M. (Figure 7).

Purification

a) Group separation

Trichloracetic acid (10%) was added (2:1; v/v) to the extract. After centrifugation the supernatant still retained it's full pharmacological activity. After ethanolic extraction and treatment with trichloroacetic acid it can be concluded that a protein is probably not responsible for the pharmacological action.
Acetone, which precipitates carbohydrates and peptides, did not inactivate the extract.
Catecholamines can be adsorbed on alumina. The alumina filtrate of the extract showed full pharmacological activity.
Biogenic amines can be extracted from alkaline solution into a mixture of toluene and isoamylalcohol (3:2; v/v). After acidification with acetic acid amines can be extracted back into the aqueous phase. Using this method, the pharmacological activity in the kidney extract was partially extracted and back-extracted.
Steroids were removed by extraction with acetic-ethylester/ether (1:1; v/v). The remaining aqueous solution showed no decrease in pharmacological activity. Chloroform extraction was equally ineffective in diminishing the pharmacological activity, although it will extract digoxin and it's cardioactive metabolites efficiently.

b) Physico-chemical behaviour

The pharmacological activity was not affected by neuramidase, chymotrypsin, and pronase (1 mg/ml, 38° C, 18 hrs.), but was inactivated by boiling (60 min.). The extracts lost activity at extreme acidic and alkaline conditions.

c) Gel-filtration

The extracts were treated with trichloroacetic acid, acetone, passed through alumina and the filtrate treated with ethyl acetate/ether (1:1; v/v). The residue was subjected to gel-filtration on Sephadex G-25 (4 × 0.5 cm, phosphate-buffer pH 7.34, UV-detection at 254 nm). The elution of the extract occurred shortly after the Dextran-blue marker. Only the front portion of the main peak exhibited pharmacological activity on the guinea-pig ileum (Figure 8). The original extract itself showed a high cross-reactivity in the digoxin radioimmunoassay (NEN) and gelfiltration did not separate this cross-reactivity from the pharmacologically active principle (Figure 9).

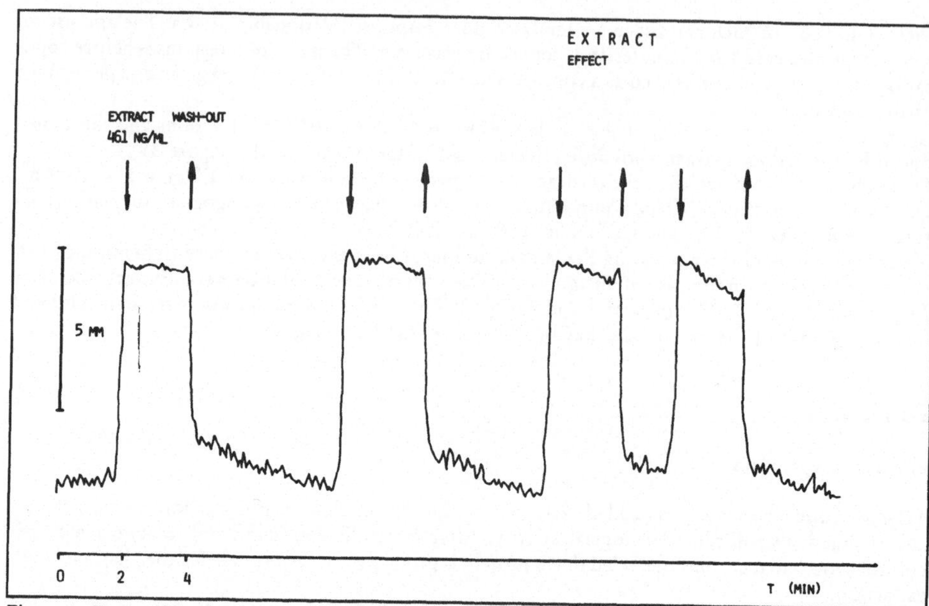

Figure 4: Extract from human kidneys (461 ng/ml, final concentration) gives a sustained spasm of the guinea-pig ileum, fully reversible after wash-out without tachyphylaxia.

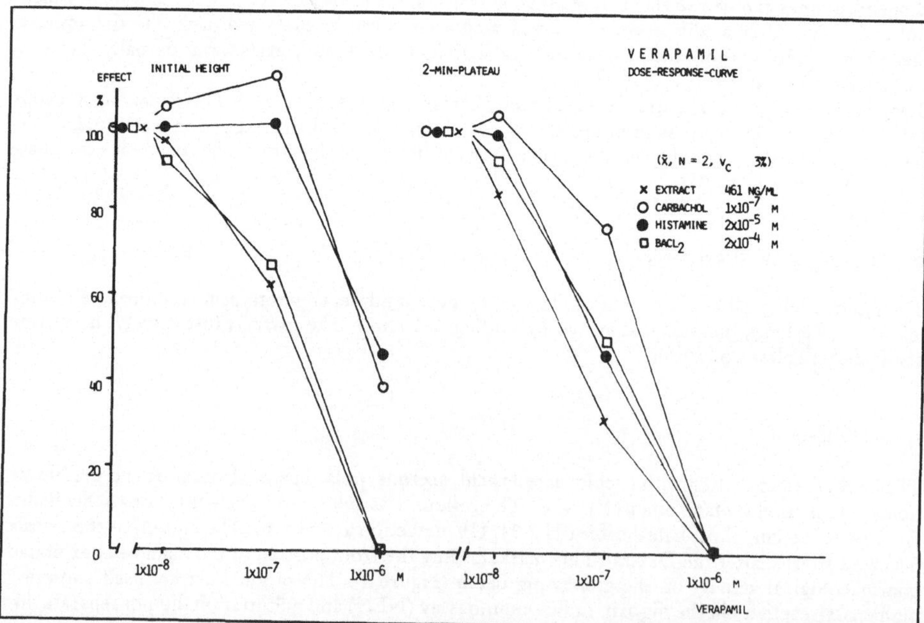

Figure 7: Antagonism of equieffective doses (given as per cent of control) of extracts from human kidneys ([X] 461 ng/ml), carbachol ([O] 1×10^{-7} M), histamine ([●] 2×10^{-5} M), $BaCl_2$ ([$\times 10^{-4}$ M) by verapamil on the guinea-pig ileum. Plateaus (2 min after application) refer to inhibition of sustained contraction (see text).

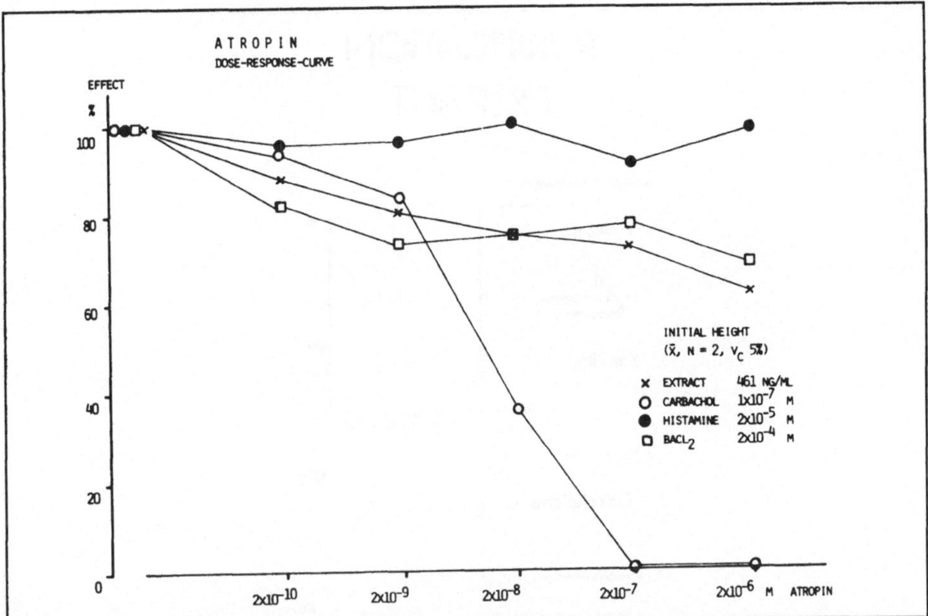

Figure 5: Antagonism of equi-effective doses (given as per cent of control) of extract from human kidneys ([X] 461 ng/ml), carbachol ([O] 1×10^{-7} M), histamine ([●] 2×10^{-5} M), $BaCl_2$ ([□] 2×10^{-4} M) by atropine on the guinea-pig ileum.

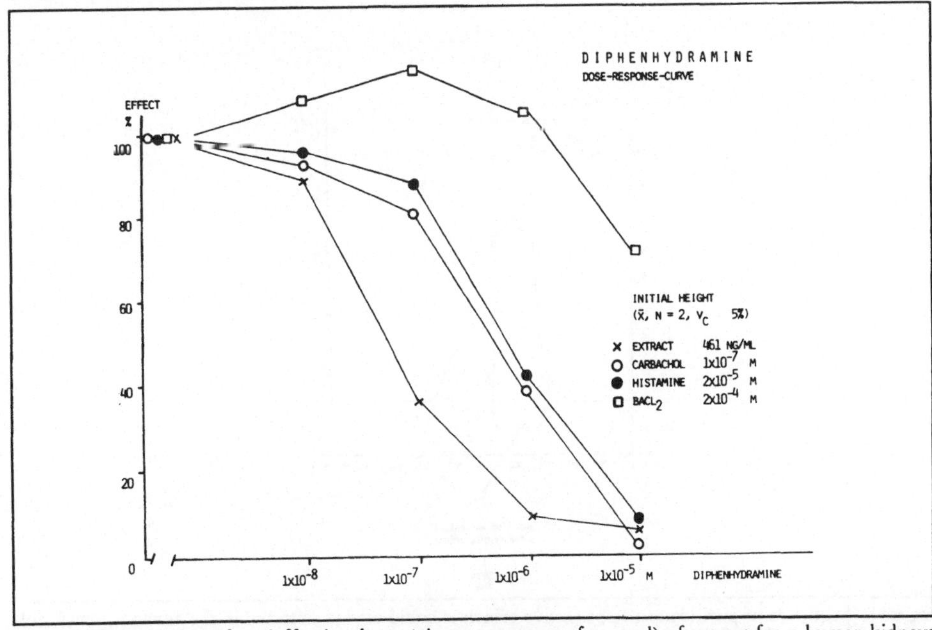

Figure 6: Antagonism of equieffective doses (given as per cent of control) of extract from human kidneys ([X] 461 ng/ml), carbachol ([O] 1×10^{-7} M), histamine ([●] 2×10^{-5} M), $BaCl_2$ ([□] 2×10^{-4} M) by diphenydramine on the guinea-pig ileum.

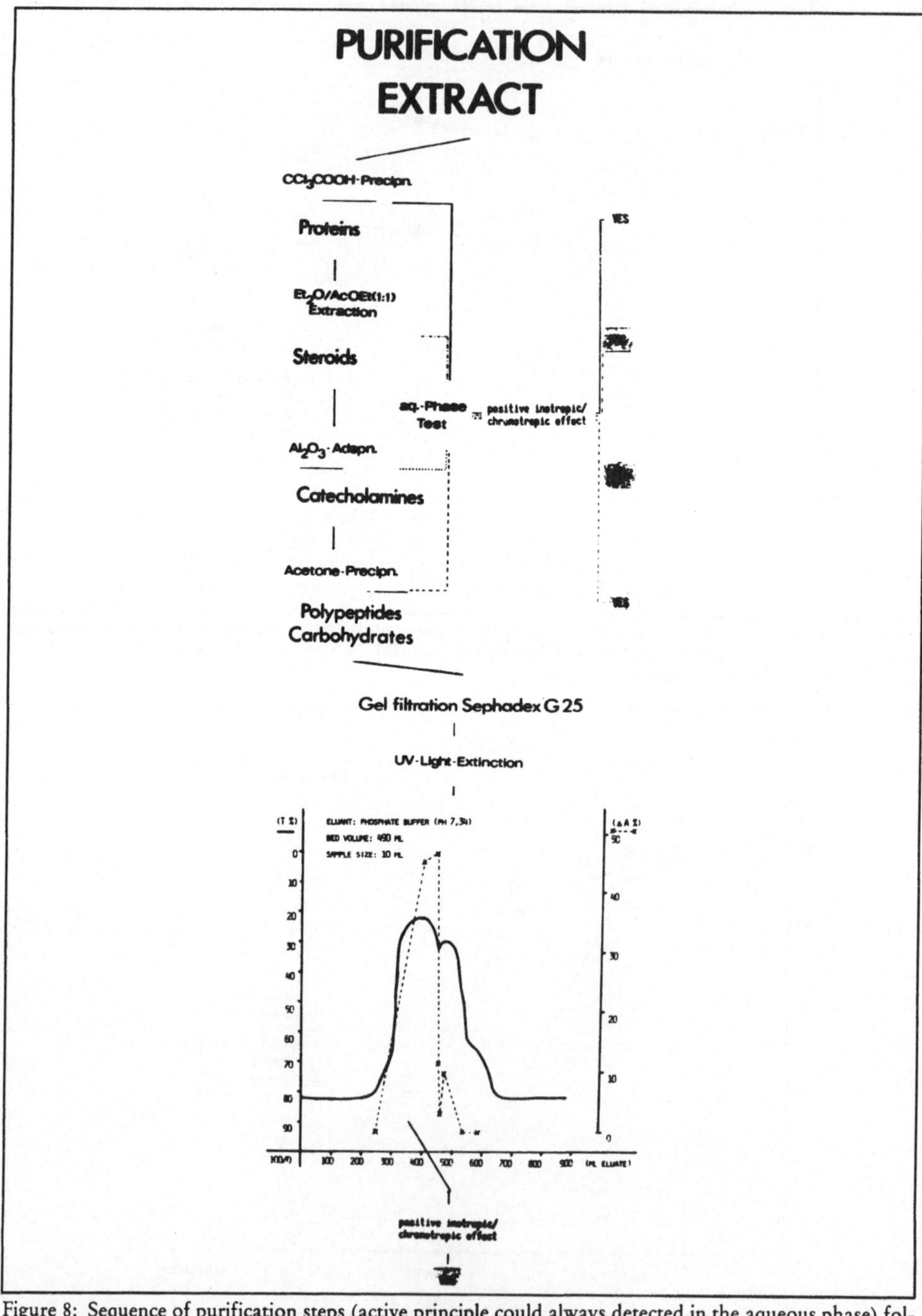

Figure 8: Sequence of purification steps (active principle could always detected in the aqueous phase) followed by gel filtration. The graph (———) gives the UV-Light extinction (T%, left ordinate), dependent on eluate ([ml], abscissa), and the corresponding positive inotropic activity (— — — — — — —) (▷ A%, right ordinate).

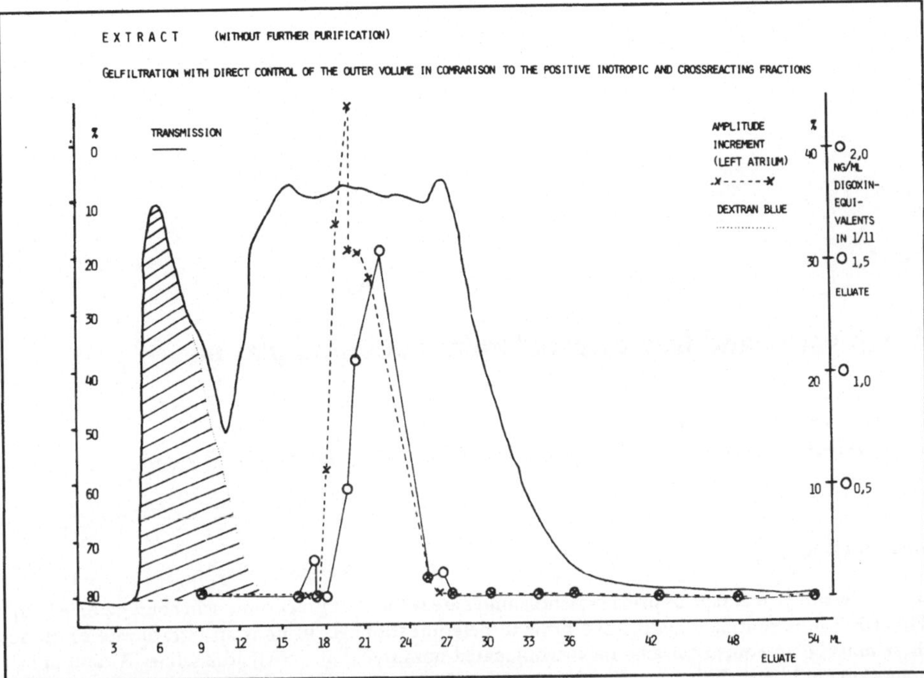

Figure 9: Gel filtration of kidney extract. Positive inotropic activity (x— — — — — —x— —, %, per cent of increment, right ordinate) could be detected in the middle part of the main peak of UV-transmission (——— = transmission) and was not separated from cross-reactivity in the digoxin radioimmunoassay (Digoxin RIA-NEN; O———O, (ng/ml) digoxin equivalents after 1/11 dilution, right ordinate). First peak is dextran blue.

Resume

Positive inotropic action and non-specific antibody binding activity prevents the direct radioimmunoassay and bioassay of digoxin in extracts from human tissues. Digoxin can be separated from substances bearing cross-reactivity and p. i. activity by chloroform extraction.

Literature

[1] Belz, G. G.: Personal communication (1978).

[2] Fühner, H.: Rektale Strophanthinvergiftung. Der „Fall Mertens—Dr. Richter".—Dtsch. med. Wschr. 55, 1408—1409 (1929).

[3] Kirsten, R., B. Heinz, K. Nelson: in preparation.

[4] Scholz, H.: Pharmakologie und Klinik tödlich verlaufender Glykosidintoxikationen: Versuch eines pharmakologischen Nachweises von Herzglykosiden in Leichenteilen, 2nd Berliner Seminar 1978.

Conjugated and free catecholamines in blood plasma

M. Nagel and H. J. Schümann
Pharmakologisches Institut der Universität Essen GHS, Hufelandstr. 55, 4300 Essen

Introduction

A considerable percentage of urine catecholamines are sulfuric or glucuronic acid conjugates [4], [6]. This fraction is routinely hydrolysed prior to determination. As urine is an ultrafiltrate of blood there must be an equivalent amount of conjugated noradrenaline (NA), adrenaline (A) and dopamine (DA) in blood. This was already shown by Häggendahl [3] and Buu *et al.* [1]. The applied methods for hydrolysis are unsatisfactory because hydrolysis is either not complete or the catecholamines are destroyed to varying degrees. The presented method yields complete hydrolysis without detectable destruction of the amines. The hydrolysate is suitable for radioenzymatic determination of NA, A and DA.

Experimental and results

Blood samples, drawn from blood donors immediately after loss of 500 ml blood, were mixed with a solution containing dithiothreitol and ethylenglycol-bis(β-aminoethyl ether) N,N'-tetraacetic acid (EGTA), cooled and centrifuged. One part of the plasma was used to measure free catecholamines. Another part was mixed with 0.6 N perchloric acid (PCA) containing EGTA. The precipitated protein was sedimented and the supernatant heated to 95° C for various times. After cooling the total (= free + conjugated) NA, A and DA were determined by our own modification of the methods of Peuler and Johnson [5] and Daprada and Zürcher [2]. For determination of free catecholamines we used non-deproteinized plasma since in deproteinized acidified samples the conjugated amines might be partially hydrolysed.
For radioenzymatic O-methylation the incubation mixture contained 25 μl sample, hydrolysed or non-hydrolysed, and 25 μl of a reaction mixture containing Tris buffer, $MgCl_2$, EGTA, catechol-O-methyltransferase, 1 μCi S-adenosyl-L-methionine-methyl-^3H (5-10 Ci/mmol) and dithiothreitol. For quantitative analysis to each sample were added 100 pg of NA, A and DA each as internal standards. The O-methylated catecholamines were extracted into diethylether and re-extracted into HCl. The aqueous phase was washed with butyl acetate and evaporated. The residue was chromatographed on Kieselgel F254 plates. The spots corresponding to normetanephrine, metanephrine and methoxytyramine were scraped into separate scintillation vials. Normetanephrine and metanephrine were oxidized to vanillin and extracted into a toluene scintillation cocktail. Methoxytyramine was dissolved in HCl and Quickszint 212^R was added.

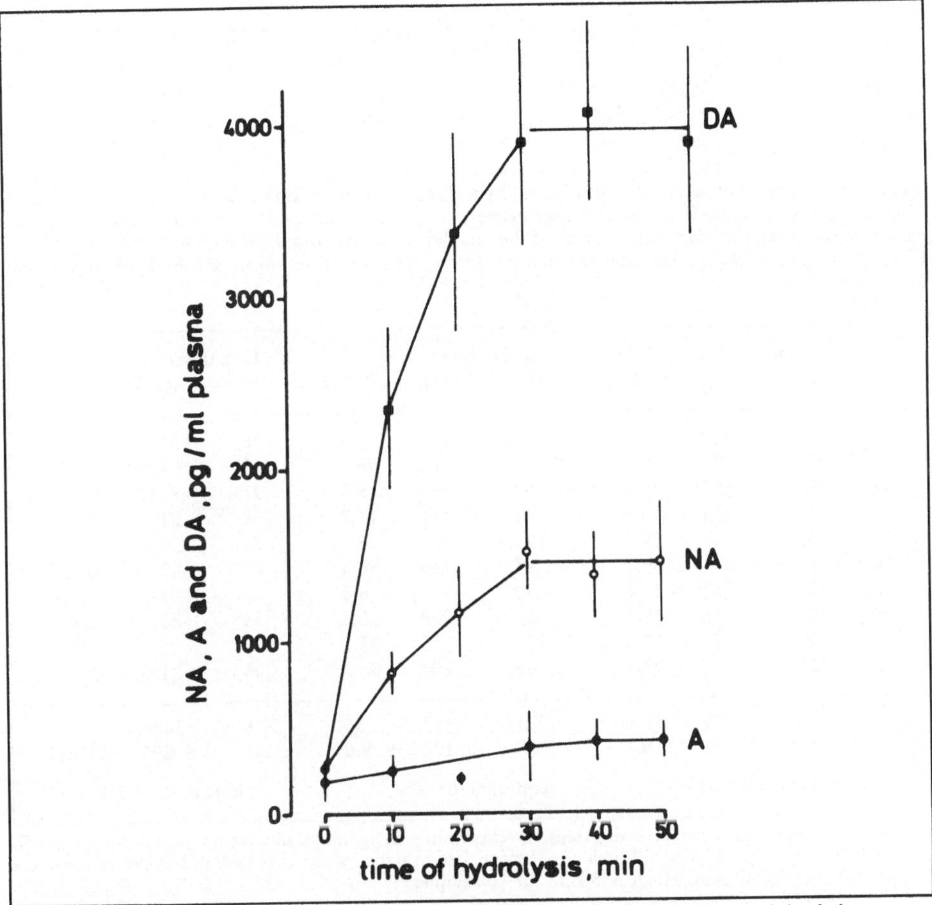

Figure 1: Rise of detectable catecholamines with increasing time of hydrolysis. Deproteinized plasma samples were heated for various times to 95° C, cooled and the catecholamines determined radioenzymatically. 0 min samples were kept at 20° C.

Complete hydrolysis was achieved after 40 min (Figure 1). The rate of destruction of catecholamines was determined after various times of hydrolysis. There was no detectable loss of NA, A and DA (Table 1). Table 2 shows the catecholamine contents of plasma samples from blood donors. The individual values for free NA vary from 10 to 60%, those for A from 5 to 95% and those for DA are usually less than 1%. Free NA and A together amount to 16% according to Buu and Kuchel [1], whereas DA was not detectable. The mean of our values is higher probably due to the moderate degree of stress caused by the loss of blood. Preliminary studies showed that the percentage of free and conjugated catecholamines vary with the intensity of stress (Figure 2).

Summary

A modified method for hydrolysis of conjugated plasma catecholamines is presented that yields complete hydrolysis without detectable destruction of noradrenaline, adrenaline and dopamine.
As there are considerable amounts of conjugated catecholamines in plasma, it is of interest whether

	CPM (before)	CPM (after)	100% = CPM before
NA	5274 ± 186	5120 ± 218	97.1 ± 4.7%
A	4299 ± 302	4199 ± 386	95.8 ± 9.0%
DA	9255 ± 441	9607 ± 511	103.4 ± 5.5%

Table 1: Destruction of catecholamines during hydrolysis. To deproteinized samples were added 100 pg NA, 100 pg A and 100 pg DA before or after hydrolysis so that the internal standard was heated together with the plasma catecholamines in one part of the samples. CPM are counts per minute of the samples plus CPM of 100 pg catecholamines after the radioenzymatic determination. Mean ± S.E.M. of 10 different plasma samples.

Age	Noradrenaline			Adrenaline			Dopamine		
	free	total	% free	free	total	% free	free	total	% free
20	79	738	10.7	49	835	5.9	26	3533	0.73
31	416	683	60.9	76	80	95	53	7877	0.68
37	356	892	39.9	92	563	16.3	27	8413	0.32
21	213	468	45.5	79	446	17.7	34	7108	0.48
23	330	1106	29.8	125	431	29	29	3095	0.94
26	345	631	54.7	81	149	54.4	27	3746	0.72
35	315	805	39.1	90	1330	6.8	30	4422	0.68
39	561	3017	18.6	81	224	36.2	35	5017	0.69
39	439	844	52.0	116	210	55.2	29	9423	0.31
40	206	903	22.8	68	204	33.3	36	2128	1.7
	326 ± 43	1008 ± 230	37.4 ± 5.2	87.5 ± 7	447 ± 122	35 ± 8.6	32.6 ± 2.5	5476 ± 800	0.73 ± 0.12
	conjugated: 62.6%			conjugated: 65%			conjugated: 99.3%		

Table 2: Free and total (free + conjugated) catecholamines in pg/ml plasma from blood donors immediately after loss of 500 ml blood. Plasma samples for determination of total NA, A and DA were routinely heated to 95° C for 40 min. Mean ± S.E.M. of 10 samples.

or not the total amount of noradrenaline, adrenaline and dopamine is a better indicator for the tone of the sympathetic nervous system than free noradrenaline and adrenaline alone. The presented method for hydrolysis is exceedingly simple such that measurement of conjugated catecholamines is no more difficult than measuring free catecholamines alone.

References

[1] N. T. Buu and O. Kuchel, J. Lab. Clin. Med. *90*, 680—685 (1977)

[2] M. Daprada and G. Zürcher, Life Sci. *19*, 1161—1174 (1976)

[3] J. Häggendahl, Acta physiol. scand. *59*, 255—260 (1963)

[4] Z. Kahane, A. H. Esser, N. S. Kine and P. Vestergaard, J. Lab. Clin. Med. *69*, 1042—1050 (1967)

[5] J. D. Peuler and G. A. Johnson, Life Sci. *21*, 625—636 (1977)

[6] H. Weil-Malherbe, Z. Klin. Chem. *2*, 161—167 (1964)

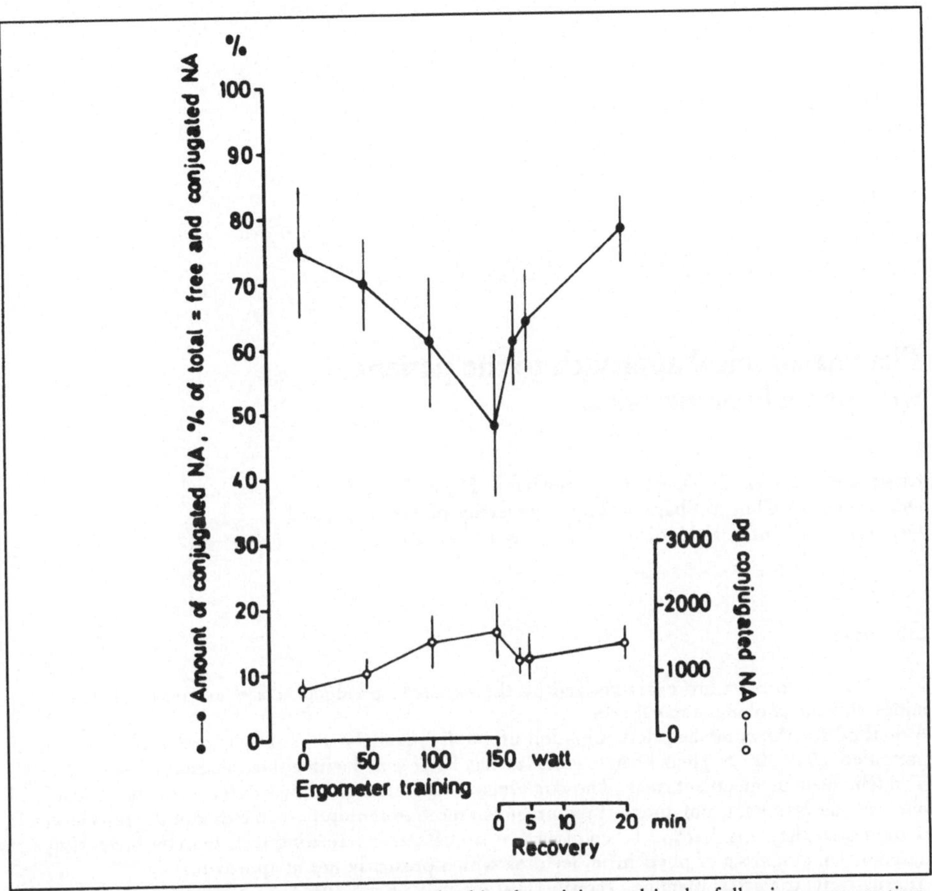

Figure 2: Conjugated plasma noradrenaline under bicycle training and in the following recovery time. Volunteers rode on an ergometer bicycle producing an output of 50, 100 and 150 watt for 5 min. At the end of each exercise, and at certain times during the following recovery, blood was drawn from the antecubital vein and free and conjugated NA was determined. The percentage of conjugated NA falls during the physical training. The amount of conjugated NA raises under physical stress.
Volunteers: 4 male and 4 female persons, 22—39 years old.

Pharmacological approach to the patient with pheochromocytoma

Kirsten, R., Heintz, B., Deeg, P., Hennemann, H., Nelson, K.
Department of Clinical Pharmacology, University of Frankfurt and
Department of Internal Medicine, University of Würzburg

Summary

Pheochromocytomata are characterized by the excessive production and excretion of catecholamines and catecholamine metabolites.
A method for the combined determination of vanillylmandelic acid and metanephrines in urine is presented. 80 to 90% of pheochromocytomata may be detected with either determination of vanillylmandelic acid or metanephrines. The combined determination allows detection of practically all pheochromocytomata, and does not require much more expenditure than either of the tests alone. It is suggested that this method be employed as an effective screening test, thereby improving the antemortem diagnosis of pheochromocytoma which presently lies at approximately 35%.
Alternatively, the catecholamine excretion in urine may be measured. 13 of 14 pheochromocytoma patients exhibited increased concentration of norepinephrine in 24 h urine samples. This study does not allow a definitive conclusion as to which method is more effective in diagnosing pheochromocytoma.
In plasma, the determination of catecholamines, using the technique of central venous blood sampling can be utilized in localizing small or poorly vascularized tumors when radiological techniques fail.

Introduction

Although pheochromocytomata account for only 0.1% of all hypertension cases [13], these tumors are life threatening, invariably leading to death when unrecognized or untreated. Diagnosis and localization of the tumor are worthwhile since surgical removal cures at least 97% of these patients [15].
The rareness and kaleidoscopic symptoms of the disease are two important reasons why the pheochromocytoma so often remains undetected. Even the hypertension is by no means an infallible symptom; occasionally patients are normotensive but death may result from a hypertensive crisis triggered by moderate stress or a surgical procedure. The "typical" paroxysmal character of the hypertension occurs in only half of all pheochromocytoma patients. The other 50% exhibit sustained hypertension, not differentiable from essential hypertension [13]. Further difficulty is encountered

in diagnosis since several disease entities such as neurofibromatosis, hemangioblastomas or medullary thyroid carcinomas may occur simultaneously with pheochromocytoma. The symptomatology of these diseases can overshadow the clinical manifestations provoked by the pheochromocytoma. Adding to the confusion is the experience that besides the most typical complaints such as headache, excessive sweating, palpitations, tachycardia and hypertension, other symptoms which may occur which are not unique to pheochromocytoma. For example, hyperglycemia and impairment of glucose tolerance may easily be mistaken for symptoms of diabetes mellitus [13]. Sweating, weight loss and tremor might suggest hyperthyroidism. Tachypnea, anxiety, anorexia or emotional lability often suggest psychiatric disorders [9].
These examples underscore why "The Great Mimic" [5], pheochromocytoma, often escapes the correct diagnosis. The only way to nonsurgically verify the diagnosis of pheochromocytoma is to demonstrate enhanced levels of catecholamines or their metabolites in the plasma or urine.
Numerous reports have emphasized the reliability of the quantitative determination of the catecholamines and their metabolites in detecting pheochromocytoma [1, 4, 6]. Provided specific and accurate methods are applied, the diagnosis can be established in most cases. Summarizing the results of four of the most advanced centres for quantitating catecholamines and catabolites, only 2 from 191 confirmed pheochromozytoma cases exhibited normal values when both vanillylmandelic acid and metanephrines were determined [8, 14]. Adding the assay of epinephrine, norepinephrine and dopamine in urine, all pheochromocytoma could be diagnosed. Two prerequisites for diagnosis must be met: first, urine from patients with paroxysmal hypertension or with intermittent clinical manifestations should be collected on several occasions to increase the chance of obtaining samples from active intervals; second, the methods should be highly reproduceable so that the normal range of urine values is kept within narrow limits.

Methods

Combined quantitative determination of vanillylmandelic acid and metanephrines (Figure 1)—A 2 ml sample of 24 h urine was hydrolyzed by adding 200 µl 3.2 N HCl, lyophilized and extracted in 2 ml ethylacetate by shaking for 1 minute [2]. The aqueous phase was frozen by dipping the tube into liquid nitrogen and decanting the unfrozen organic phase into a clean tube. 100 µl of 1 mM NaOH was added to the ethylacetate. The tube was shaken 1 minute, the aqueous phase again frozen and the organic phase decanted and discarded. The aqueous phase was adjusted to pH 1 and lyophilized. The residue was dissolved in 20 µl ethanol and applied to TLC plates (silica gel 60 F_{254} with concentrating zone, precoated layer thickness 0.25 mm, Merck 11798). The plates were developed twice in the following solvent system: isopropanol-ethylacetate-ammonia-water, (45:30:17:8) [17], drying between developments. The separated spots (Figure 2) were quantitated (Figure 3) at 254 mµ employing fluorescence quenching (remission) with a Zeiss Chromatogram Spectralphotometer KM 3 [10].
Catecholamines—The catecholamines (Figure 4) were determined according to the radioenzymatic method first described by Axelrod [3]. One ml blood samples, obtained by vena-cava catheterization were mixed with 20 µl of a stabilizing solution containing 95 mg EGTA and 60 mg glutathione per ml. The samples were immediately centrifuged (30 seconds at 12000 rpm), and the plasma frozen in liquid nitrogen. 50 µl plasma or 50 µl 1:10 diluted urine were then incubated with catechol-O-methyltransferase (COMT) and ^3H marked S-adenosyl-L-methionine (SAM). A radioactive methyl group is transferred from the ^3H-SAM to the catecholamines during incubation. The products of this reaction are methylated analogs of the catecholamines (metanephrines) which are stable, readily separable and measurable. The metanephrines were extracted into a 3:2 toluol/isoamylalcohol mixture, applied to thin layer chromatography aluminum cards and developed in the following solvent system: t-amylalcohol/ethanol/propanol/benzol/methylamine (2:1:2:5:5). The separated metanephrine spots were visualized under UV light, cut out and transferred to liquid scintillation vials where the radioactivity was measured. The assay range is between 0.006 and 10 pmol with a variation coefficient of 3%. Interference between the three catecholamines lies under 1%. Figure 5 shows the separated metanephrines [11].

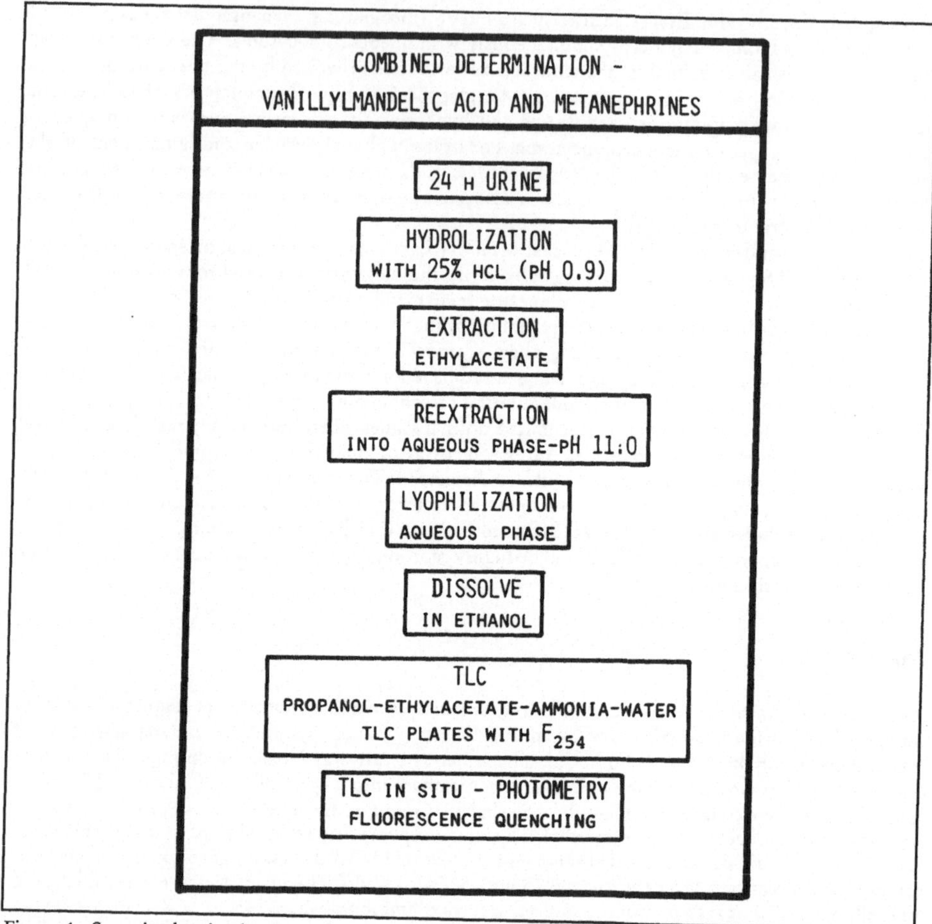

Figure 1: Steps in the simultaneous determination of vanillylmandelic acid and metanephrines.

Results

Diagnosis based on vanillylmandelic acid and metanephrines in urine—Table 1 shows the means and ranges of vanillylmandelic acid and metanephrines from 48 non-pheochromocytoma patients (20—60 years) and 37 pheochromocytoma patients. No pheochromocytoma patient exhibited less than 11.6 nmol metanephrines/mg creatinine in urine. Only 1 of 48 non-pheochromocytoma patients exhibited more than 11.6 nmol metanephrines/mg creatinine. None of these patients had more than 23.7 nmol metanephrines/mg creatinine, whereas 80% of the pheochromocytoma patients exhibited values higher than 23.7 nmol metanephrines/mg creatinine.

Vanillylmandelic acid in urine ranged from 6.70—26.0 nmol/mg creatinine in non-pheochromocytoma patients with a mean of 7.22 nmol/mg creatinine. The range for the pheochromocytoma patients was 18.04—284 nmol/mg creatinine with a mean of 91 nmol/mg creatinine. 97% of pheochromocytoma patients revealed a concentration of more than 26 nmol/mg creatinine in urine.

Diagnosis based on catecholamines in urine—Table 2 compares the excretion values and range for norepinephrine, epinephrine and dopamine in 48 non-pheochromocytoma and 14 pheochromocytoma patients. 13 pheochromocytoma cases exhibited higher values of norepinephrine, 5 of the cases more epinephrine and 8 cases more dopamine than those from non-pheochromocytoma patients.

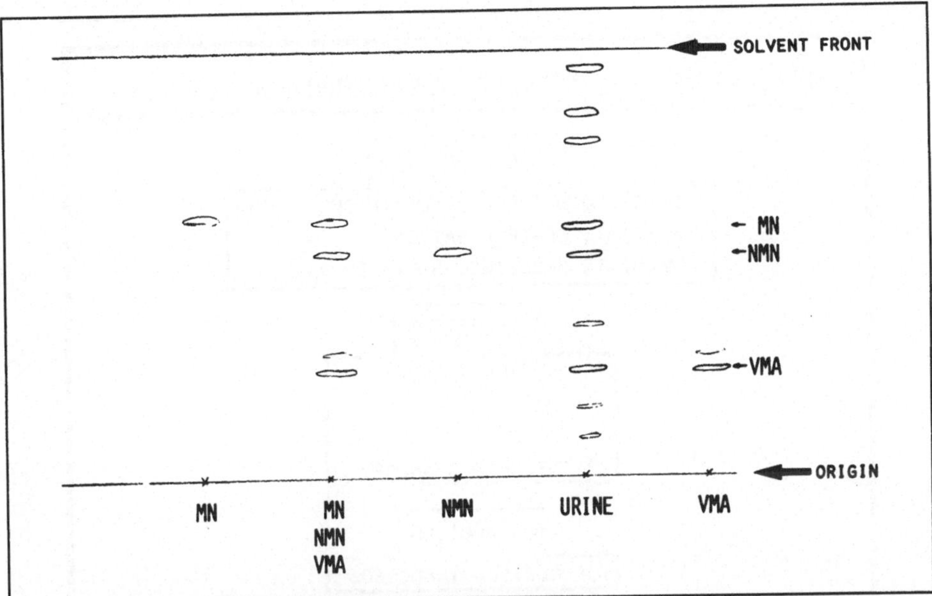

Figure 2: Thin-layer-chromatogram pattern of vanillylmandelic acid and metanephrines. Spots marked with pencil under u-v-lamp. Solvent system: iso-propanol—ethylacetate—ammonia—water. MN = metanephrine, NMN = normetanephrine, VMA = vanillylmandelic acid.

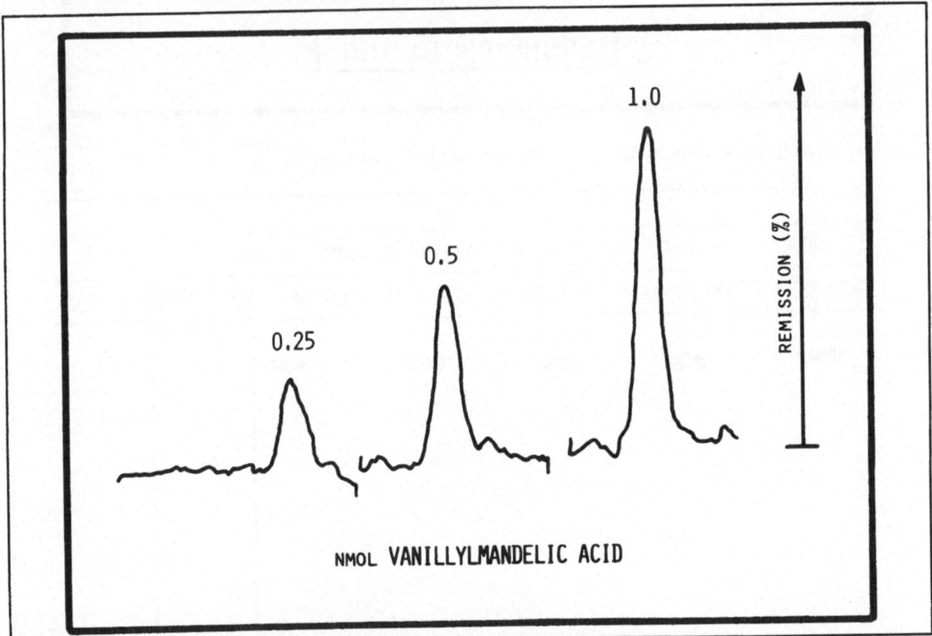

Figure 3: Remission recording of 3 standards (0.25, 0.5 and 1 nmoles) of vanillylmandelic acid after thin-layer-chromatography. $\lambda_{Exc.}$ = 254 nm; $\lambda_{Em.}$ = 484 nm; sec. filter: 325—2500 nm; recording speed: 120 mm/min; slit: 0.1 nm. Area under peak is proportional to amount of vanillylmandelic acid.

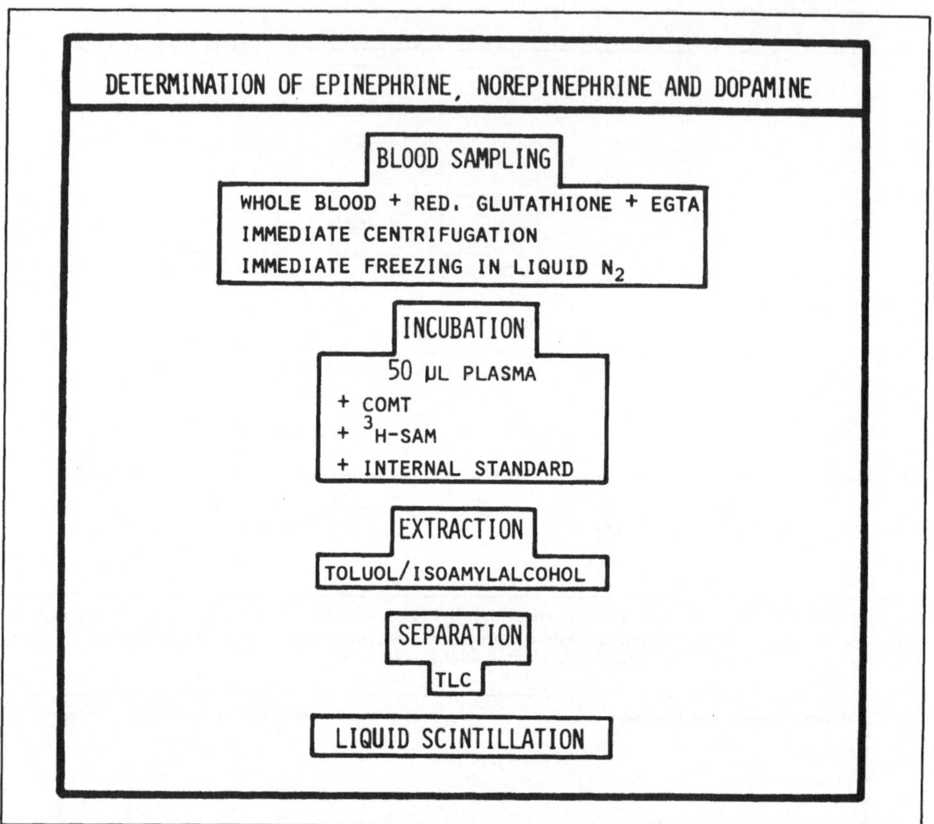

Figure 4: Steps in the determination of catecholamines in blood samples.

TLC-CARDS SILICA GEL F_{254} 0.20 MM DEVELOPING TIME : 45 MIN.

PROPANOL + ETHANOL + t-AMYLALCOHOL + BENZOL + METHYLAMINE

SUBSTANCE	R_f-VALUE
MT	0.66
MN	0.48
NMN	0.35

Figure 5: Thin-layer-chromatogram pattern from blood samples of methylated catecholamines. Original: spots darkened under day light. MT = methoxytyramine, MN = metanephrine, NMN = normetanephrine.

URINARY VALUES OF CATECHOLAMINE METABOLITES (NMOL / MG CREATININE)			
		CONTROLS	PHEOCHROMOCYTOMA
METANEPHRINES	RANGE	4.75 - 19.5	11.6 - 296
	MEAN	8.95	82.1
	BORDER VALUE & FREQUENCY	<11.6 (98%) <23.7 (100%)	>11.6 (100%) >23.7 (80%)
VANILLYL-MANDELIC ACID	RANGE	6.70 - 26.0	18.04 - 284
	MEAN	7.22	91.8
	BORDER VALUE & FREQUENCY	<26 (100%)	>26 (97%)

Table 1: Urinary values of catecholamine metabolites (nmol/mg creatinine) from 48 non-pheochromocytoma adults (controls) and 37 pheochromocytoma patients.

Tumor localization by determination of plasma catecholamines—Table 3 lists the concentration of catecholamines in plasma obtained via venous catheterization from various levels of the vena cava from a patient with confirmed pheochromocytoma. The elevation of the catecholamines in the plasma of the vein draining the left adrenal coincided with the tumor site.

Discussion

Methods—Considering that only every third pheochromocytoma patient is diagnosed antemortem [9, 18], emphasis must be put on reliable diagnosis. Since only 0.1% of all hypertonic patients carry a pheochromocytoma, diagnosis should be inexpensive, fast, reliable and simple. The combined method described for vanillylmandelic acid and metanephrines fulfills these requirements as a screening test and should be able to close the "diagnosis gap" [7].
For combined determination of vanillylmandelic acid and metanephrines preliminary extraction with ethylacetate is necessary to eliminate urinary substances interfering in the subsequent thin-layer separation. Simple colorimetric tests based on transformation of vanillylmandelic acid to vanillin are less exact for two reasons: first, urinary substances other than vanillylmandelic acid may be converted to vanillin or vanillin like compounds and are responsible for the large range of values found. Usage of such methods may allow tumors secreting smaller amounts of vanillylmandelic acid or a higher percentage of catecholamines to remain undetected due to the wide "normal" range; second, methods based on measuring the vanillin produced from vanillylmandelic acid are influenced by the varying content of vanillin in the diet [16].
The radioenzymatic micromethod for quantitative determination of catecholamines in plasma is reproducable and requires only 10 ml blood for a total of 30 different samples—sufficient for safe tumor localization [11].
Results—80 to 90% of pheochromocytomata may be detected with any single method; either determination in urine of vanillylmandelic acid, metanephrines or catecholamines. At least one of these three urine components was above the normal range in 48 pheochromocytoma patients. The three tests are equally reliable with the determination of vanillylmandelic acid and metanephrines being

URINARY EXCRETION OF CATECHOLAMINES (NMOL/MG CREATININE)			
		NON-PHEOCHROMOCYTOMA	PHEOCHROMOCYTOMA
NOREPINEPHRINE	MEAN (± SD)	230 ± 96	3900 ± 6450
	RANGE	80 - 305	290 - 36100
	BORDER VALUE & FREQUENCY (%)	< 305 (100%) < 290 (80%)	> 305 (92.9%) > 290 (100%)
EPINEPHRINE	MEAN (± SD)	45 ± 28	630 ± 1120
	RANGE	5 - 84	5 - 5600
	BORDER VALUE & FREQUENCY (%)	< 84 (100%)	> 84 (35.7%)
DOPAMINE	MEAN (± SD)	1080 ± 44	4630 ± 5200
	RANGE	280 - 1620	630 - 22400
	BORDER VALUE & FREQUENCY (%)	< 1620 (100%)	> 1620 (57.1%)

Table 2: Urinary excretion of catecholamines (nmol/mg creatinine) from 48 non-pheochromocytoma adults and 14 pheochromocytoma patients.

easier to carry out than the determination of catecholamines. This study does not allow a definitive conclusion as to which method is more effective in diagnosing pheochromocytoma.
The combined determination of vanillylmandelic acid and metanephrines presented here has the advantage of requiring approximately the same amount of time and material as either test alone. This combination makes an excellent screening test which allows detection of practically all pheochromocytomata, obviating the need for the more complicated determination of urine catecholamines.
Due to diurnal variation and the paroxysmal secretion pattern of the catecholamine producing tumor, a 24 h sample of the urine is recommended.
Before the final diagnosis of pheochromocytoma is drawn as a result of one or more of the above mentioned tests, other disease entities accompanied by increased excretion of catecholamines must be excluded. Traumatological conditions with intracranial lesions, autonomic hyperflexia, eclampsia, hypoglycemia, acrodynia, porphyria, lead poisoning and tetanus are all conditions where increased catecholamine excretion has been observed [13].

SAMPLE LOCATION	NOREPINEPHRINE	EPINEPHRINE (PMOL/ML PLASMA)	DOPAMINE
VENA JUGULARIS DEXTRA	3.17	0.23	0.06
" SUBCLAVIA DEXTRA	4.30	0.28	0.08
" " SINISTRA	4.63	0.22	0.03
" CAVA SUPERIOR, LEVEL T_{10}	4.68	0.19	0.09
" " " , LEVEL T_{12}	5.15	3.26	1.68
ATRIUM DEXTRUM	4.99	0.88	0.36
VENTRICULUM DEXTRUM	6.47	1.13	1.19
VENA HEPATICA	2.88	0.79	3.46
" SUPRARENALIS DEXTRA	5.46	2.14	0.79
" " SINISTRA	24.53	60.68	2.46
" RENALIS DEXTRA	8.79	6.47	1.79
" " SINISTRA	4.93	0.66	0.99
" CAVA INFERIOR, LEVEL L_2	3.87	0.24	0.09
" " " , LEVEL L_4	4.32	0.31	0.16
" ILIACA COMMUNIS DEXTRA	4.98	0.19	0.05
" " " SINISTRA	4.11	0.13	0.08
" " INTERNA DEXTRA	4.89	0.21	0.07
" " " SINISTRA	3.57	0.09	0.09
" " EXTERNA DEXTRA	4.49	0.26	0.04
" " " SINISTRA	3.33	0.08	0.12

Table 3: Catecholamine concentrations in plasma samples drawn from various sites of the vena cava: distinct increase of epinephrine *in vena* suprarenalis sinistra.

The case shown in Table 3 is an example of the possibility for employing vena cava catheterization for localization of an established tumor. More examples demonstrating reliability of this localization technique have recently been described in detail [12]. Pheochromocytomata vary from 3 to more than 3000 grams [13] and vascularization varies considerably, making some tumors impossible to locate with radiological techniques. Small, poorly vascularized tumors which cannot be radiologically localized may be localized using vena cava catheterization and determination of catecholamines in plasma samples [12].
This pharmacological approach to the suspected pheochromocytoma patient enables the physician to confirm or exclude the diagnosis of a catecholamine secreting tumor, and when confirmed, to localize the pheochromocytoma as well.

References

[1] Amery, A., Conway, J.: A critical review of diagnostic tests for pheochromocytoma. Am. Heart J. *73*, 129—133 (1967).

[2] Armstrong, M. D., Shaw, K. N. F., Wall, P. E.: The phenolic acids in human urine. Paper chromatography of phenolic acids. J. Biol. Chem. *218*, 293—303 (1956).

[3] Axelrod, J.: O-methylation of epinephrine and other catechols in vitro and in vivo. Science *126*, 400—401 (1957).

[4] Crout, J. R., Sjoerdsma, A.: Catecholamines in the localization of pheochromocytoma. Circulation *22*, 516—525 (1960).

[5] Decourcy, J. L., Decourcy, C. B.: Pheochromocytomas and the General Practitioner. Cincinnati, Barclay Newman (1952).

[6] Engel, A., v. Euler, U. S.: Diagnostic value of increased urinary output of noradrenaline and adrenaline in pheochromocytoma. Lancet II, 387 (1950).

[7] Engelman, K.: Principles in the diagnosis of pheochromocytoma. Bull. N. Y. Acad. Med. *45*, 851—858 (1969).

[8] Gitlow, S. E., Mendlowitz, M., Bertani, L. M.: The biochemical techniques for detecting and establishing the presence of a pheochromocytoma. Am. J. Cardiol. *26*, 270—279 (1970).

[9] Hermann, H., Mornex, R.: Human Tumours secreting catecholamines: Clinical and physiopathological study of the pheochromocytomas. Oxford, New York, Pergamon Press (1964).

[10] Kirsten, R., Heintz, B., Heintz, St., Ullrich, St.: Combined quantitative determination of vanillylmandelic acid and metanephrines in urine. In preparation.

[11] Kirsten, R., Heintz, B., Nelson, K.: Optimized radioenzymatic determination of catecholamines. In preparation.

[12] Kirsten, R., Hennemann, H., Heintz, B., Nelson, K.: Methoden zur Lokalisations-Diagnostik von Katecholamin-Sezernierenden Tumoren. In: Hierholzer, K., Rietbrock, N., Eds.: Physiologische und pharmakologische Grundlagen der Therapie, Berliner Seminar 3, Braunschweig, Vieweg (1980).

[13] Manger, W. M., Gifford, R. W., Jr.: Pheochromocytoma. New York, Heidelberg, Berlin, Springer-Verlag (1977).

[14] Pertsemlidis, D., Gitlow, S. E., Siegel, W. C., Kark, A. E.: Pheochromocytoma: 1. Specificity of laboratory diagnostic tests, 2. Safeguards during operative removal. Ann. Surg. *169*, 376—385 (1969).

[15] Remine, W. H., Chong, G. C., van Heerden, J. A., Sheps, S. G., Harrison, E. G., Jr.: Current management of pheochromocytoma. Ann. Surg. *179*, 740—748 (1974).

[16] Sandler, M., Ruthven, C. R. J.: The measurement of 4-hydroxy-3-methoxymandelic acid and homovanillic acid. Pharmacol. Rev. *18*, 343—351 (1966).

[17] Schmid, E., Henning, N.: Über den Nachweis der 3-Methoxy-4-Hydroxy-Mandelsäure im Harn. Klin. Wschr. *41*, 566—567 (1963).

[18] Smithwick, R. H., Greer, W. E. R., Robertson, C. W., Wilkins, R. W.: Pheochromocytoma; a discussion of symptoms, signs and procedures of diagnostic value. New Engl. J. Med. *242*, 252—257 (1950).

Chapter 11

Assessment of interactions and side effects

Beidellite (an aluminium silicate) and digoxin, checking of a suspected drug interaction by *in vivo* and *in vitro* assays

E. Albengres*, J. C. Le Parco**, and J.-P. Tillement*

* Département de Pharmacologie, Faculté de Médecine de PARIS XII, 8 rue du Général Sarrail, F 94010 CRETEIL

** Service de Médecine Interne, Hôpital Albert Chennevier, 40 rue de Mesly, F 94020 CRETEIL

Introduction

Drug-drug interactions where gastric protecting drugs impair the absorption of simultaneously orally administered drugs are well known [1, 7, 9, 10, 12, 15]. However there is no general rule since only a lower absorption rate [8] or no obvious interaction [4] can sometimes be observed. Moreover, when drugs are not simultaneously administered but given in different chronological sequences, the occurrence of such a drug interaction could be modified [13].
Beidellite (*) is a smectite widely used in France as a gastric protecting drug. It is an aluminium silicate (Si_4O_{10}) (Al_2) (OH_2) with a layered crystalline structure. Each layer is composed of three folias, two tetraedrics with aluminium and one octaedric with silicate. The layers are repetitively disposed including between them cationic substances: K^+, Na^+, Ca^{++} which weakly bind to the oxygens of the folias, and constitutive H_2O. Previous *in vitro* studies [12] showed that beidellite can interact with different neutral drugs mainly by physical absorption and possibly by OH-binding.
As digoxin is a non-ionizable, i. e. neutral and an incompletely absorbed drug even after oral administration of aqueous-alcoholic solution [6], it seemed to be a good model to check a possible beidellite interaction. This was done by both *in vivo* and *in vitro* studies. The first studies involved a comparison in humans of the bioavailability of digoxin tablets, given alone or in combination with beidellite in different sequences. Later studies were to measure the amount of digoxin bound to beidellite and to check the reversibility of the binding.
Two main questions were to be answered: does beidellite significantly impair digoxin absorption? Could an *in vitro* experiment be a valuable predicting test for such a drug interaction?

(*) *Smecta*®, I.P.S.E.N.

Materials and methods

In vivo assay

This consisted of a four way cross over study conducted in twelve healthy volunteers (21 to 29 years), nine men and three women, weighing 58 to 73 kg. They took no medication in the period 12 hours prior to the study and received a light lunch 4 hours after ingestion of the drugs. The relative absorption of a single dose of digoxin (*) 0.5 mg, was checked after the following four treatments: digoxin and beidellite (3000 mg) simultaneously administered, digoxin 0.5 hour before beidellite, digoxin 0.5 hour after beidellite, digoxin alone. The subjects received their second, third and fourth treatment at two week intervals. The sequence of the four treatments was randomized for each subject.

Blood samples were taken at different times; 0 (before digoxin intake), 5, 10, 15, 20, 30, 45, 60 minutes and at 1.25, 1.5, 1.75, 2, 4, 6, 8, 24, 48 hours, and urine samples were collected for four days as follows: 0—2, 2—4, 4—6, 6—8, 8—24, 24—48, 48—72, 72—96 hours.

Relative bioavailability was estimated by means of four parameters [14]: areas under the plasma concentration versus time curves, maximum plasma concentrations, times to the maximum plasma concentrations, amounts of drug excreted unchanged in the urine as percentage of total. Results were compared either using mean values (M ± SD) in the Student-t-test, or using the different values obtained with the four treatments in the same subject with the non-parametric WILCOXON matched pairs signed ranks test.

The plasma and urine samples were analyzed by radio immunoassay (*CEA*).

In vitro assays

The fraction of the digoxin dose adsorbed by the beidellite was estimated in the following way: samples were prepared in 3 ml tubes by adding beidellite 100 mg and 1 ml of a digoxin solution of 2.5 μg/ml of unlabelled compound into which was incorporated 5 ng/ml of labelled digoxin (^3H, Amersham®, 10.6 Ci/mole). pH adjustments were made either to 2.0 or to 5.5. The samples were agitated (stirring = 50 per minute) in a water bath for different time-intervals, 0.5, 1, 1.5, 2.5, 3, 4, 5, 15, 30 and 60 minutes and four samples were carried out for each time-interval. The samples were then centrifugated for 15 minutes at 3000 rpm and the concentrations of free labelled digoxin were measured in the supernatant by liquid scintillation counting. The adsorption reversibility was checked as follows:

samples were prepared as already described but after incubation for 2 minutes and centrifugation for 15 minutes at 3000 rpm, the supernatant was removed and 3 ml of a buffered solution (pH 2.0 or 5.5) were added. The mixture was then resuspended and incubated with stirring for 2 minutes as described above. This was repeated 2 more times, each 2 minutes for a total of 6 minutes washing. 8 samples for each time-period were performed.

Results

In vivo assay

The mean values ($M \pm SD$) of the four parameters previously mentioned are summarized in Table I. It is clear that no statistically significant differences were found between the four treatments, and this is confirmed by the results of the non-parametric WILCOXON test as shown in Table II. T is the smallest sum of like signed ranks, N is the number of matched pairs minus the number of equal pairs. If an observed T is equal or less than the values given in the proper table under a particular significance level for the observed value of N, the null hypothesis may be rejected at that level of significance. At a 0.05 level the observed T must be equal or less than 2 if $N = 7$, 4 if $N = 8$, 6 if $N = 9$, 11 if $N = 11$, 14 if $N = 12$. None of the present T values is small enough to reject the null hypothesis. The mean plasma digoxin concentrations versus time curves obtained with digoxin alone or associated with beidellite are shown in Figure 1. Although the mean values do not differ significantly, the slight difference between the maximum levels as shown in that figure and the slight delay in time to maximum level which was found for each subject comparing digoxin alone versus digoxin plus beidellite results, suggest a decrease in the absorption rate which was analyzed by *in vitro* experiments.

(*) two tablets of *Digoxine Nativelle®*

In vitro assays

Within 2 minutes, about 45% of the digoxin dose is fixed by beidellite and remained adsorbed during the time of the experiment, 60 minutes (Figure 2). This was observed at pH = 2.0 and pH = 5.5. At both pH values, more than half of the digoxin remains free when in contact with the corresponding dose of beidellite.
The adsorption phenomenon is quickly reversible as indicated on table III. The adsorbed digoxin is almost completely released in 6 minutes.

Treatment	AUC µg ml−1h	*C*max ng/ml	*TC*max min.	$\frac{U}{T} \times 100$
Digoxin alone	27.36 ± 15.88	3.68 ± 1.32	52.5 ± 13.57	44.19 ± 13.62
Digoxin + Beidellite	21.1 ± 10.5	3.18 ± 0.70	51.92 ± 14.16	47.16 ± 14.96
Digoxin before Beidellite	27.57 ± 12.64	3.55 ± 1.42	46.92 ± 16.36	39.51 ± 7.85
Beidellite before Digoxin	21.72 ± 10.62	3.1 ± 1.11	56.92 ± 11.77	38.47 ± 6.96

Table 1: Parameters of digoxin bioavailability

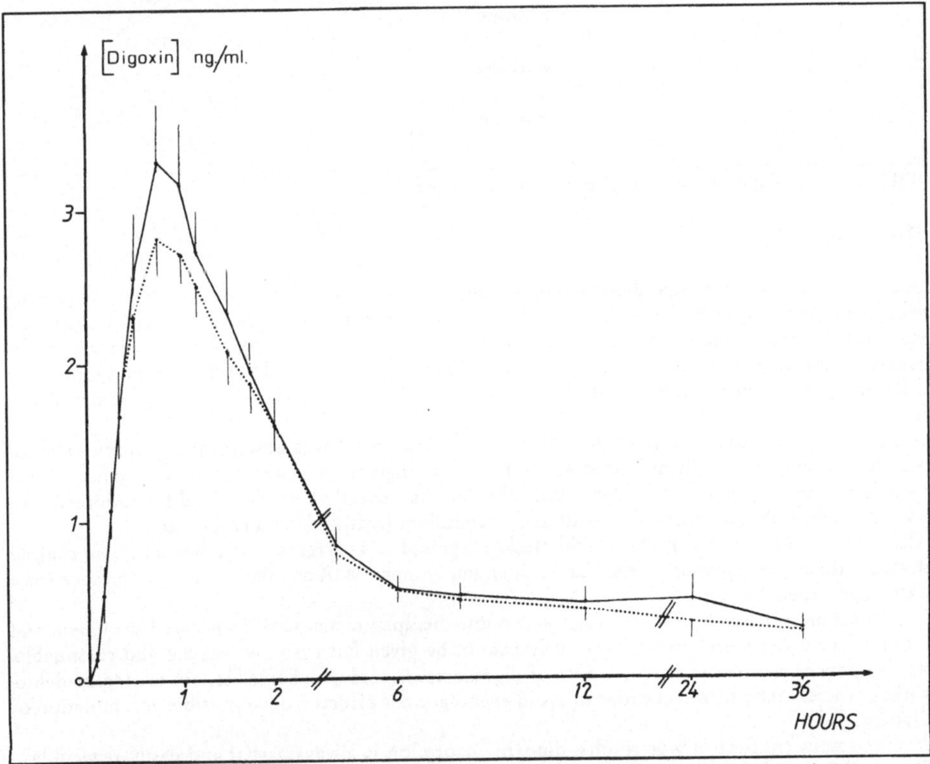

Figure 1: *Mean (M ± SD) plasma digoxin concentrations obtained with digoxin given alone* (full line) *or in association with beidellite* (dotted line)

Parameters \ Treatments	Digoxin alone *versus* Digoxin before beidellite	Beidellite before digoxin	Digoxin and beidellite
AUC	$T+ = 38$ $N = 12$	$T- = 30$ $N = 12$	$T- = 24$ $N = 12$
C max	$T+ = T- = 39$ $N = 12$	$T- = 23$ $N = 11$	$T- = 15$ $N = 11$
T max	$T- = 9$ $N = 8$	$T+ = 9$ $N = 7$	$T- = 22$ $N = 9$
Elimination levels	$T- = 27$ $N = 12$	$T- = 23$ $N = 12$	$T- = 34$ $N = 12$

Table 2: Non parametric WILCOXON matched pairs signed ranks test results

Time in minutes		Free digoxin (cumulated in % of total dose)
2		53.6 ± 2.6
	washing	
4		75.9 ± 3.4
	washing	
6		88.4 ± 4.2
	washing	
8		95.8 ± 5.0

Table 3: Reversibility of digoxin adsorption by beidellite *in vitro*

Discussion

Both statistical tests show that digoxin bioavailability is not impaired by beidellite whatever the drug sequences used. Digoxin plasma kinetics show marked interindividual variations which raises the standard deviations and decreases the sensitivity of the parametric tests applied to mean values. However, the non parametric WILCOXON test is not limited in this way. Thus the lack of a significant difference, when this test is used, clearly shows that beidellite does not impair digoxin bioavailability.

It is generally claimed that gastric protecting compounds impair drug absorption [2] and this phenomenon has been specifically discussed with reference to digoxin [5]. The results obtained here therefore seem unusual; however the same lack of effect has already been described for indomethacin with a mixture of aluminium hydroxide and magnesium hydroxide and carbonate [5].

Although not statistically significant, the study suggested to us (Figure 1) that beidellite can slightly decrease the digoxin plasma levels. Can such an impairment be of any therapeutic importance for a particular patient?

This question is directed towards drugs with a low therapeutic index, as is the case for digoxin and indomethacin. A general answer obviously cannot be given but it seems sensible and reasonable, when a patient receives an effective dose of digoxin associated with beidellite, not to stop beidellite without careful monitoring in order to avoid eventual toxic effects from a possible accumulation of digoxin.

In vitro assays confirm *in vivo* results: digoxin adsorption is always partial and easily reversible. Digoxin adsorption by another group of smectites, namely montmorillonites has been reported [11]. This binding induces some degradation of digoxin [12] specially at pH = 2.0, and for this reason, it

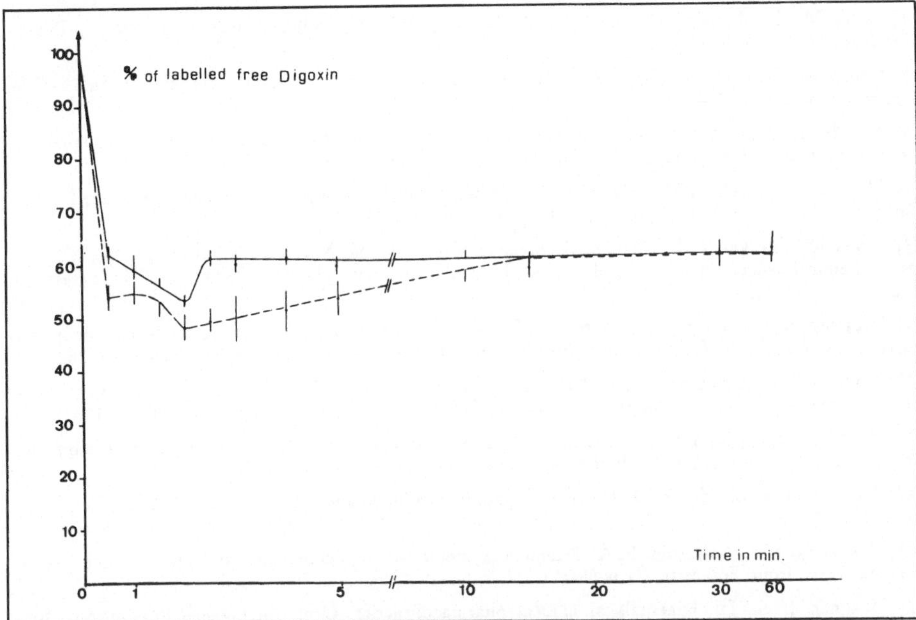

Figure 2: *Digoxin adsorption by beidellite in vitro* at pH = 2, full line and pH = 5.5., dotted line.

was suggested by these authors that combination of clays and digoxin should be avoided. These experiments however were performed using incubation times of several hours cf. 1 hour in the present study, and this could explain why digoxin degradation was observed. Our *in vivo* results showed that all the maximum plasma levels were reached in less than one hour and did not significantly differ when digoxin is administered alone or in combination with beidellite. Digoxin degredation therefore does not seem to be a problem *in vivo*.
The last question is to know if these *in vitro* experiments could be valuable as Prediction Test to forecast other similar drug interactions. In this study, they illustrate clearly that digoxin adsorption is quantitatively small and rapidly reversible thus indicating that impairment of digoxin absorption is unlikely. This was verified by the *in vivo* experiments.
These tests should be checked with other gastric protecting compounds and with other acidic and basic drugs so as to establish the value of the technique and its range of applicability.

Acknowledgments

Calculations and statistical interpretation of results have been done by P. d'Athis and N. Le Rumeur of Département d'Informatique Médicale, Hôpital du Bocage, Dijon Cedex (Pr. ag. L. Dusserre).

Reference

[1] Barr, W. H., Adir, J., Garretson, L.: Decrease of tetracycline absorption in man by sodium bicarbonate.—Clin. Pharmacol. Ther. 12, 779—784 (1971).

[2] Doherty, J. E.: Digitalis glycosides. Pharmacokinetics and their clinical implications.—Ann. Intern. Med. 79, 229—278 (1973).

[3] Galeazzi, R. L.: The effect of an antiacid on the bioavailability of indomethacin.—Europ. J. Clin. Pharmacol. 12, 65—68 (1977).

[4] Gault, M. H., Charles, J. D., Sugden, D. L., Kepkay, D. C.: Hydrolysis of digoxin by acid.—J. Pharm. Pharmac. 29, 27—32 (1976).

[5] Greenblatt, D. J., Smith, T. W., Koch-Weser, J.: Bioavailability of drugs: the digoxin dilemma.—Clin. Pharmacokinetics. 1, 36—51 (1976).

[6] Hauffman, D. H., Manion, C. V., Azarnoff, D. L.: Absorption of digoxin from different oral preparations in normal subjects during steady-state.—Clin. Pharmacol. Ther. 16, 310—317 (1974).

[7] Hurwitz, A., Sheehan, M. B.: The effect of antacids on the absorption of orally administered pentobarbital in the rat.—J. Pharmacol. Exp. Ther. 179, 124—131 (1971).

[8] Lewis, R. J., Trager, W. F., Chan, K. K., Breckenridge, A., Orme, M., Rowland, M., Shary, W.: Warfarin stereochemical aspects of its metabolism and the interaction with phenylbutazone.—J. Clin. Invest. 53, 1607—1617 (1974).

[9] Lucarotti, R. L., Colaizzi, J. L., Barry, H., Poust, R. I.: Enhanced pseudoephedrine absorption by concurrent administration of aluminium hydroxide gel in humans.—J. Pharm. Sci. 61, 903—905 (1952).

[10] Paul, H. E., Harrington, C. M.: Adsorption characteristics of adriamycin and terramycin on aluminium hydroxide gel and on bismuth subsalicylate preparation.—J. Amer. Pharm. Ass. 41, 50 (1952).

[11] Porubcan, L. S., Born, S. G., White, J. L., Hem, S. L.: Interaction of digoxin and montmorillonite: mechanism of adsorption and degradation.—J. Pharm. Sci. 68 [3], 358—361 (1979).

[12] Sternson, L. A, Shaffer, R. D.: Kinetics of digoxin stability in aqueous solution.—J. Pharm. Sci. 67 [3], 327—330 (1978).

[13] Tillement, J. P., Albengres, E. A.: Interactions médicamenteuses in Pharmacologie Clinique I.—Expansion Scientifique Francaise, Paris (1978).

[14] Wagner, J. G.: Fundamentals of clinical pharmacokinetics. Drug Intelligence Publications, Inc., Hamilton, Illinois, 1975.

[15] Waisbren, B. A., Hueckel, T. S.: Reduced absorption of aureomycin caused by aluminium hydroxide gel.—Proc. Soc. exp. Biol. Med. 73, 73—74 (1950).

In situ measurement of left ventricular pressure and cardiac output in rat heart after acute and chronic Adriamycin application*

B. Höfling and H.-D. Bolte
Medizinische Klinik I, Klinikum Großhadern der Universität München,
Marchioninistr. 15, 8000 München 70, W.-Germany

Introduction

Adriamycin is one of the most effective antitumor drugs [1]. Its clinical use is limited by cardiotoxic side effects [2, 3, 4]. Various cardioprotective agents such as digitalis, ubiquinone, coenzyme Q10, Vit. E, EDTA, carnitine and tocopherol are suggested [5, 6, 7, 8]. In our laboratory experiments were carried out in rats with simultaneous measurements of muscle-mechanical, hemodynamic and biochemical parameters with the following aims:

a) to define more precisely an experimental model;
b) to contribute to knowledge on the pathogenic mechanism in the development of the Adriamycin-cardiomyopathy;
c) to use this experimental model as a test-model to investigate cardioprotective effects of above mentioned drugs.

In this study the emphasis of our experiments was laid on hemodynamic changes following acute and chronic Adriamycin-application.

Method

Experiments were performed in thoracotomized adult Wistar rats during barbital or ether anesthesia. Cardiac output (minus coronary flow) was measured with an electromagnetic flowmeter around the ascending aorta. Left ventricular pressure curves were obtained by means of a steel-cannula in the left ventricle connected to statham transducers. In addition, ECG, heart rate, arterial pressure and venous pressure were monitored continuously and the heart was paced via the ventricle-cannula (see diagram). To study acute hemodynamic effects of Adriamycin, increasing doses of the drug were given intravenously. To study the chronic action of Adriamycin rats were pretreated with two to six courses of Adriamycin (each course was 1 mg drug/kg b.w., i. p., on 3 consecutive days followed by a rest of 4 days). After pretreatment, changes in left ventricular pressure, maximum rate of left ventricular pressure rise and heart frequency following maximally effective dobutamine doses were measured and compared with analogous data obtained in control rats.

* Supported by Wilhelm Sander-Stiftung

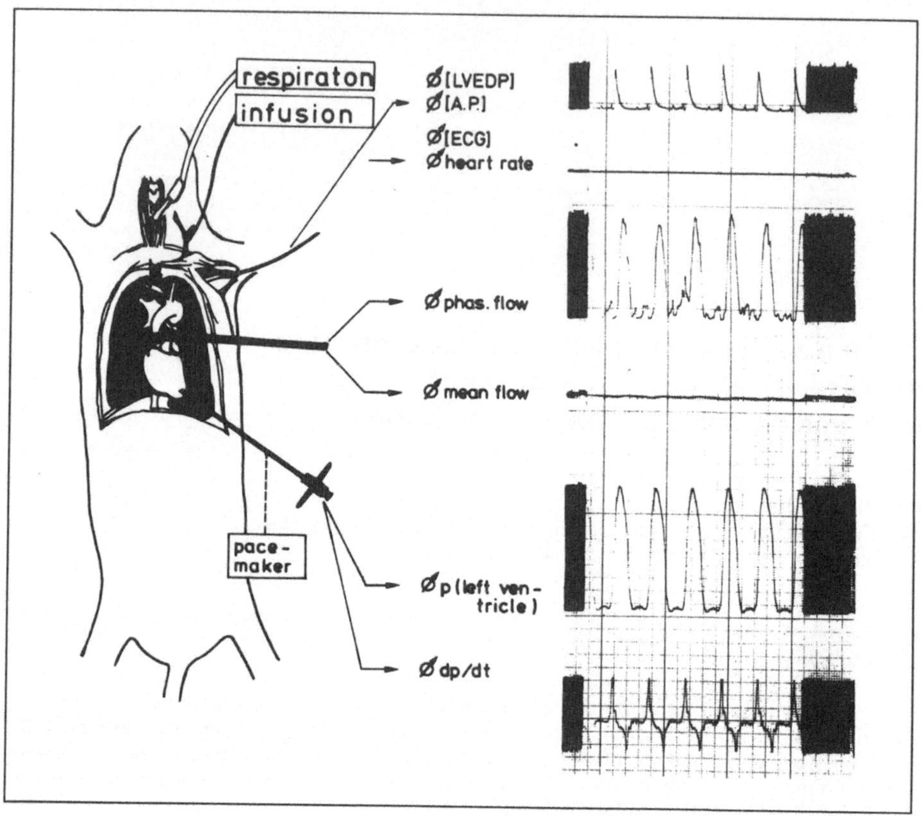

Results

Acute action of Adriamycin:

Figure 1 shows that Adriamycin causes a dose-dependent reduction of maximum left ventricular pressure. The cardio-depressive effect is 23.5 ± 14.8% of pre-drug value after a dose of only 2.5 mg/kg b.w. Further reduction of left ventricular pressure occurs with increasing doses until the lethal dose is reached around 30 mg/kg b.w. The maximum rate of left ventricular pressure rise (dp/dt_{max}) and the cardiac output are effected in a similar dose-dependent manner. The cardio-depressive effect develops within a few minutes and is spontaneously reversible in the early stages. In our experiments no ECG-changes could be observed.
These data demonstrate that there is an acute myocardial effect of Adriamycin which is not ECG-related.

Chronic action of Adriamycin:

Pretreated animals (4—6 courses) show bradycardias of 182 ± 21 beats/min in comparison to control rats under ventilation and thoracotomy having 283 ± 38 beats/minute. Left ventricular pressure, cardiac output and rate of left ventricular pressure rise in pretreated animals were not significantly different in comparison to control rats. Figure 2 demonstrates a myocardial dysfunction of pretreated animals which becomes evident after maximal dobutamine stimulation. Whereas dobuta-

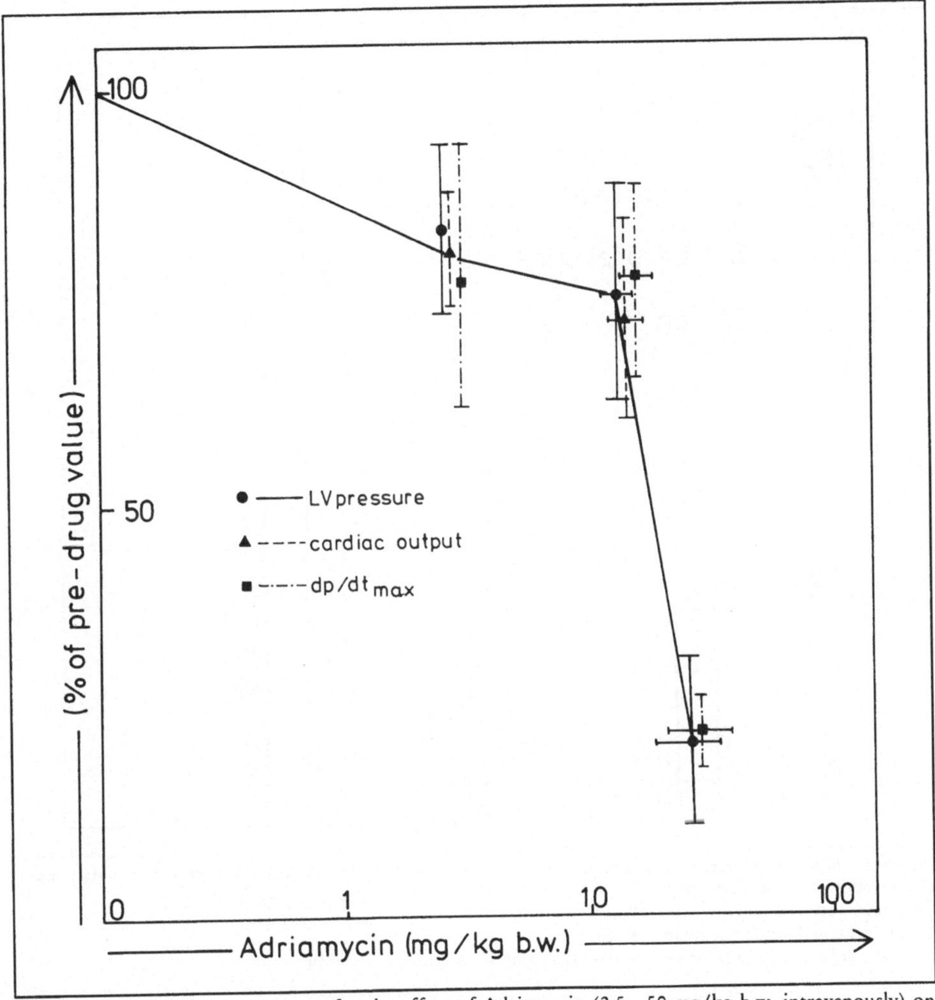

Figure 1: Log-dose-response-curve for the effect of Adriamycin (2.5—50 mg/kg b.w. intravenously) on maximum left ventricular pressure, cardiac output and left ventricular pressure rise of rat heart in situ (n = 8).
Ordinate: left ventricular pressure, cardiac output and left ventricular pressure rise as % of pre-drug values.

mine increases heart rate, left ventricular pressure and dp/dt_{max} above control values in normal animals by 41 ± 14.5, 75.1 ± 28 and 152 ± 29% respectively, the corresponding increases in Adriamycin-pretreated animals were only 10 ± 5.9, 19.5 ± 14 and 71.5 ± 32% respectively.
These data demonstrate that the myocardial effect of chronic Adriamycin might be latent with regard to basal functions and that myocardial dysfunction becomes apparent when a stimulatory test is used to evaluate maximal myocardial performance.

Acknowledgments

We gratefully acknowledge the skillful technical assistance by Mr. M. Rupff and Ms. K. Pichler.

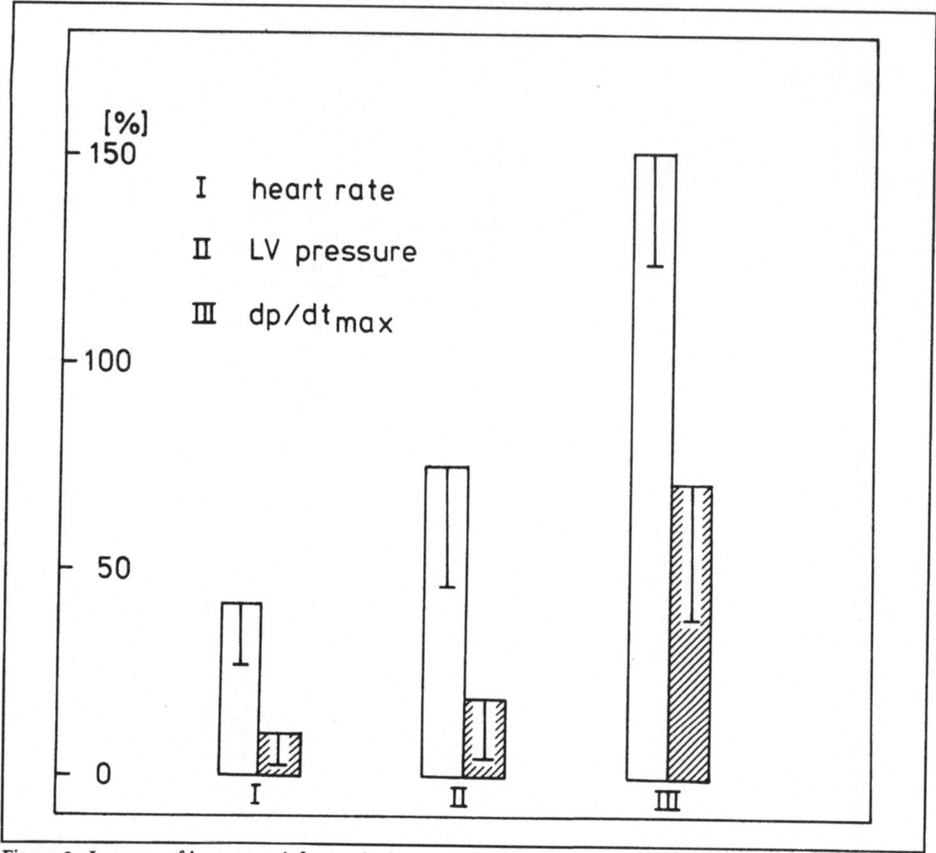

Figure 2: Increase of heart rate, left ventricular pressure and max. left ventricular pressure rise after maximum dobutamine stimulation.
Ordinate: Increase as % of control values
Open columns = control rats (n = 8)
Hatched columns = Adriamycin pretreated rats; 4—6 courses (n = 8)

References

[1] Blum, R. M., Carter, S. K. Adriamycin: A new anticancer drug with significant clinical activity, Ann. Intern. Med. *80* (249—259) 1974.

[2] Lefrak, E. A., Pitha, J., Rosenheim, S., Gottlieb, J. A. A clinicopathological analysis of Adriamycin cardiotoxicity, Cancer *32* (302—314) 1973.

[3] Lenaz, L., Page, J. Cardiotoxicity of Adriamycin and related anthracyclines, Cancer Treatment Rev. *3* (111—120) 1976.

[4] Ferrans, V. J., Herman, E. H. Cardiomyopathy induced by Antineoplastic Drugs, (Eds. Kaltenbach, Loogen, Olson), Springer Verlag Berlin, Heidelberg, New York, 1978, pp 12—26.

[5] Guthrie, D., Gibson, A. L. Doxorubicin cardiotoxicity: Possible role of digoxin in its prevention, Brit. Med. J. *2* (1447—1449) 1977.

[6] Herman, E. H., Mhatre, R. M., Lee, I. P., Waravdekar, V. S. Prevention of the cardiotoxic effects of Adriamycin and Daunomycin in the isolated dog heart, Proc. Soc. exp. Biol. Med. *140* (234—239) 1972.

[7] Cortes, E. P., Gupta, M., Chou, C., Amin, V. C., Folkers, K. Coenzyme Q10 (CoQ10) and the prevention of Adriamycin (ADM) cardiotoxicity, Proc. 14th Ann. Meet. ASCO Abstracts No. C-139, 623, 590 (1978).

[8] Henderson, I. C., Frei, E. Adriamycin and the heart, New Engl. J. Med. *300* (310—312) 1979.

Excretion profiles of L-alanine-aminopeptidase in normal subjects; a method for the evaluation of nephrotoxicity in man

F. Sörgel*, H.-G. Grigoleit, and H. Groetsch
Hoechst AG, Frankfurt/Main, and Pharma Research, Frankfurt/Main

Introduction

Possible nephrotoxicity of a drug has to be established in the very early phases of its development. Nephrotoxicity is predominantly manifested in the tubular system and only becomes clinically evident when damage has reached a relatively advanced stage. It is therefore necessary to look for variables which would allow an early detection of pathological changes within the kidney. Mondorf *et al.* [1] have shown that alanine-aminopeptidase (AAP) is a marker of tubular damage. This enzyme was shown to be released from the brush border cells of the kidney. After treatment with cephalosporines these authors have shown increases of AAP excretion and they therefore advised that AAP should be measured during treatment with drugs like cephalosporines which act on the proximal tubule.

Aim of these investigations

As each drug excreted by the kidney and the kidney tubule system is potentially toxic to this system, it is useful to have a routinely available test for this severe side effect. We have therefore planned two studies of four days duration to show the excretion pattern of this enzyme in healthy subjects. The subjects had standardized diet and fluid intake and lived under similar conditions so that real interindividual variations could be related to physiological variations and not to different environmental conditions.

Methods

Alanine-aminopeptidase (AAP) was measured according to Mondorf *et al.* [2]. Urine was concentrated by dialysis before measurement.

* Institut für Gerontologie der Universität Erlangen-Nürnberg (Present address)

Subjects

Eight healthy volunteers participated in this study. Prior to admission into the trial each subject was subjected to medical examination including hematological, clinical chemistry examination and urine analysis. Creatinine clearance was measured during the whole trial. Diet and fluid intake were strictly standardized and it was made certain that subjects lived under the same conditions.

Results

Urine concentration and excretion of AAP during weeks one and two are shown; Figures 1 and 2. AAP excretion was constant for the two weeks of the trial, there being no differences between weeks one and two. Creatinine clearance was constant during the whole trial. Urinary volume did not show any fluctuations, urine osmolality and urinary pH were within the normal range (Figure 3). There was evidence of a circadian rhythm in AAP excrĕtion. AAP excretion was high in the morning after the first fluid intake and low at night during bedrest (Figure 4). There were considerable inter-individual variations in AAP excretion.

Discussion

We show that AAP-excretion in urine is a constant factor within the subject and does not fluctuate from day to day under the standardized conditions used in this trial. There was high AAP excretion in the morning, which could partly be explained by the fluid intake. This was also the case after a 12 hour abstention from any fluid. The reduced excretion rate during bedrest may possibly be explained by reduced glomerular filtration as shown by decreasing GFR in the evening. Our results on the daily urinary AAP excretion were in good agreement with data from Mondorf [1]. We are able to conclude that there are no essential differences in the measurements of this enzyme by different laboratories. The simplicity of the assay may mean that measurement of AAP can be useful for clinical research and safety control with drugs known to act on the proximal tubule.

Literature:

[1] Mondorf, A. W., Zegelman, M., Klose, J., Maske, L., Scherberich, J. E., Stefanesan, T., Miller, H., Schoeppe, W., Europ. J. clin. Pharmacol. *13*, 357—363 (1978).

[2] Mondorf, A. W., Breier, J., Hendus, J., Scherberich, J. E., Mackenrodt, G., Shah, P. M., Stille, W., Schoeppe, W., Europ. J. clin. Pharmacol. *13*, 133—142 (1978).

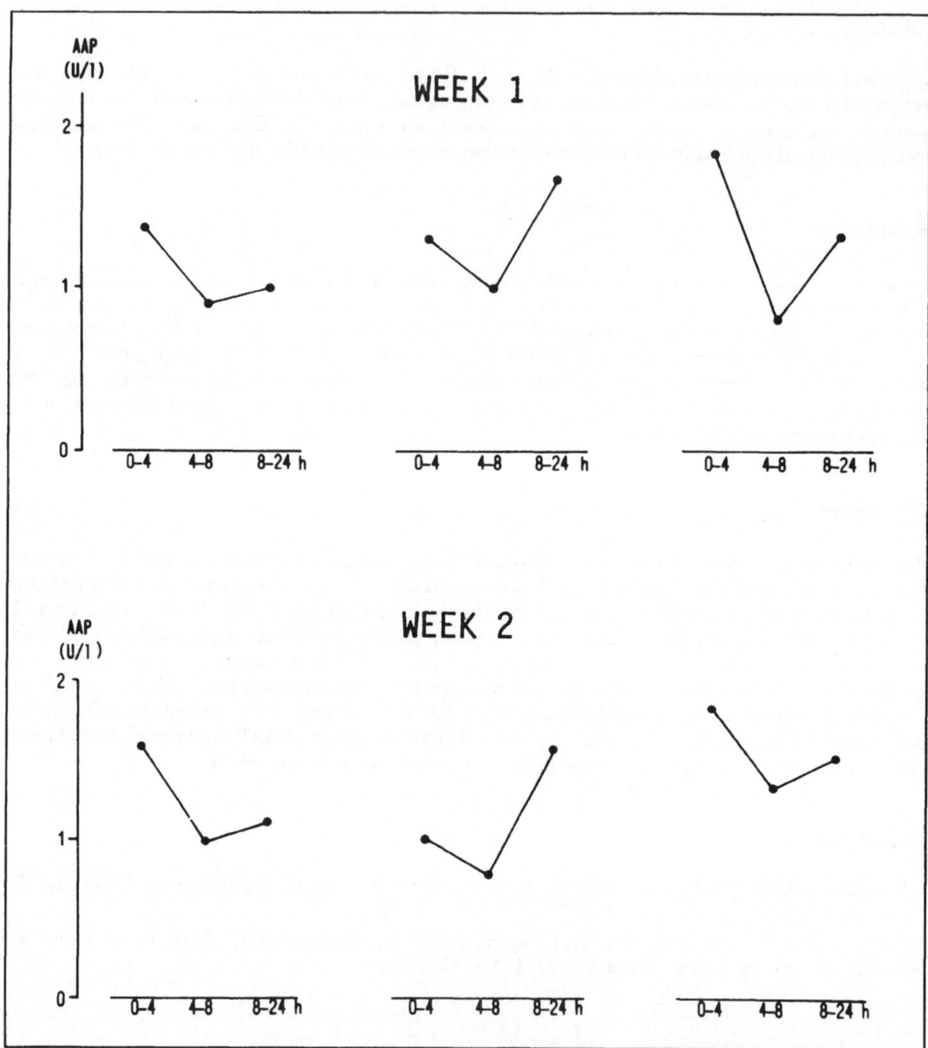

Figure 1: Urinary concentration of AAP in healthy volunteers on three consecutive days ($\bar{x}$, n = 8)

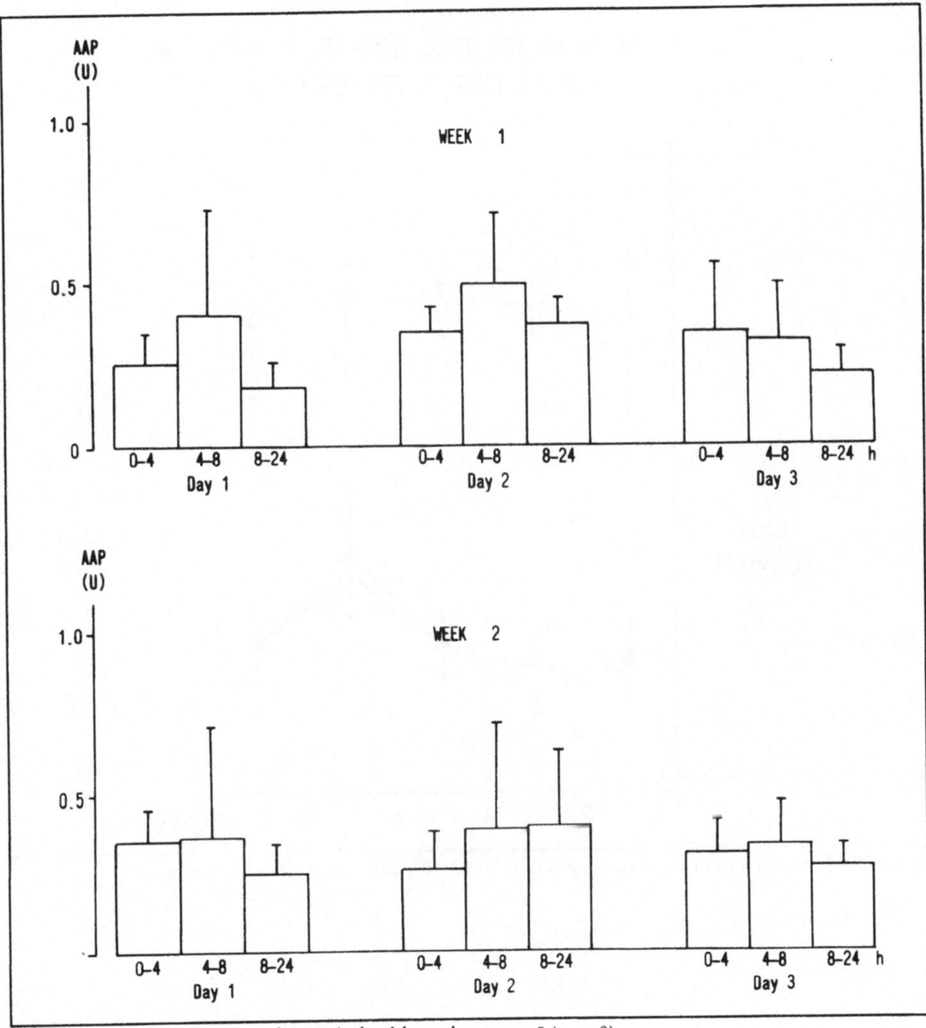

Figure 2: Urinary excretion of AAP in healthy volunteers, $\bar{x}$ (n = 8)

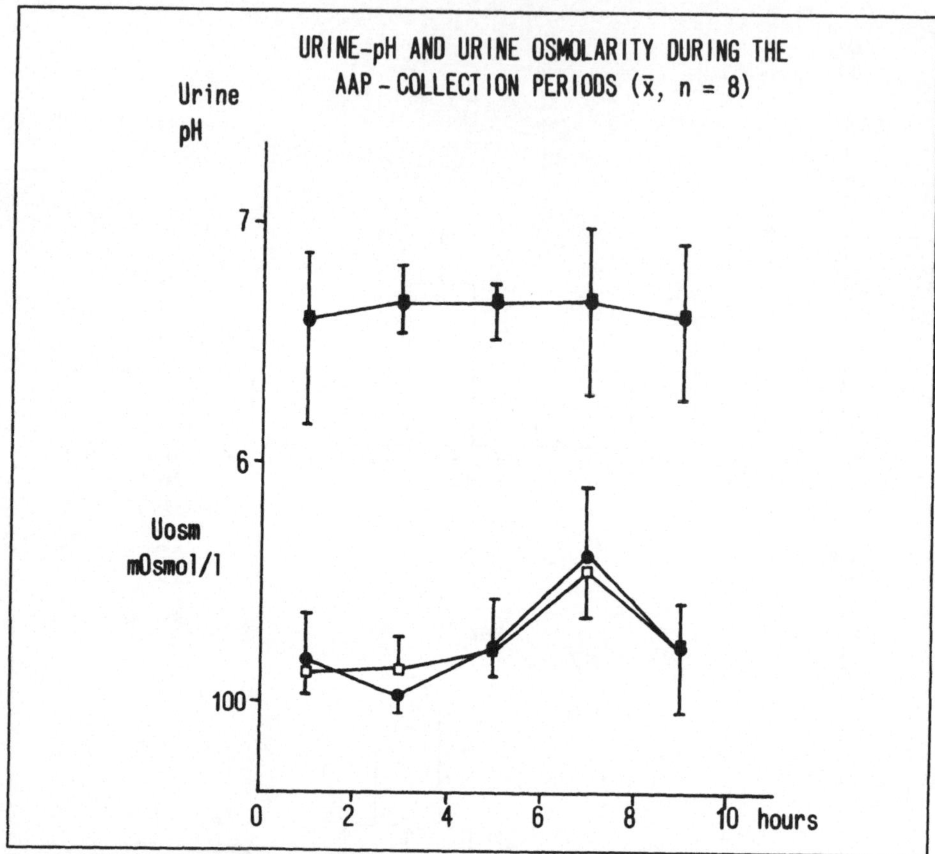

Figure 3: Urine-pH and urine osmolality during the AAP-collection periods ($\bar{x}$, $n = 8$)

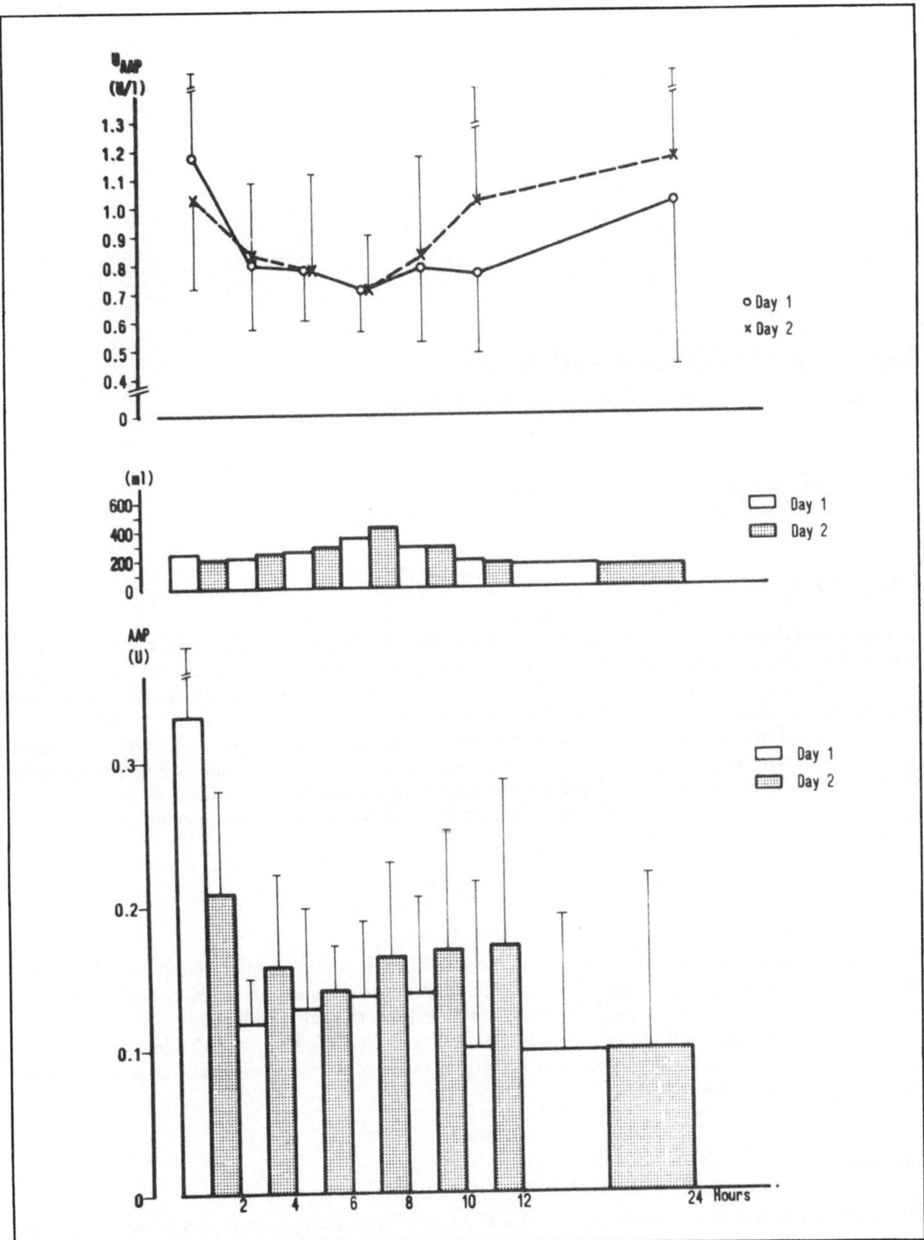

Figure 4: Urinary AAP concentration and excretion in comparison to urine volume during the day.

Influence of hydrochlorothiazide on uric acid excretion in normal subjects

F. Sörgel*, E. E. Dagrosa, and H.-G. Grigoleit
Hoechst AG, Frankfurt/Main

Introduction

It is supposed that phase-I studies in healthy volunteers are of limited predictive value in the evaluation of side effects of new compounds in man. This may partly be explained by the fact that the drugs are often studied in single-dose trials only. After multiple dosing in patients, however, side effects may become evident, which would not have been observed in a single dose phase-I trial.
Early studies of oral diuretics showed reduced urate excretion, which can provoke attacks of gout in patients with elevated plasma urate levels at the beginning of therapy. Another side effect of some antihypertensives is the increase of plasma cholesterol after long term treatment of hypertension. The calcium retention side effect of hydrochlorothiazide treatment, however, may be used in hypercalciuria.

Aim of the trials

The aim of these trials in healthy subjects was to test whether the above mentioned side effects can also be established in a typical phase-I study with single-dose administration. Hydrochlorothiazide was administered as a single 50 mg dose and as multiple doses to healthy subjects. Problems of reaching steady state plasma levels of urate as well as plasma/saliva correlation were also investigated. The effects of hydrochlorothiazide on calcium excretion, calcium plasma levels and cholesterol plasma levels were further investigated.

Methods

The electrolytes were measured by standard procedures. Uric acid in plasma and urine were measured enzymatically according to Kageyama [1]. Plasma cholesterol levels were analysed by the method of Röschlan [2].

* Institut für Gerontologie der Universität Erlangen-Nürnberg (Present address)

Subjects

Only male healthy volunteers participated in these trials. All had medical examinations, including clinical chemistry and urine tests for abnormal urine protein and glucose. As the evaluation of the hyperuremic effect of hydrochlorothiazide was the main aim of these investigations, only subjects in whom plasma urate levels were at the upper end of the normal uric acid levels range were chosen.

Fluid intake:	2475 ml
Sodium intake:	229 mMol
Potassium intake:	78 mMol

Results

After administration of 50 and 200 mg hydrochlorothiazide, plasma levels of urate increased within 24 hours after administration. There was, however, no dose-dependent increase in urate plasma levels. After placebo there was a slight decrease in urate plasma levels (Figure 1). Hydrochlorothiazide was shown to have a dual effect on urinary uric acid excretion. During the first three hours after drug administration, there was an increase in uric acid excretion as compared to placebo, and this was followed by decreased urinary uric acid excretion (Figure 2). Over 24 hours dose dependent retention of uric acid after hydrochlorothiazide as compared to placebo took place. After administration 50 mg of hydrochlorothiazide for ten consecutive days uric acid plasma levels were raised, the most marked rise being observed 24 hours after the first dose. No correlation could be established between the concentrations of uric acid in plasma and saliva (Figure 3). Calcium excretion was also increased during the first hours after administration. This was similarly followed by decreased calcium excretion (Figure 4) which led to an increase of serum calcium (Figure 5). Calcium excretion is therefore different from the excretion of other electrolytes which did not even show a rebound effect during the first 24 hours after drug administration (Figure 4).

Plasma cholesterol levels were increased 24 hours after drug administration. The increase was not dose-dependent and was statistically significant in comparison to placebo (Figure 6).

Discussion

It has been clearly shown that three of the major side-effects of hydrochlorothiazide in man could be reproduced in healthy volunteers after a single dose. The increase of uric acid levels in plasma resulted from decreased urinary uric acid excretion. Although there was dose-dependent retention of uric acid, there was no dose-dependent elevation of plasma uric acid levels. The time course of uric acid excretion did not support the thesis that elevation of plasma uric acid after thiazides is due to inhibition of uric acid secretion in the proximal tubule.

Urinary calcium excretion also behaved in two different ways: an increase during the first hours after administration, followed by a more pronounced retention, such that over 24 hours an elevation of serum calcium levels was observed in comparison to placebo. The different excretion of calcium in contrast to other ions could be at least partly explained by different hormonal control.

Hypercholesterolemia being a well-recognised risk factor in the development of atherosolerosis, it is important to study the influence of diuretics on lipid metabolism in detail, especially high density lipoproteins (HDL) and low density lipoproteins (LDL). If diuretics influence lipoprotein metabolism in a negative way, then the benefit which results from their antihypertensive action could, to a certain extent, be impaired.

Literature:

[1] Kageyama, N., Clin. chim. Acta, *31*, 421 (1971).

[2] Röschlan *et al.*, J. Clin. Chem. Clin. Biochem., *12*, 403 (1974).

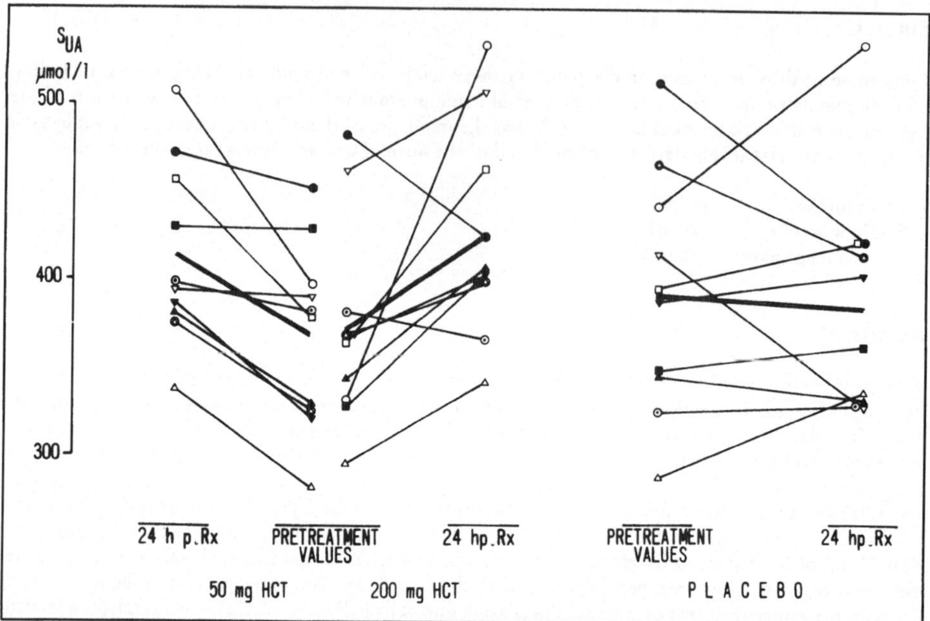

Figure 1: Serum uric acid levels after administration of hydrochlorothiazide and placebo to healthy volunteers ($n = 10$)

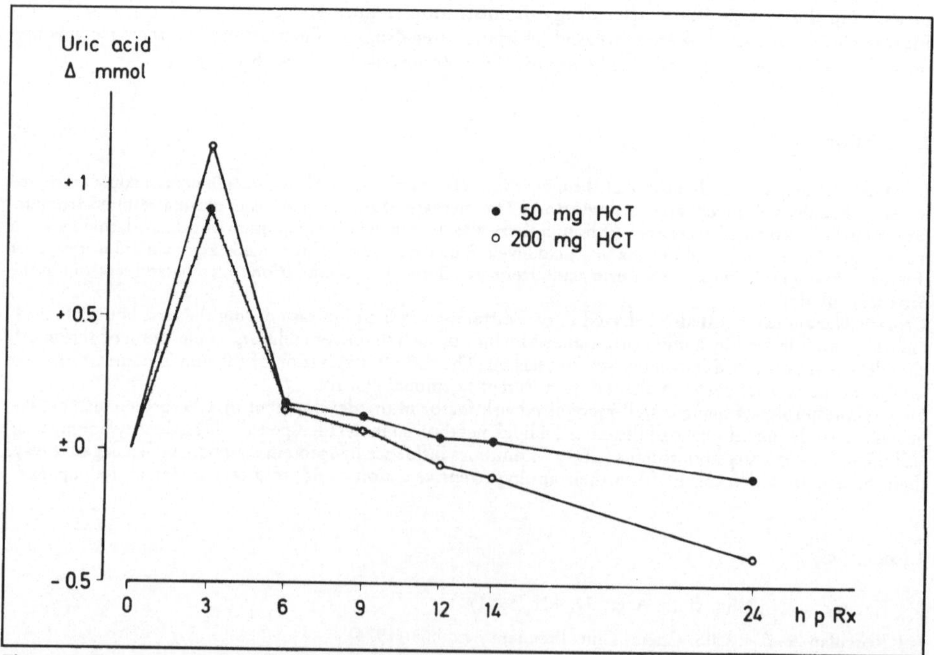

Figure 2: Cumulative uric acid excretion after hydrochlorothiazide in healthy volunteers ($n = 9$) (difference compared to placebo)

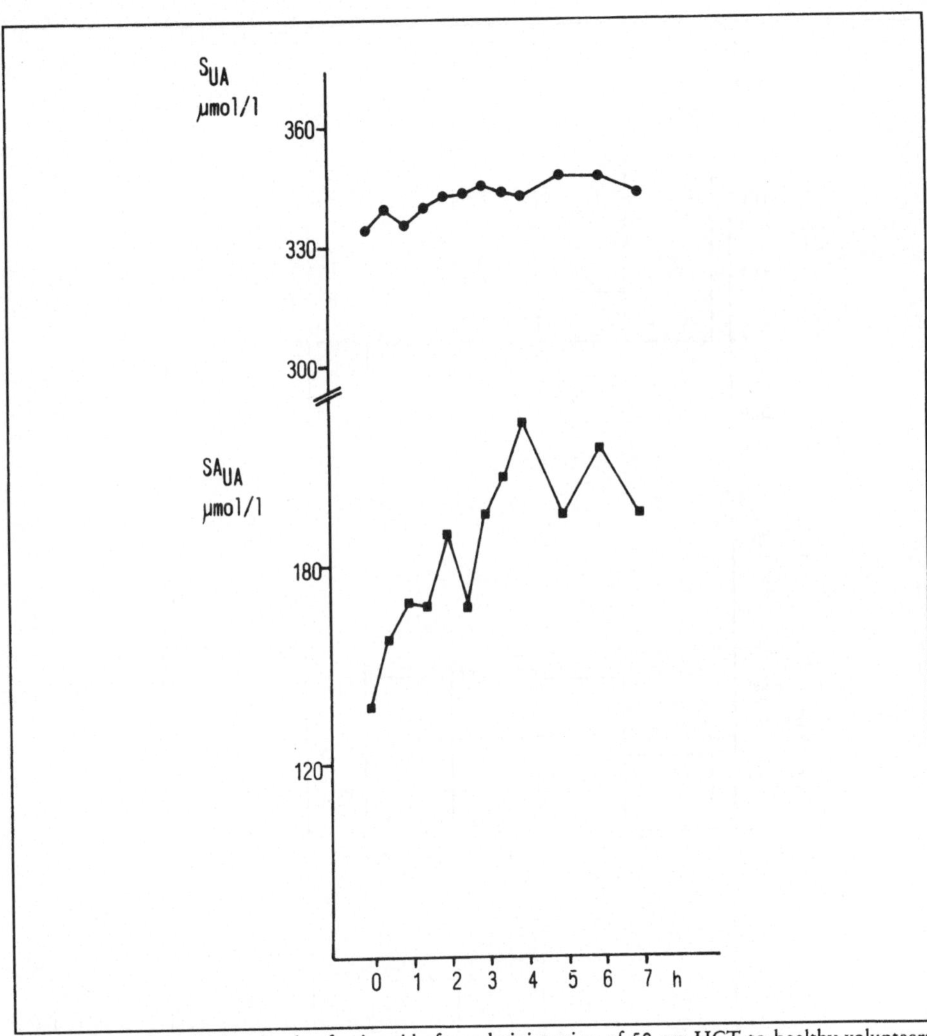

Figure 3: Serum and saliva levels of uric acid after administration of 50 mg HCT to healthy volunteers ($n = 8$)

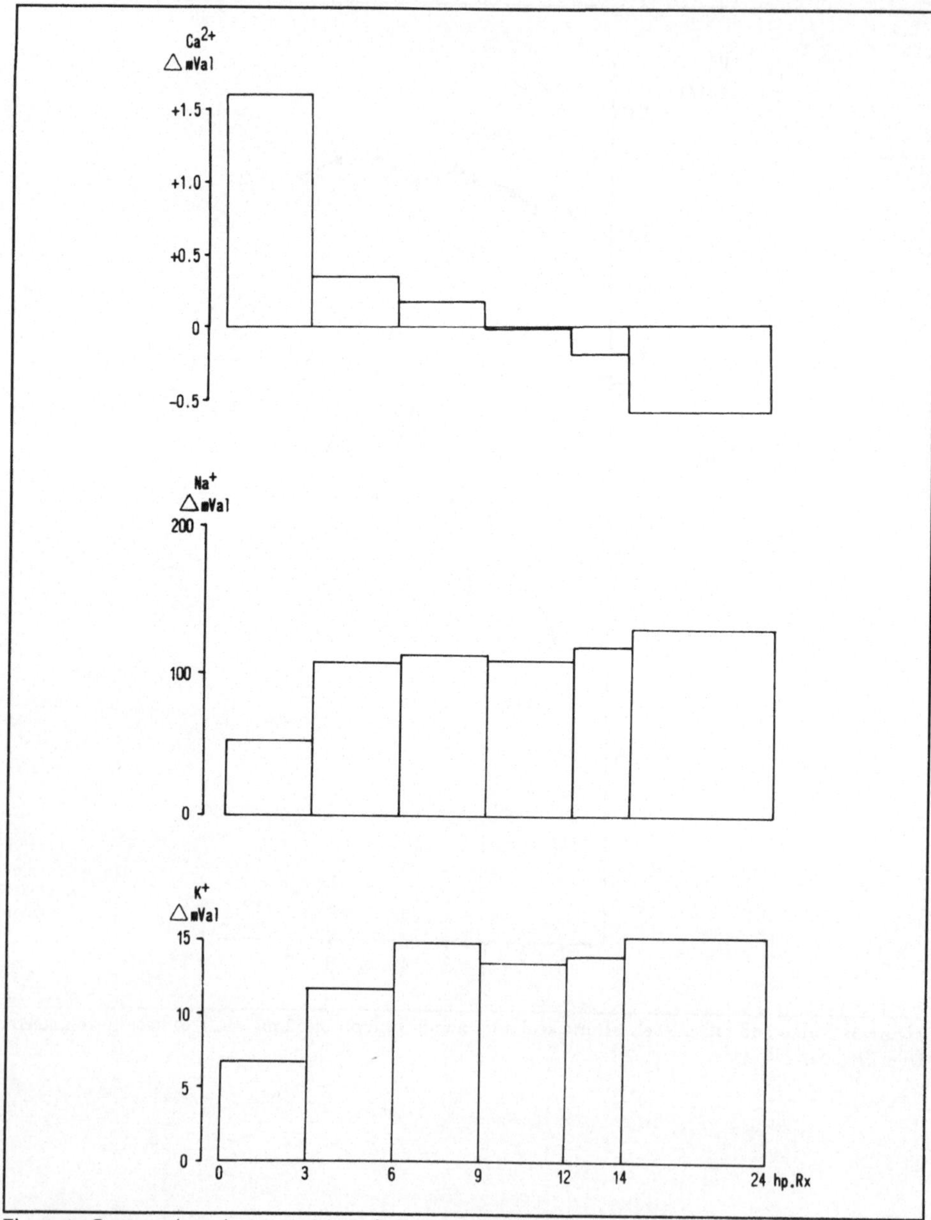

Figure 4: Comparative urinary excretion of calcium, sodium and potassium after administration of 50 mg hydrochlorothiazide to healthy volunteers (n = 10) (Difference to placebo)

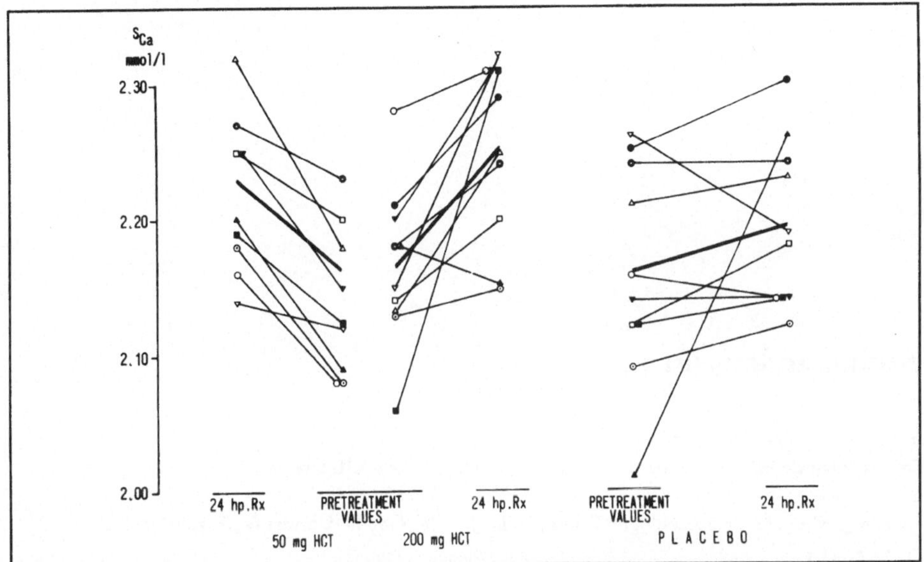

Figure 5: Serum calcium levels after administration of hydrochlorothiazide and placebo to healthy volunteers ($n = 10$)

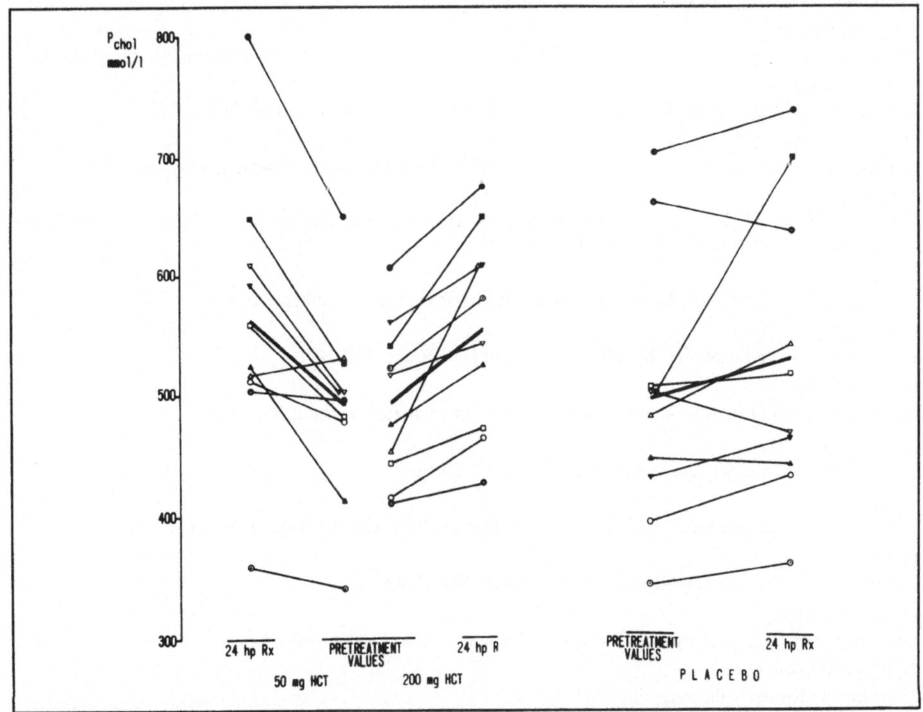

Figure 6: Serum cholesterol levels after administration of hydrochlorothiazide and placebo to healthy volunteers ($n = 10$)

Author address list

E. ALBENGRES,
Département de Pharmacologie, Faculté de Médecine de Paris XII, Creteil

R. G. ALKEN,
Abteilung Klinische Pharmakologie, Klinikum der Joh. W. Goethe-Universität, Frankfurt/Main

D. ARNDTS,
C. H. Boehringer Sohn, Ingelheim

P. ARNOLD,
Byk Gulden Lomberg, Research Division, Konstanz

J. K. ARONSON,
MRC Unit and University Department of Clinical Pharmacology, Radcliffe Infirmary, Oxford, U. K.

T. H. M. ARTS,
Central Animal Laboratory, Sint Radboud Hospital, University of Nijmegen, Nijmegen

N. D. S. BAX,
Department of Therapeutics, University of Sheffield, The Hallamshire Hospital, Sheffield, U. K.

S. BEAL,
Division of Clinical Pharmacology, Department of Medicine, and Department of Laboratory Medicine, University of California, San Francisco, California

R. BENDER,
Hoechst AG, Medizinische Abteilung, Klinische Pharmakologie, Frankfurt/Main

L. BENEDIKTER,
Department of Medicine, Dr. Karl Thomae GmbH, Biberach/Riß

H.-D. BOLTE,
Medizinische Klinik I, Klinikum Großhadern der Universität München, München

G. v. BOMHARD,
Medizinische Klinik der Universität Würzburg, Würzburg

K. BORNER,
Institut für Klinische Chemie und Klinische Biochemie der Freien Universität Berlin, Berlin

D. BRACHTEL,
Department of Medicine, University of Würzburg, Würzburg

D. D. BREIMER,
Department of Pharmacology, University of Leiden, Sylvius Laboratories, Leiden

D. BROCKMEIER,
Zentrum für Kinderheilkunde, Gießen

J. BUSCHMANN,
Department of Medicine, University of Würzburg, Würzburg

J. V. COLLINS,
Department of Clinical Pharmacology, Cardiothoracic Institute, Brompton Hospital, London

E. E. DAGROSA,
Hoechst AG, Medizinische Abteilung, Klinische Pharmakologie, Frankfurt/Main

R. VAN DALEN,
Intensive Care Unit, Sint Radboud Hospital, University of Nijmegen, Nijmegen

M. DANHOF,
Department of Pharmacology, University of Leiden, Sylvius Laboratories, Leiden

P. DEEG,
Department of Internal Medicine, University of Würzburg, Würzburg

J. EPPING,
Med. Klinik der Universität Würzburg, Würzburg

G. FACHINGER,
Zentrum der Inneren Medizin, Abt. für Pneumologie, Klinikum der Johann-Wolfgang-Goethe-Universität, Frankfurt/Main

C. I. FLASCH,
Medizinische Forschung, Beiersdorf AG, Hamburg

F. FOLLATH,
Clinical Pharmacology Division, Department of Medicine, Kantonsspital, Basel

A. S. E. FOWLE,
Wellcome Research Laboratories, Beckenham, Kent, U. K.

R. L. GALEAZZI,
University of Berne, Department of Medicine, Inselspital, Bern

J. S. F. GIMBRÈRE,
Intensive Care Unit, Sint Radboud Hospital, University of Nijmegen, Nijmegen

H.-G. GRIGOLEIT,
Hoechst AG, Frankfurt/Main

G. GROETSCH,
Hoechst AG, Frankfurt/Main

R. GUGLER,
Department of Medicine, University of Bonn, Bonn

R. HAEGLSPERGER,
Gustav-Embden-Zentrum der Biologischen Chemie, Abteilung Zellchemie, Frankfurt/Main

J. C. M. HAFKENSCHEID,
Laboratory for Clinical Chemistry, Department of Internal Medicine, Sint Radboud Hospital, University of Nijmegen, Nijmegen

H. M. von HATTINGBERG,
Zentrum für Kinderheilkunde, Gießen

K.-O. HAUSTEIN,
Section of Clinical Pharmacology, Institute of Pharmacology and Toxicology, Medical Academy Erfurt, Erfurt

B. HEINTZ,
Department of Clinical Pharmacology, University of Frankfurt

N. HEINZ,
Medizinische Forschung, Beiersdorf AG, Hamburg

H. HENNEMANN,
Department of Internal Medicine, University of Würzburg, Würzburg

H. HEUSLER,
Department of Medicine, University of Würzburg, Würzburg

B. HÖFLING,
Medizinische Klinik I, Klinikum Großhadern der Universität München, München

H.-J. HOHORST,
Gustav-Embden-Zentrum der Biologischen Chemie, Abteilung Zellchemie, Frankfurt/Main

M. HROPOT,
Hoechst AG, Frankfurt/Main

F. T. M. HUYSMANS,
Department of Internal Medicine, Division of Nephrology, Sint Radboud Hospital, University of Nijmegen, Nijmegen

R. JOERES,
Department of Medicine, University of Würzburg, Würzburg

G. KAISER,
Zentrum der Pharmakologie, Klinikum der Johann-Wolfgang-Goethe-Universität, Frankfurt/Main

A. KELMAN,
Department of Clinical Physics and Bio-Engineering, West of Scotland Health Boards, Glasgow

R. KIRSTEN,
Department of Clinical Pharmacology, University of Frankfurt, Frankfurt/Main

E. VAN DER KLEIJN,
Department of Clinical Pharmacy, Sint Radboud Hospital, University of Nijmegen, Nijmegen

U. KLOTZ,
Dr. Margarete Fischer-Bosch-Institut für Klinische Pharmakologie, Stuttgart

A. LASSMANN,
Department of Clinical Pharmacology, Klinikum der Johann-Wolfgang-Goethe-Universität, Frankfurt/Main

G. LAZARUS,
Institute of Anaesthesiology, Klinikum der Julius-Maximilians-Universität, Würzburg

K. LEHMANN,
Kreiskrankenhaus Main-Taunus, Bad Soden/Ts.

M. S. LENNARD,
Department of Therapeutics, University of Sheffield, The Hallamshire Hospital, Sheffield U. K.

G. LEOPOLD,
Medical Research, Human Pharmacology Centre, E. Merck, Darmstadt

J. LICHEY,
Medizinische Klinik und Poliklinik, Klinikum Steglitz der Freien Universität Berlin, Berlin

W. E. LINDUP,
Department of Pharmacology and Therapeutics, University of Liverpool, Liverpool

R. LISSNER,
Zentrum der Pharmakologie, Klinische Pharmakologie der Johann-Wolfgang-Goethe-Universität, Frankfurt/Main

G. LUDWIG,
Byk Gulden Lomberg, Research Division, Konstanz

V. MARATHE,
School of Business Administration, University of California, Berkeley, California

W. A. C. McALLISTER,
Department of Clinical Pharmacology, Cardiothoracic Institute, Brompton Hospital, London

G. E. MAWER,
Department of Pharmacology, Materia Medica and Therapeutics, University of Manchester, Manchester

R. MERGET,
Zentrum der Inneren Medizin, Abt. für Pneumologie, Klinikum der Johann-Wolfgang-Goethe-Universität, Frankfurt/Main

K. H. MOLZ,
Klinikum der Universität Frankfurt, Zentrum der Pharmakologie, Abteilung Klinische Pharmakologie, Frankfurt/Main

J. MORLEY,
Department of Clinical Pharmacology, Cardiothoracic Institute, Brompton Hospital, London

P. W. MULLEN,
Department of Pharmacology, Materia Medica and Therapeutics, University of Manchester, Manchester

R. MUSCHAWECK,
Hoechst AG, Frankfurt/Main

E. MUTSCHLER,
Pharmakologisches Institut für Naturwissenschaftler, Universität Frankfurt, Frankfurt/Main

M. NAGEL,
Pharmakologisches Institut der Universität Essen, Essen

K. NELSON,
Department of Clinical Pharmacology, University of Frankfurt, Frankfurt/Main

J. OSTROWSKI,
Pharmaforschung Cassella AG, Frankfurt/Main

J. PABST,
Medical Research, Human Pharmacology Centre, E. Merck, Darmstadt

D. PALM,
Zentrum der Pharmakologie, Klinikum der Johann-Wolfgang-Goethe-Universität, Frankfurt/Main

J. PARASKEVOVA,
Klinikum der Johann-Wolfgang-Goethe-Universität, Abteilung für klinische Pharmakologie, Frankfurt/Main

J. C. LE PARCO,
Service de Médecine Interne, Hôpital Albert Chennevier, Creteil

A. W. PECK,
Wellcome Research Laboratories, Beckenham, Kent, U. K.

K. RESAG,
Pharmaforschung Cassella AG, Frankfurt/Main

E. RICHTER,
Medizinische Klinik der Universität Würzburg, Würzburg

I. RIETBROCK,
Institute of Anaesthesiology, Klinikum der Julius-Maximilians-Universität Würzburg, Würzburg

N. RIETBROCK,
Klinikum der Johann-Wolfgang-Goethe-Universität, Abteilung für klinische Pharmakologie, Frankfurt/Main

D. RÖHL,
Kreiskrankenhaus Main-Taunus, Bad Soden/Ts.

B. ROSENBERG,
School of Business Administration, University of California, Berkeley, California

T. ROYEN,
Hoechst AG, Medizinische Abteilung, Klinische Pharmakologie, Frankfurt/Main

M. SCHÄFER,
Pharmakologisches Institut für Naturwissenschaftler, Universität Frankfurt, Frankfurt/Main

H. J. SCHÜMANN,
Pharmakologisches Institut der Universität Essen, Essen

G. SCHULTZE-WERNINGHAUS,
Zentrum der Inneren Medizin, Abt. für Pneumologie, Klinikum der Johann-Wolfgang-Goethe-Universität, Frankfurt/Main

D. SCHUPPAN,
Zentrum der Pharmakologie, Klinische Pharmakologie der Johann-Wolfgang-Goethe-Universität, Frankfurt/Main

F. L. SHAND,
Department of Experimental Immunobiology, Wellcome Research Laboratories, Beckenham, Kent, U. K.

L. B. SHEINER,
Division of Clinical Pharmacology, Department of Medicine, and Department of Laboratory Medicine, University of California, San Francisco, California

F. SÖRGEL,
Institut für Gerontologie der Universität Erlangen—Nürnberg

A. SOMOGYI,
Department of Medicine, University of Bonn, Bonn

P. SPRING,
Clinical Pharmacology Division, Department of Medicine, Kantonsspital, Basel

H. STÄHLE,
C. H. Boehringer Sohn, Ingelheim

A. H. STAIB,
Zentrum der Pharmakologie, Klinische Pharmakologie der Johann-Wolfgang-Goethe-Universität, Frankfurt/Main

I. H. STEVENSON,
Department of Pharmacology and Therapeutics, Ninewells Hospital and Medical School, Dundee

C. J. STRUCK,
C. H. Boehringer Sohn, Ingelheim

T. A. THIEN,
Department of Internal Medicine, Division of Nephrology, Sint Radboud Hospital, University of Nijmegen, Nijmegen

J. P. TILLEMENT,
Département de Pharmacologie, Faculté de Médecine de Paris XII, Creteil

H. TROUVAIN,
Dr. Karl Thomae GmbH, Biberach/Riß

G. T. TUCKER,
Department of Therapeutics, University of Sheffield, The Hallamshire Hospital, Sheffield, U. K.

W. UNGETHÜM,
Medical Research, Human Pharmacology Centre, E. Merck, Darmstadt

N. P. E. VERMEULEN,
Gorlaeus Laboratories, Leiden

D. VOEGELE,
Pharmaforschung Cassella AG, Frankfurt/Main

H. F. VÖHRINGER,
Schloßparkklinik, Berlin

G. VOELCKER,
Gustav-Embden-Zentrum der Biologischen Chemie, Abteilung Zellchemie, Frankfurt/Main

S. VOZEH,
Clinical Pharmacology Division, Department of Medicine, Kantonsspital, Basel

T. B. VREE,
Department of Clinical Pharmacy, Sint Radboud Hospital, University of Nijmegen, Nijmegen

M. WENK,
Clinical Pharmacology Division, Department of Medicine, Kantonsspital, Basel

B. WHITING,
Department of Materia Medica, University of Glasgow, Glasgow

B. G. WOODCOCK,
Department of Clinical Pharmacology, University Clinic, Frankfurt/Main

H. F. WOODS,
Department of Therapeutics, University of Sheffield, The Hallamshire Hospital, Sheffield, U. K.

R. M. ZAPF,
Hoechst AG, Medizinische Abteilung, Klinische Pharmakologie, Frankfurt/Main

K. ZECH,
Byk Gulden Lomberg, Research Division, Konstanz

W. ZILLY,
Medizinische Klinik der Universität Würzburg, Würzburg

A. ZIMMER,
Dr. Karl Thomae GmbH, Biberach/Riß